Studies in Computational Intelligence

Volume 1018

The series "Studies in Computational Intelligence" (SCI) publishes new developments and advances in the various areas of computational intelligence—quickly and with a high quality. The intent is to cover the theory, applications, and design methods of computational intelligence, as embedded in the fields of engineering, computer science, physics and life sciences, as well as the methodologies behind them. The series contains monographs, lecture notes and edited volumes in computational intelligence spanning the areas of neural networks, connectionist systems, genetic algorithms, evolutionary computation, artificial intelligence, cellular automata, self-organizing systems, soft computing, fuzzy systems, and hybrid intelligent systems. Of particular value to both the contributors and the readership are the short publication timeframe and the world-wide distribution, which enable both wide and rapid dissemination of research output.

Indexed by SCOPUS, DBLP, WTI Frankfurt eG, zbMATH, SCImago.

All books published in the series are submitted for consideration in Web of Science.

Fabio Crestani · David E. Losada · Javier Parapar
Editors

Early Detection of Mental Health Disorders by Social Media Monitoring

The First Five Years of the eRisk Project

Springer

Editors
Fabio Crestani
Faculty of Informatics
Università della Svizzera Italiana (USI)
Lugano, Switzerland

David E. Losada
Centro Singular de Investigación en
Tecnoloxías Intelixentes (CiTIUS)
Universidade de Santiago de Compostela
Santiago de Compostela, Spain

Javier Parapar
Centro de Investigación en Tecnoloxías da
Información e as Comunicacións (CITIC)
Universidade da Coruña
A Coruña, Spain

ISSN 1860-949X ISSN 1860-9503 (electronic)
Studies in Computational Intelligence
ISBN 978-3-031-04430-4 ISBN 978-3-031-04431-1 (eBook)
https://doi.org/10.1007/978-3-031-04431-1

This Springer imprint is published by the registered company Springer Nature Switzerland AG
The registered company address is: Gewerbestrasse 11, 6330 Cham, Switzerland

Foreword

Early in 2013, my wife Rebecca and I were out on a "date night" having food and wine at a restaurant named—pragmatically, but uninspiringly—Food And Wine. We found ourselves discussing some work being done recently by my tribe, computational linguists, that might potentially be interesting to her tribe, clinical psychologists. By the time dessert arrived we had hatched the idea of a workshop that would bring the two tribes together. Not too long afterward I pitched the idea to Meg Mitchell, who had been involved in a number of interesting studies on language analysis in connection with mental health conditions like autism and cognitive impairment with Brian Roark, Emily Prud'hommeaux, and others.[1] The three of us led the organization of the first Workshop on Computational Linguistics and Clinical Psychology, at the 2014 ACL conference. CLPsych, as it is known, has taken place every year since then, except for what I sincerely hope will be just a single break during a global pandemic.[2]

We organized CLPsych because we could see that there were an increasing number of people interested in bringing the tools of natural language processing and machine learning to the problems of mental health and well-being, but they were

[1] See for example:

- Emily T. Prud'hommeaux, Margaret Mitchell, and Brian Roark. 2011. Using patterns of narrative recall for improved detection of mild cognitive impairment. International Conference on Technology and Aging (ICTA) 2011, Toronto, Ontario.
- B. Roark, M. Mitchell, J. -P. Hosom, K. Hollingshead and J. Kaye, "Spoken Language Derived Measures for Detecting Mild Cognitive Impairment," in IEEE Transactions on Audio, Speech, and Language Processing, vol. 19, no. 7, pp. 2081-2090, Sept. 2011.
- Van Santen, J. P., Prud'Hommeaux, E. T., Black, L. M., & Mitchell, M. (2010). Computational prosodic markers for autism. Autism, 14(3), 215-236.
- Roark, B., Mitchell, M., & Hollingshead, K. (2007, June). Syntactic complexity measures for detecting mild cognitive impairment. In Proceedings of the ACL 2007 Workshop on Biomedical Natural Language Processing (BioNLP), Prague, pp. 1-8, June 2007.

[2] Proceedings can be found at CLPsych.org.

scattered, presenting their work in a wide range of different journals, conferences, and workshops. There was critical mass, and it was time to start building a community.

The book you're holding (or, these days, viewing, or perhaps listening to), emerges from a similar recognition—a recognition of real-world needs, of a range of capable people with the right skills to tackle those needs, and of an opportunity to bring that body of intelligence and enthusiasm and energy together. The organizers of eRisk identified a common thread running through a range of concerns for human well-being: the value of identifying risks and threats sooner rather than later. This has given rise to the concept of *early risk detection systems* as a coherent, interdisciplinary research area.

The application areas for early risk detection are numerous. These include risks directly associated with mental health, such as major depression and suicidality, but they also go further, to include risks from sexual predators, for example, or cyberbullying, or political radicalization, or addiction.

What makes all this possible is the ever-increasing availability of online evidence about people's thoughts and behaviors—what Lazer and colleagues, introducing the field of computational social science, referred to as "digital traces that can be compiled into comprehensive pictures".[3]

Similarly, Coppersmith and his colleagues talk about the "clinical whitespace" in the context of mental health; this describes the long periods of time that intervene in between attention from clinical providers, periods that used to be entirely opaque to providers of care, but which now hold the potential for yielding valuable or even crucial signal about people's mental state and, as such, new opportunities for early intervention.[4]

This notion of time is really central, and one of eRisk's most distinguishing and innovative features. It's very easy for us, as technologists, to define "tasks" and their associated evaluation metrics in whatever way we find intuitively plausible or easy to execute. But tasks and metrics, if they are to be *relevant*, are not stand-alone things. Rather, progress needs to be made using faithful abstractions of the real-world problems the technology is eventually intended to help address, and that means thinking about real-world use cases. One obvious example of this is in speech recognition, where the tasks worked on by the community have progressed, over the decades, from isolated words, to speech read by broadcasters, to conversations, to meetings, all with an increased awareness of the need for tolerance in the face of noise and variation among speakers. Another is information retrieval, where standard thinking about evaluation in terms of precision and recall has now been updated with more relevant metrics in the context of how people actually search for information on a day-to-day basis. What sense does it make to evaluate systems as if we care about every single relevant document they return, for example, in a world where

[3] Lazer, D., Pentland, A., Adamic, L., Aral, S., Barabasi, A. L., Brewer, D., ... & Van Alstyne, M. (2009). Social science. Computational social science. Science (New York, NY), 323(5915), 721–723.

[4] Coppersmith, G., Leary, R., Crutchley, P., and Fine, A. (2018). Natural language processing of social media as screening for suicide risk. Biomedical Informatics Insights, 10, 117822261879286.

most searches are done on the web and almost nobody looks past the first ten hits? Measuring precision-at-10, the number of relevant hits among the first ten returned, is a better abstraction for assessing the extent to which a system will satisfy that real-world need.

Correspondingly, in settings where proactive intervention is the ultimate real-world goal, data don't arrive all at once. Much of time, datapoints arrive in a stream over time. The question, therefore, is not just how to do good classification, it's about *when* a system should raise a flag saying that an individual or a situation merits attention. The eRisk tasks are, therefore, designed from the ground up with chronological considerations in mind, from an incremental data release strategy to evaluation metrics that consider not only the accuracy but also the speed with which choices are made.

As another key thing to consider, better technology is not a goal in and of itself. Even if a technology genuinely performs well in formal evaluations, that doesn't necessarily mean that it can be deployed in a way that actually represents progress. Most technologists are familiar with the distinction between intrinsic and extrinsic evaluations, the latter category meaning that what is measured is the performance of the entire system in which the to-be-evaluated technology is embedded. For example, you can evaluate a natural language parser intrinsically, by looking at the parse trees it produces, or you can consider it extrinsically in the context of a machine translation system, looking at how different parsing approaches improve, or don't improve, the overall quality of the translations being produced.[5]

When it comes to risk, systems like the ones described in this volume are being evaluated intrinsically in the eRisk tasks, but it's important to remember that ultimately what matters most is how they will perform extrinsically—embedded not just in some other automatic system, like machine translation, but in an entire ecosystem that involves not just technologies but also human beings providing care or assistance.[6] This gives rise to some challenges for the typical ways technologists gather data for technological development and evaluation; for example, Ernala and colleagues have pointed out some of the downsides of using online self-reports and other proxies as a stand-in for clinically valid diagnoses.[7] It's notable and important, therefore, that eRisk's criteria go further and require explicit mention of a *diagnosis of* a condition like depression, not just a statement about having depression; this is a credible way of balancing the goal of collecting data at reasonable scale against

[5] Resnik, P., and Lin, J. (2013). Evaluation of NLP systems. In Clark, A., Fox, C., & Lappin, S. (Eds.) (2010). The Handbook of Computational Linguistics and Natural Language Processing. Wiley-Blackwell.

[6] Resnik, P., Foreman, A., Kuchuk, M., Musacchio Schafer, K., and Pinkham, B. (2021). Naturally occurring language as a source of evidence in suicide prevention. Suicide and Life Threatening Behavior, 51(1), 88–96.

[7] Ernala, S. K., Birnbaum, M. L., Candan, K. A., Rizvi, A. F., Sterling, W. A., Kane, J. M., and De Choudhury, M. (2019, April). Methodological gaps in predicting mental health states from social media: Triangulating diagnostic signals. In Proceedings of the 2019 ACM CHI conference on human factors in computing systems (p. 134).

the goal of defining ground-truth categories that will actually matter to clinicians or other relevant subject matter experts.

The chapters in this volume do a great job providing a comprehensive understanding of these and other considerations. The technology-oriented reader will find clear rationales for the choices being made, detailed discussions of the best work so far in eRisk tasks, and thorough contemplation of findings.

Even more important, though, this volume is a milestone setting the stage for the next generation of eRisk. In looking at the future of eRisk, the discussion of expanding the range of problems is exciting, particularly the idea of selecting new challenges to focus on based on broad social relevance—for example, anxiety disorders are trending upward as a result of COVID-19 pandemic, and digital evidence may be one of the most important ways to help clinical professionals handle the mental health tsunami following in its wake.[8] Similarly, the ability to improve early detection of dementia may have a dramatic impact on well-being for large swaths of the world's aging population.

Equally exciting is eRisk's more recent and continuing push in the direction of prediction not just for a single class (at-risk or not), but for symptom-level responses of the kind reported in clinical questionnaires. Particularly for mental health providers, the yes-or-no question of a diagnosis matters, but it's far from the end of the story: finer-grained information is needed in order to really understand what's going on with patients, and in fact there are efforts underway in the mental health community to improve the organization, description, and measurement of psychopathology via data-driven, empirically based organization of signs and symptoms.[9] The move toward obtaining ground-truth data from validated questionnaires, and defining the goals of prediction tasks accordingly, is a move toward bridging more effectively between the things technologies can provide and the things clinicians need.

In the end, whether we are talking about mental health risks in particular, or other risks more generally, that kind of bridging—creating momentum and community among technologists, combined with relevance for the non-technologists—is the way real progress is going to be made. The work in this book is an important contribution to that enterprise.

October 2021

Philip Resnik
Department of Linguistics and Institute
for Advanced Computer Studies
University of Maryland
College Park, Maryland, USA

---

[8] Inkster, B. and Digital Mental Health Data Insights Group (DMHDIG) (2021). Early warning signs of a mental health tsunami: A coordinated response to gather initial data insights from multiple digital services providers. Frontiers in Digital Health, 2, 64.

[9] Kotov, R., Krueger, R. F., Watson, D., Achenbach, T. M., Althoff, R. R., Bagby, R. M., ... & Zimmerman, M. (2017). The Hierarchical Taxonomy of Psychopathology (HiTOP): A dimensional alternative to traditional nosologies. Journal of Abnormal Psychology, 126(4), 454-477.

Preface

This book presents the best of the first five years of eRisk. eRisk[10], which is a shortening of *Early Risk Prediction on the Internet*, is concerned with the exploration of techniques for the early detection of certain health problems which manifest in the way people write and communicate on the internet, in particular in user generated content. eRisk is also concerned with the evaluation methodology for such techniques, in particular with effectiveness metrics where early detection is an important issue. The eRisk project was proposed as part of the Conference and Lab of the Evaluation Forum (CLEF) in 2016 and started as a lab in 2017. Thus, 2020 was the fifth year of eRisk.

Proud of what we achieved after five years and excited for what the future will bring to this endeavor, we decided to compile this book to present the best of what was achieved in these first five years of this interesting and challenging task. We hope this book will be of interest not just to the many past and future participants of the lab but also to other researchers and practitioners involved in similarly challenging endeavors.

Lugano, Switzerland | Fabio Crestani
Santiago de Compostela, Spain | David E. Losada
A Coruña, Spain | Javier Parapar
October 2021

[10] See: https://erisk.irlab.org/.

Contents

Early Risk Prediction of Mental Health Disorders

Fabio Crestani, David E. Losada, and Javier Parapar

Abstract The monitoring of social media use and postings to discern users' mental health is not a novel application of Information Retrieval, Text Mining, and Natural Language Processing. Yet, the evaluation of the proposed solutions has only recently started to be properly addressed. The eRisk project aims at stimulating research on such topic by providing an experimental framework that enables the proper development and testing of tools that not only can detect signs of failing mental health, but that can also track such signs over time and flag a warning when they become serious. This book provides the context in which this project was developed and presents the best results achieved so far. This chapter introduces the book and gives an overview of its content.

1 Introduction

This book presents the best of the first five years of eRisk. eRisk,[1] which stands for *Early Risk Prediction on the Internet*, is concerned with the exploration of techniques for the early detection of mental health problems which manifest in the way people write and communicate on the internet, in particular in user generated content. eRisk is also concerned with the development of test collections and the design of

[1] See: https://erisk.irlab.org/.

F. Crestani
Università della Svizzera italiana (USI), Lugano, Switzerland
e-mail: fabio.crestani@usi.ch

D. E. Losada (✉)
Centro Singular de Investigación en Tecnoloxías Intelixentes (CiTIUS), Universidade de Santiago de Compostela, Santiago de Compostela, Spain
e-mail: david.losada@usc.es

J. Parapar
Centro de Investigación en Tecnoloxías da Información e as Comunicacións (CITIC), Universidade da Coruña, A Coruña, Spain
e-mail: javierparapar@udc.es

F. Crestani et al. (eds.), *Early Detection of Mental Health Disorders by Social Media Monitoring*, Studies in Computational Intelligence 1018,
https://doi.org/10.1007/978-3-031-04431-1_1

a suitable evaluation methodology for such techniques, in particular with the design of effectiveness metrics where early detection is an important issue.

Early detection technologies can be employed in different areas, particularly those related to health and safety. For instance, early alerts could be sent when the writing of a teenager starts showing increasing signs of depression or some other psychological disorder, or when a social media user starts showing suicidal inclinations, or again when a potential offender starts publishing antisocial threats on a blog, forum or social network. In fact, our main goal, when we started the project, was to pioneer a new interdisciplinary research area that would be potentially applicable to a wide variety of situations and to many different problems and personal profiles.

The eRisk project started in 2015 in the context of a three month long research visit by Prof. Losada at the Universitá della Svizzera Italiana (USI), to work with Prof. Crestani. The visit was funded by the Swiss National Science Foundation (SNSF) under the International Short Visits program (Grant N. IZK0Z2_160614). During that visit the idea of creating a test collection that could be used for fostering research in the above areas was conceived, following the example of similar collections developed in the context of the well-known TREC series (Text REtrieval Conference).[2] The following year was spent in that effort of creating such test collection and in the design of suitable evaluation methodologies for the tracking of early risks in the internet. The idea, presented in a paper at the Conference and Lab of the Evaluation Forum (CLEF) 2016, attracted a lot of attention and pushed us to continue it as a lab that became part of that series of conferences. So, the eRisk series of labs started in 2017 and, since then, it has attracted an increasing number of participants engaged in different tasks that were proposed in a yearly basis.

In 2017 eRisk included an exploratory task on the early detection of signs of depression. This shared task was defined using the test collection and evaluation metrics we proposed. The interactions between depression and natural language use was an intriguing problem and the eRisk participants approached the challenge from multiple perspectives testing a number of different approaches. The 2017 task was demanding both for the participants and the organisers because, in line with the idea of evaluating early risk detection, it had ten successive releases of data, and, after each release, the teams had just one week to submit their predictions. Furthermore, the eRisk collection was new to all participants, making it difficult to use machine learning techniques given the lack of training data. In addition, the involved research groups were not familiar with the novel evaluation metrics and could not adjust the many parameters of their models for the optimisation of their performance. As a result, only eight teams (out of 30 registered participants) were able to submit their runs for evaluation.

In 2018 two shared tasks were organised. The first was on early detection of signs of depression (which was a continuation of the 2017's pilot task), while the second was on early detection of signs of anorexia. The two tasks had the same overall organisation and used the same evaluation methodology of the previous year. eRisk 2018 had 11 active participants (out of 41 registered teams) who submitted

[2] See: https://trec.nist.gov/.

45 and 35 system variants, for the two tasks respectively. The increasing numbers of participants and runs submitted suggested that eRisk was rapidly becoming an experimental reference for early risk research. This realisation made us think that we needed a larger team, so we included Prof. Parapar in the organisation of the event.

In 2019 three shared tasks were organised. Two of them were oriented to the same early detection task, addressing anorexia and self-harm. The third one was a new task oriented to automatically filling a depression questionnaire based on user interactions in social media. The idea was to capture in more detail the type and level of depression with a screening tool that is used by professionals, easier to interpret, yet in a fully automatic way. The 2019 edition had 14 active participants (out of 62 registered teams).

In 2020 only two shared tasks were organised. The first task was a continuation of the 2019s task on the early detection of signs of self-harm, while the second was a continuation of 2019s task on depression level estimation. In 2019, these two tasks were really challenging and the participants had no training data, but in 2020, participants could use the 2019 data for training their machine learning algorithms, attempting to detect new cases. This brought a good increase in results, that were still low anyway from being optimal and suggesting that new approaches needed to be tested. The edition had 12 active participants (out of 52 registered teams), which was a small decrease compared to the previous year, but still a large effort for the organisers. In fact, we introduced a new way of delivering data to participants. The user-generated submissions were not delivered anymore in "sets", but as a proper "stream", as the idea of the early detection was originally intended. This enabled participants to analyse the postings one by one, as if they were published by users, making the task more realistic.

We reached the present. In 2021, while starting the organisation of the current edition of eRisk, we decided to compile this book to report on the first five years of this interesting and challenging project. We hope this book will be of interest not just to the many past and, possibly, future participants, but also to other researchers involved in similarly challenging endeavours.

2 Book Content

This book presents a selection of the best eight participants to the first four tasks we introduced in eRisk. The papers were selected based on the evaluation that we, the organisers, carried out at the end of each of the first four yearly editions of CLEF of which eRisk was part, so far. That is, they were selected from 45 active participants (out of 185 registered teams) of the 2017-2020 editions of CLEF eRisk. Authors were asked to extend the papers they presented for inclusion in the eRisk Proceedings (published online in the CEUR Workshop proceedings,[3]) including a more detailed explanation of their models, more experiments, and a better analysis

[3] See: http://ceur-ws.org/.

of their results. Papers were reviewed by at least two external reviewers before being accepted for inclusion in the book.

The book is divided in three parts. Part I, titled "The eRisk Initiative" provides an overview of the eRisk initiative. First, in the chapter titled *The Challenge of Early Risk Prediction on the Internet*, we provide an overview of how the challenge is organised, explaining the datasets, the tasks, and the evaluation design an metrics. In the second chapter, titled *A Survey of the First Five Years of eRisk: Findings and Conclusions*, we present a detailed overview of the findings of the first five years of eRisk, detailing the different approaches presented by all the participants over the years. The chapter should also provide the motivations for the choice of the papers included in the following part of the book.

Part II presents the invited contributions from the best eight approaches presented in the four tracks (thus, two each) that were part of eRisk since 2017. The first two papers deal with early risk detection of depression.

The chapter titled *From Bag-of-Words to Transformers: A Deep Dive into the Participation in the eRisk Early Risk Detection of Depression Tasks with Classical and new Approaches* describes how the participants extended the work carried out in the context of eRisk to further explore the use of language models for the detection of early risks of depression. In particular, they combined hand-crafted features based on linguistic metadata and emotion and sentiment lexica. In addition, they present their work with new word embedding ensembles to explore possible improvements as detected with the new and alternative early detection evaluation metrics proposed in later editions of eRisk.

The chapter titled *Comparison of Machine Learning Models for Early Depression Detection from Users' Posts* reevaluates the models the authors developed for their participation at eRisk over the years and carries out a more robust comparison of results. The authors also include new models and perform an ablation study to analyze the most important features for each one of them, comparing their performance with BERT.

The second two papers deal with the early risk detection of *anorexia*. The chapter titled *Quick and (maybe not so) Easy Detection of Anorexia in Social Media: to Explainability and Beyond* uses several attention-based neural sub-models to extract features and predict class probabilities, which are later used as input features to a Support Vector Machine (SVM), making the final classification. The chapter also includes additional experiments performed on the model in order to evaluate it in terms of explainability.

The chapter titled *Two Simple and Domain-independent Approaches for Early Detection of Anorexia* presents two distinct domain-independent approaches to address the early risk detection of anorexia. The first approach is based on a temporal-aware document representation, whereas the second one consists of a simple, interpretable text classification model specifically designed for addressing early risk detection scenarios.

The third group of two papers deals with early risk detection of *self-harm*. The chapter titled *Early Risk Detection of Self-Harm using BERT-based Transformers* describes how the authors use a BERT-based classifier to achieve their excellent results, but more interestingly they present further work on the refining of the training scheme, and the tuning of the scoring mechanism to deal with other mental health disorders, such as pathological gambling and suicide detection.

The chapter titled *Detecting Traces of Self-harm on Reddit through Emotional Patterns* describes an approach based on a new text representation method called Bag of Sub-Emotions (BoSE), which considers fine-grained emotions for the detection of users suffering from self-harm. The paper extends the work presented in eRisk to better model and capture the emotional changes expressed by social media users through their posts.

Finally, the fourth group of two papers presents the two best approaches on the *automatic filling of the Beck Depression Inventory (BDI)* from text found on social media. The chapter titled *On the Estimation of Depression through Social Mining* presents an approach that leverages both standard machine learning algorithms and behavioral and linguistic patterns identified in specialized literature for the estimation of mental health conditions, as captured by questionnaires like the BDI. The paper rightly advocates the use of social monitoring of users' mental health as a digital complement to other standard public health surveillance and intervention practices.

Lastly, the chapter titled *Automatically Estimating the Severity of Multiple Symptoms Associated with Depression* presents how the authors used a combination of Latent Dirichlet Allocation (LDA), topic modelling, and the analysis of the user's writing styles to achieve their excellent results in the automatic filling of the BDI questionnaire from social media text.

Part III of the book reports on two approaches that somehow complement the work carried out in eRisk and that use different text collections, in addition of those developed by eRisk. The choice of these two papers was motivated by our intention to stimulate new initiatives directed to the automatic detection of mental health disorders from social media, in particular those that provide an attempt to explaining results. This is a direction of research that we find very interesting and that we plan to further explore in future editions of eRisk at CLEF.

The chapter titled *Beyond risk: Individual Mental Health Trajectories from Large-Scale Social Media Data* presents the work of the authors in the field of "precision mental health". Their work leverages large-scale data of the behavioral, cognitive, emotional and social traces to explore the possibility of modelling individualized mental health trajectories at population scale to identify high-precision targets for the detection, intervention, and mitigation of internalizing disorders.

The chapter titled *Explainability of Depression Detection on Social Media: from Deep Learning Models to Psychological Interpretations and Multimodality* explores the explainability of neural network models for mental health disorder detection in social media to make decisions more reliable, easier to trust, and more helpful for the identification of specific patterns in the data which are indicative of mental disorders. Particularly interesting is the collection and use a new multimodal dataset: *multiRedditDep*, consisting of social media data including texts and images posted by depressed users. With this, the authors present their attempts at automatically discovering signs of depression in a multimodal setting.

Finally, Part IV that concludes the book presents our current plans for the future of eRisk and perhaps for another five or more years of this initiative. In the chapter titled *The Future of eRisk* we reflect on the lessons learned from each of the challenges and editions of eRisk so far, integrating them into design decisions on the future of the project.

The eRisk Initiative

The Challenge of Early Risk Prediction on the Internet

David E. Losada, Fabio Crestani, and Javier Parapar

Abstract Internet provides massive amounts of data. Millions of users publish contents and interact in a daily fashion. This opens the opportunity for developing and deploying a wide range of applications, including commercial tools and public surveillance services. By analising online data one can extract valuable cues about specific individuals, segments of users, geographic communities or the society as a whole. The eRisk campaigns have focused on stimulating research in extracting signs of different types of risk from Internet data. This chapter describes the main features of this experimental framework that, over the years, has brought together dozens of research teams to tackle different challenges related to early risk detection on the Internet.

1 Introduction

As any major innovation brought to our lives, the Internet has unquestionable advantages but it also comes with challenges. For example, online tools, such as Social Networks or Internet fora, are able to break traditional communication barriers at the cost of a reduced control on the quality of contents and interactions. There is a huge variety of users and online publications and, in some cases, the Internet can be a source of risk (e.g., when a user sends, posts or shares harmful contents about some-

D. E. Losada (✉)
Centro Singular de Investigación en Tecnoloxías Intelixentes (CiTIUS), Universidade de Santiago de Compostela, Santiago de Compostela, Spain
e-mail: david.losada@usc.es

F. Crestani
Università della Svizzera italiana (USI), Lugano, Switzerland
e-mail: fabio.crestani@usi.ch

J. Parapar
Centro de Investigación en Tecnoloxías da Información e as Comunicacións (CITIC), Universidade da Coruña, A Coruña, Spain
e-mail: javierparapar@udc.es

F. Crestani et al. (eds.), *Early Detection of Mental Health Disorders by Social Media Monitoring*, Studies in Computational Intelligence 1018,
https://doi.org/10.1007/978-3-031-04431-1_2

one else); the Internet can also be reflective of risks that happen offline (e.g., when a teenager is developing depression and starts posting suicidal thoughts online).

Text analysis methods—e.g., based on techniques from text retrieval/classification and natural language processing—are valuable tools to exploit Internet data in an attempt to gain an understanding about users, contents, and the related risks. The eRisk shared-task campaigns [9–12], together with previous efforts to create benchmarks on language use and psychological conditions [8], have become a reference on this area. Over the last five years, this evaluation framework has contributed to set the experimental foundations of early risk detection technology and, within eRisk, a number of early detection and related challenges have been organised and successfully executed.

The eRisk lab has intended to design an experimental framework potentially applicable to multiple types of risks. Two core elements that are common across multiple types of risks are the availability of online data and the fact that the data come in a chronological way. For example, if we want to track the occurrence of cyberbullying behaviour then there are multiple Internet sources (e.g., Social Networks or certain Internet fora) where such offensive attitudes are public and explicit. Furthermore, the signs of harassment do not typically appear all at once, but rather show up gradually (e.g., as a thread of posts or comments that increasingly become more offensive). Another example relates to individuals at risk of developing a psychological disorder, such as depression. Again, there are numerous Internet platforms (e.g., Social Networks or support discussion groups) where signs of these psychological risks become explicit and these signs come as a stream of publications posted at different times (e.g., initial posts might be indicative of minor psychological issues or personal concerns while publications at more advanced stages might be much more concerning and even life-threatening).

Since its inception, eRisk aimed at instigating the development of *proactive* technologies able to do risk detection based on early traces. We understood that the temporal dimension was crucial because, in most application domains, appropriate intervention at early stages can reduce or minimise the problems. We did not want to promote the development of algorithms that merely react to the presence of explicit signals (e.g., criminal threats or suicidal thoughts). On the contrary, eRisk's main goal has been to gain an understanding on the onset of the risks and to instigate the design of innovative algorithms that are proactive and can make decisions based on early cues. Related to this, eRisk's data release strategy was by itself an innovation. Rather than setting a standard one-time release strategy, where participants get the whole dataset in a single release, we opted for sequential (and chronologically ordered) releases of data. In this way, the early detection algorithms could be evaluated in terms of how effectively and rapidly they respond to the existing evidence. More details on the evaluation process and effectiveness metrics are given in Sect. 4.

The rest of the chapter is organised as follows. Section 2 presents text analysis as a promising means to infer risk signals from user's data. The main datasets built under eRisk are presented in Sect. 3 and the evaluation design is explained in Sect. 4.

Section 5 is dedicated to report the specific characteristics of an eRisk task, initiated in 2019, centered on automatically estimating the answers of a depression questionnaire. The chapter ends with some concluding remarks.

2 Text as a Source of Risk Evidence

The topics that people discuss and the way in which we employ words that are seemingly mere lexical connectors can be highly revealing. Using innovative text analytics techniques we can, for example, analyse online conversations and try to detect inappropriate behaviour, such an adult interacting with children for sexual purposes (sexual predation identification [7]) or criminals recruiting new members to terrorist groups [1]. Risk detection can also be done from textual data published by individual users (e.g., analysing a user's thread of Social Media submissions). As argued by [18], the words people use reveal crucial aspects of their psychological and social worlds. There is substantial evidence linking the usage of natural language (including subtleties in linguistic styles and part-of-speech particles) and multiple psychological dimensions, such as personality, situational factors, emotional state and mental health [17, 18].

The link between language use and different psychologically-related risks has been studied for decades [18]. Over the years, this has resulted in a wide range of empirical investigations and clinical case studies oriented to disorders such as schizophrenia, depression, paranoia, or somatisation disorder, just to name a few. For example, the association between depression and a higher use of first person singular pronouns was already found nearly thirty years ago [3]. Early studies in these areas have been confined to clinical settings (e.g., based on analysing spontaneous speech or written essays). With the increased use of online media, a significant proportion of the society has adopted new forms of communication. Millions of interactions happen in a daily basis and Internet data provide new challenges and opportunities. Ríssola et al. [19] and Skaik and Inkpen [21] recently published surveys on the use of computational methods that employ social media for mental health analysis. In the last decade, there is a steady stream of contributions where, for example, several teams have attempted to predict or analyse depression using analytical methods [4, 5, 15, 16].

Commonly, Text or Social Analytics studies work with two groups of Internet users: a positive group, which contains users suffering from a given psychological condition, and a control group, which contains users who do not suffer from such condition. In some cases, the positive users are recruited using, for example, crowd-sourcing. In other cases, the positive group is obtained by searching for explicit mentions of diagnosis on Social Media. In any case, many studies in the literature focus on the language difference between the two groups, ignoring the temporal dimension of the data.

The eRisk campaigns organised so far have mostly focused on risks related to psychological problems (depression, anorexia and self-harm, for example) and the shared-tasks posed early detection challenges where the participants had not only to differentiate between risk and non-risk users. The teams had to work from chronologically ordered streams of user data, where submissions become available at different points in time and delays in alerts are penalised. The eRisk collections represent a seminal attempt to build benchmarks where a large chronological sequence of writings leading to a certain type of risk (e.g., diagnosis of a psychological disorder) is properly stored and analysed.

In the context of psychologically-related risks, timely actions or interventions are essential. Over the years, eRisk has aimed at instigating research on innovative early detection solutions able to identify the states of those at risk of developing major disorder episodes. To this end, we have stimulated the development of algorithms that computationally treat language as a meaningful tracker of the evolution of risks.

The next section explains the main features of the created datasets and Sect. 4 describes the evaluation design.

3 Datasets

Although multiple data sources were considered for building the eRisk datasets, all the collections produced so far contain publications (posts and comments) from a single source, Reddit.

Reddit is an open-source Social Media website where its members (the so-called *redditors*) submit content in the form of posts, comments or direct links. Any user can vote submissions, and Reddit's contents are organised into *subreddits*, which are subcommunities that define areas of interests. There is a wide range of subreddits. Some of them are quite general (e.g., news) while others are quite specific (e.g., subreddits on specific movies or TV series).

Reddit has been a valuable source for creating the eRisk collecions. It has a large group of users and many of them have published a large thread of submissions (typically, covering several years of interactions within the platform). This facilitates the construction of risk-related collections were evolution over time is an important factor. Another interesting characteristic of this Social Media website is that it contains substantial contents related to certain types of psychologically-related risks. For example, there are some subreddits about different disoders, such as depression and anorexia. Furthermore, the terms and conditions of Reddit allow researchers to use the published contents for research purposes[1]. Reddit has therefore a number of features that make it attractive for creating collections for early risk detection.

[1] At the time of building the eRisk collections, the policy of Reddit stated explicitly that the posts and comments users make are not private and would still be accessible after the user account is deleted. Reddit does not permit "unauthorized commercial use of its contents or redistribution, except as permitted by the doctrine of fair use". Research is considered an example of fair use.

3.1 Positive Group

The early risk collections constructed under the umbrella of the eRisk lab are all organised into two classes of users: risk users and non-risk users. The first class is typically referred to as the positive group and contains subjects for whom there is evidence that they suffer some type of risk. The second class of users is the control group, which contains users who are estimated to be *risk-free*.

For risks related to psychological disorders, a fundamental problem is how to determine the users to be included into the positive group. To this end, some past studies, e.g. [5], have employed medical questionnaires. However, relying on such clinical surveys is cumbersome, as it requires to individually contact with every potential participant. Furthermore, the volume and quality of data obtained in this way is limited. The eRisk lab, instead, adopted the proposal made by Coppersmith and colleagues [6], who proposed a method to identify people diagnosed with depression in Twitter. Their technique was based on searching for self-expressions of depression diagnoses. For example, users suffering from depression can be identified by running specific searches (e.g. "I was diagnosed with depression") against the Social Media platform.

This somehow automatises the process of finding candidate users for the positive set. However, it still requires manual inspection of the retrieved posts, in order to verify that the diagnoses look really genuine. We employed this strategy on Reddit and our confidence on the quality of the data is high. In Reddit, texts are often long and discussions about diagnosis are explicit. In fact, many of the matched entries are from psychologically-related subreddits (e.g., the depression subreddit), which are supportive spaces for people struggling with certain psychological issues. The individuals who are active on these subreddits tend to be very open about their clinical condition.

This is therefore a semi-automatic method (because it still requires manual intervention), but it is simple and effective. Following this approach, we have been able to extract large sets of people that explicitly declare having being diagnosed with a given psychological condition. The manual assessments were strict. For example, when creating a positive group for the depression tasks, expressions like "I think I have depression", "I have depression", or "I am depressed" were not considered as explicit expressions of a depression diagnosis. A user was included into the depression group if and only if there was an explicit and unquestionable mention of a diagnosis (e.g., "In may, I was diagnosed with depression", "After struggling with depression for many months, last week I was diagnosed").

The strategy sketched above was employed for extracting the positive groups of the following eRisk tasks: eRisk 2017 T1 task (depression), eRisk 2018 T1 task (depression), eRisk 2018 T2 task (anorexia), eRisk 2019 T1 task (anorexia), eRisk 2019 T2 task (self-harm), and eRisk 2020 T1 task (self-harm). Of course, the search expressions changed depending on the task.

3.2 Control Group

Following standard practice, the positive group was complemented with a control group composed of non-risk users. To this end, we extracted from the Social Media platform a large set of random users and, in most of the eRisk collections, we also included in the control group users who were active on psychologically-related subreddits (e.g., the depression subreddit) but had no psychological issues. For example, psychologists giving support to people or people interested in psychological disorders because they have some relative suffering from certain disorder. This type of control users makes the datasets realistic and challenging because their topics of interest are highly related to those of the positive group. In this way, the automatic methods designed to detect signs of psychological risks should not be merely based on topic-like classification but, instead, they need to incorporate more subtle forms of evidence.

It cannot be ruled out that the control group might contain some positive case (i.e., risk user). And it cannot be ruled out that the positive group might contain some negative case (because a user's claim about being diagnosed might be deceitful). However, we expect the impact of such cases to be negligible and, in any case, other extraction strategies (e.g. depression screening based on questionnaires) can also incorporate such type of noise in the collections.

3.3 Extraction of the User's Submissions

For each user, the maximum number of posts and comments that Reddit's API supplies is 1000 posts and 1000 comments. We extracted as many user's posts and user's comments as possible and, as a consequence, the eRisk collections contain up to 2000 submissions. Indeed, it is common that the most active users get to the 2000 limit. The user's submissions include textual entries (posts, comments to posts made by other users, and links) submitted to any subreddit. We collected the user's submissions made to any subreddit. Users often interact on a variety of subreddits and we were interested in extracting a whole representation of each individual. In this way, the collections contain a complete view of the user's language, which includes discussions and concerns about a wide range of topics.

The resulting collections have submissions from many subreddits such as games, politics, news, memes, etc. Redditor's submissions were organised in chronological order, from the oldest post or comment to the newest post or comment. In most cases, the resulting set of submissions covers a large period of time and, thus, enables to examine not only the language differences between risk and non-risk redditors, but also the evolution of the use of the language.

Within our extraction process, we also stored the link to the post or comment where the positive users made the explicit mention to their diagnosis. Although this information might be useful for further experiments, we did not include this post or comment into the user's list of submissions. The reason for such decision is that, otherwise, the participants of the eRisk challenges could overfit their technology to the specific phrases that we employed to search for risk cases.

The eRisk datasets were stored as a set of XML files, one per user. Each user file contains the user's submissions (one XML entry per submission). Each submission represents a post or comment and stores its title (if any, as comments have no title), its text and the date. No other metadata is available.

Regarding the recency of diagnosis, we have a wide range of cases. Sometimes, the diagnosis was recent (e.g., "Last month", "Two days ago") and, as a consequence, most of the submissions extracted for such positive users are *pre-diagnosis*. In other cases, the diagnosis was long time ago (e.g., "In 2018", "1 year ago") and, thus, most of the user's submissions are *post-diagnosis*. In any case, we did not include in the collections those users whose diagnosis was done long time ago. The collections also have cases in between, with some extracted submissions being *pre-diagnosis* and some extracted submissions being *post-diagnosis*. There is often some uncertainty about the specific date of the diagnosis but this approximate information about the diagnosis date is valuable and can be potentially used in future experiments in a variety of ways.

The extraction of user's comments and posts was done with PRAW, the Python Wrapper for Reddit's API[2]. All users with less than 10 submissions were removed, as we think there would be not enough evidence to be able to track the evolution of the risks.

In 2020, we introduced Beaver, a new tool to automate users' extraction for the positive group [13]. This tool implements the methodology we presented in [14] to ease the building of new collections. In particular, this tool automates the search of diagnoses self-expressions to find the candidate users. Then, by employing a technique called pooling, which is widely standardized and used in the Information Retrieval field, the tool selects which candidates have greater chances of being positive based on their posts' content. In this way, we can make the most of the annotation effort and mainly dedicate this time to inspect candidates that are most likely to be positive. We hope that this tool will help us extract larger sets of data in the future and, thus, improve the results of the challenge.

3.4 eRisk Collections

The statistics of the resulting collections are reported in Table 1.[3] The collections contain a reasonably large number of users and a large average of submissions per user. In most cases, the data was split into a training set of users, whose complete

[2] https://praw.readthedocs.org/en/v3.1.0/.

[3] The number of words per submission were counted after text pre-processing using the scikit-learn Python toolkit, *scikit-learn.org*. We employed no stopword processing and no vocabulary pruning based on document frequency.

Table 1 Main statistics of the eRisk collections

eRisk 2017 T1 (depression)				
	Train		Test	
	Depressed	*Control*	*Depressed*	*Control*
Num. subjects	83	403	52	349
Num. submissions (posts & comments)	30,851	264,172	18,706	217,665
Avg num. of submissions per subject	371.7	655.5	359.7	623.7
Avg num. of days from first to last submission	572.7	626.6	608.31	623.2
Avg num. words per submission	27.6	21.3	26.9	22.5
eRisk 2018 T1 (depression)				
	Train		Test	
	Depressed	*Control*	*Depressed*	*Control*
Num. subjects	135	752	79	741
Num. submissions (posts & comments)	49,557	481,837	40,665	504,523
Avg num. of submissions per subject	367.1	640.7	514.7	680.9
Avg num. of days from first to last submission	586.43	625.0	786.9	702.5
Avg num. words per submission	27.4	21.8	27.6	23.7
eRisk 2018 T2 (anorexia)				
	Train		Test	
	Anorexia	*Control*	*Anorexia*	*Control*
Num. subjects	20	132	41	279
Num. submissions (posts & comments)	7,452	77,514	17,422	151,364
Avg num. of submissions per subject	372.6	587.2	424.9	542.5

(continued)

list of submissions was made available to the eRisk participants at the beginning of the evaluation cycles, and a test set of users, which was only used for the official test stage.

The average lapse of time between the user's first submission (i.e., oldest interaction) and the user's last submission (i.e., newest interaction) covers more than a year. This is a nice feature of the collections, since it facilitates the analysis of the evolution of the risks. There is a high variation in the length of the posts or comments. Some submissions are short (e.g., replies to another submission), while other

Table 1 (continued)

eRisk 2018 T2 (anorexia)

	Train		Test	
	Depressed	*Control*	*Depressed*	*Control*
Avg num. of days from first to last submission	803.3	641.5	798.9	670.6
Avg num. words per submission	41.2	20.9	35.7	20.9

eRisk 2019 T1 (anorexia)

	Train		Test	
	Anorexia	*Control*	*Anorexia*	*Control*
Num. subjects	61	411	73	742
Num. submissions (posts & comments)	24,874	228,878	17,619	552,890
Avg num. of submissions per subject	407.8	556.9	241.4	745.1
Avg num. of days from first to last submission	≈ 800	≈650	≈510	≈930
Avg num. words per submission	37.3	20.9	37.2	21.7

eRisk 2019 T2 (self-harm)

	Train		Test	
	Self-Harm	*Control*	*Self-Harm*	*Control*
Num. subjects	–	–	41	299
Num. submissions (posts & comments)	–	–	6,927	163,506
Avg num. of submissions per subject	–	–	169.0	546.8
Avg num. of days from first to last submission	–	–	≈495	≈500
Avg num. words per submission	–	–	24.8	18.8

eRisk 2020 T1 (self-harm)

	Train		Test	
	Self-Harm	*Control*	*Self-Harm*	*Control*
Num. subjects	41	299	104	319
Num. submissions (posts & comments)	6,927	163,506	11,691	91,136
Avg num. of submissions per subject	169.0	546.8	112.4	285.6
Avg num. of days from first to last submission	≈ 495	≈500	≈270	≈426
Avg num. words per submission	24.8	18.8	21.4	11.9

submissions—typically posts—are lengthy. The average submission length is relatively low (around 30 words after pre-processing) because the number of comments is higher than the number of posts.

These collections were created with the firm intention to support research on these topics. As a consequence, the collections are available for research purposes under proper user agreements.[4,5,6,7]

4 Evaluation Design

The early risk detection challenges consisted of sequentially processing pieces of evidence (in the form of Social Media posts) and detect early traces of risk as soon as possible. At the test stage, the Social Media posts (or comments) had to be processed by the participants in the chronological order the posts or comments were created. In this way, the early detection systems that effectively perform this task could be applied in practice to sequentially track publications on Social Media.

In eRisk 2017 and eRisk 2018, the user data was released in a weekly basis. We had 10 releases of data (during ten weeks) and each week a chunk of user data was made available (the first chunk contains the oldest 10% of the posts and comments, and so forth). Since 2019, we moved from the chunk-based release of data to a item-by-item release of data. To this end, we configured a REST server that iteratively gives user posts or comments to the participating teams and waits for the team's responses. More details about the server can be found at the eRisk website.[8]

For most of the early risk detection tasks (see Table 1), we provided training data, meaning that we supplied the entire history of user posts and comments together with the user labels (risk vs non-risk users). In this way, the participating systems could be tuned with some training cases. The training data was released a couple of months before the beginning of the official test stage. The test stage consisted of a period of time where the participating teams had to connect to the REST server and iteratively get user posts/comments and send responses. Each team had the opportunity to stop at any point of the user chronology and make an alert.[9]

After processing each user post or comment, each participant had to choose between: (i) emitting an alert of risk on the user, or (ii) making no risk alert on the user. In the eRisk tasks, the alerts were considered as final (i.e. further decisions about the user are ignored), while *no alerts* were considered as non-final (i.e. the teams could later send an alert if they detected the appearance of signs of risk). This

[4] eRisk 2017:https://tec.citius.usc.es/ir/code/eRisk2017.html.

[5] eRisk 2018:https://tec.citius.usc.es/ir/code/eRisk2018.html.

[6] eRisk 2019:https://tec.citius.usc.es/ir/code/eRisk2019.html.

[7] eRisk 2020:https://tec.citius.usc.es/ir/code/eRisk2020.html.

[8] http://erisk.irlab.org/server.html.

[9] In eRisk 2017 and 2018 there was no REST server and, thus, the participants could only stop and make alerts after reading an entire chunk of data.

election had to be made for each user in the test set. The participating systems were evaluated based on the accuracy of the decisions and the number of user posts or comments required to take the decisions. The REST server provided no new user data until the system said alert/no alert.

The early risk detection tasks had two main types of evaluation, decision-based evaluation metrics and ranking-based evaluation. These two forms of evaluation are explained next.

4.1 Decision-Based Metrics

This type of evaluation focuses on the binary decisions (risk vs non-risk) taken by each system for each user. The eRisk evaluation reports included standard classification measures, such as Precision, Recall and F1[10]), and also new evaluation metrics designed for the early risk detection tasks. In [8], we proposed ERDE, an early risk detection error measure that introduces a penalty for late and correct alerts (true positives). The penalty grows with the delay in emitting the alert, and the delay is measured as the number of user posts or comments that had to be analysed before making the alert. This measure is explained in the next section and Sect. 4.1.2 describes new evaluation metrics incorporated in 2019.

4.1.1 Early Risk Detection Error (ERDE)

Standard classification metrics, such as F1, can be used to evaluate the system's responses against golden truth assessments that inform about what users are at risk (respectively non-risk cases). However, standard classification metrics are time-unaware and, thus, we needed to complement them with new measures that reward early alerts.

ERDE stands for *Early Risk Detection Error* and it takes into account the correctness of the binary decision and the delay taken by the system to make the decision. The delay was measured by counting the number (k) of user posts or comments analysed before giving the answer.

Another important issue is that risk data are often unbalanced (many more non-risk cases than risk cases). As a consequence, we also needed to weight false negative and false positive errors in a different way.

Consider a binary decision d taken by a system with delay k. Given golden truth judgments, the prediction d can be a true positive (TP), true negative (TN), false positive (FP) or false negative (FN). Given these four cases, the ERDE measure is defined as:

[10] Computed with respect to the positive class.

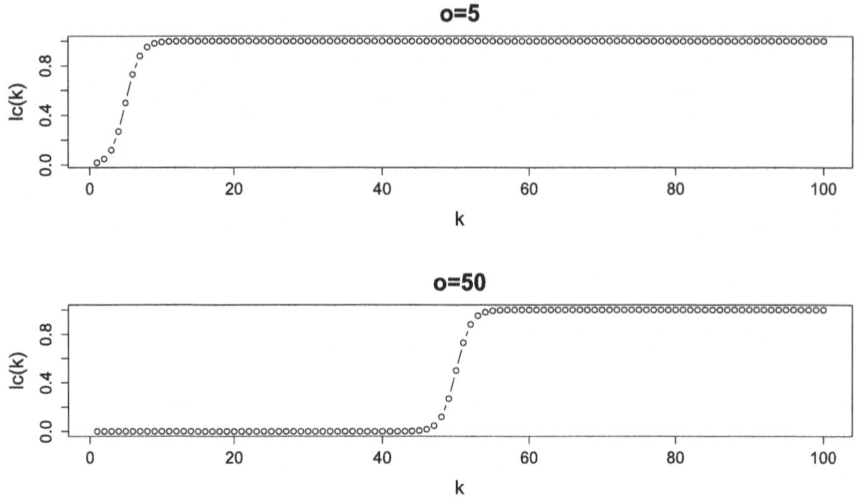

Fig. 1 Latency cost functions: $lc_5(k)$ and $lc_{50}(k)$

$$ERDE_o(d,k) = \begin{cases} c_{fp} & \text{if } d = \text{positive and ground truth=negative (FP)} \\ c_{fn} & \text{if } d = \text{negative and ground truth=positive (FN)} \\ lc_o(k) \cdot c_{tp} & \text{if } d = \text{positive and ground truth=positive (TP)} \\ 0 & \text{if } d = \text{negative and ground truth=negative (TN)} \end{cases}$$

How to set c_{fp} and c_{fn} depends on the application domain and the implications of FP and FN decisions. We will often face detection tasks where the number of non-risk cases is several orders of magnitude greater than the number of risk cases. In order to avoid building trivial systems that always catalog a user as a non-risk case, we need to have $c_{fn} >> c_{fp}$. In the eRisk tasks, we fixed c_{fn} to 1 and set c_{fp} according to the proportion of positive cases in the test data.[11] We set c_{tp} to c_{fn} (i.e. c_{tp} was set to 1) because, in practice, late detection can have severe consequences (i.e. late detection is considered equivalent to not detecting the case at all).

The function $lc_o(k) (\in [0, 1])$ represents the cost associated to the delay in detecting true positives. It is a monotonically increasing function of k that is parameterised by o, which controls the place in the X-axis where the cost grows more quickly:

$$lc_o(k) = 1 - \frac{1}{1 + e^{k-o}} \tag{1}$$

Figure 1 plots $lc_5(k)$ and $lc_{50}(k)$.

The latency-based penalty was only introduced for the true positives because we considered that late detection was not an issue for true negatives. True negatives are non-risk cases that, in practice, would not demand early intervention. The non-

[11] For example, in eRisk 2017 we set c_{fp} to 0.1296.

risk cases just need to be effectively filtered out from the positive cases. Algorithms should therefore focus on early detecting risk cases and detecting non-risk cases (regardless of when these non-risk cases are detected).

All cost weights are in [0, 1] and, thus, ERDE is in the range [0, 1]. Systems had to take one decision for each subject and the overall error is the mean of all ERDE values (one per subject).

4.1.2 Latency-Weighted F Measure

Since 2019, we complemented the eRisk evaluation toolkit with additional decision-based metrics that try to capture additional aspects of the problem. These metrics try to overcome the following limitations of ERDE:

- the penalty associated to true positives goes quickly to 1. This is due to the functional form of the cost function (sigmoid).
- in eRisk 2017 and 2018, which had a chunk-based release of test data, a perfect system that detects a true positive case right after the first round of messages (first chunk), did not get error equal to 0.
- with a chunk-based release of data, the contribution of each user to the performance evaluation has a large variance (different for users with few writings per chunk vs users with many writings per chunk).
- ERDE is not interpretable.

Some eRisk participants analysed these issues and proposed alternative ways for evaluation. Trotzek and colleagues [22] proposed $\text{ERDE}_o^{\%}$. This is a variant of ERDE that does not depend on the number of user posts or comments seen before the alert but, instead, it depends on the *percentage* of user writings seen before the alert. In this way, the user's contribution to the evaluation is normalised. However, there is an important limitation of $\text{ERDE}_o^{\%}$. In real-life applications, the overall number of user posts or comments is not known in advance. Social Media users post contents online and screening tools have to make predictions with the evidence seen so far. In practice, you do not know when (and if) a user's thread of message is exhausted. Thus, the performance metric should not depend on such lack of knowledge about the total number of user postings.

Another proposal of an alternative evaluation metric for early risk prediction was done by Sadeque and colleagues [20]. They proposed $F_{latency}$, which is described next. Imagine a user $u \in U$ and an early risk detection system that iteratively analyses u's posts and comments. By $g_u \in \{0, 1\}$, we refer to the user's golden truth label. A measure of delay was defined by Sadaque and colleagues as follows[12]:

[12] Observe that Sadeque et al. (see [20], p. 497) computed the latency for all users such that $g_u = 1$. We argue that latency should be computed only for the true positives. The false negatives ($g_u = 1$, $d_u = 0$) are not detected by the system and, therefore, they would not generate an alert.

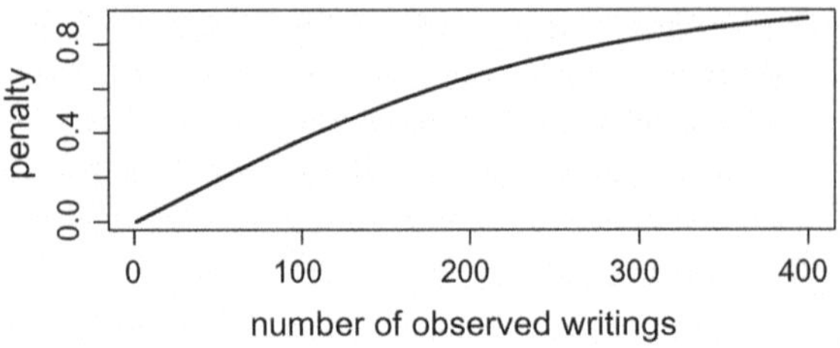

Fig. 2 Latency penalty increases with the number of observed writings (k_u)

$$\text{latency}_{TP} = \text{median}\{k_u : u \in U, d_u = g_u = 1\} \tag{2}$$

This measure of latency goes over the true positives detected by the system and assesses the system's delay based on the median number of writings that the system had to process to detect such positive cases. Following that, Sadeque et al. proposed a measure, $F_{latency}$, which combines the effectiveness of the decision (estimated with the F measure) and the delay.[13] This is based on multiplying F by a penalty factor based on the median delay. More specifically, each individual (true positive) decision, taken after reading k_u writings, is assigned the following penalty:

$$penalty(k_u) = -1 + \frac{2}{1 + \exp^{-p \cdot (k_u - 1)}} \tag{3}$$

where p is a parameter that determines how quickly the penalty should increase. In [20], p was set such that the penalty equals 0.5 at the median number of posts of a user.[14] Observe that a decision right after the first writing has no penalty ($penalty(1) = 0$). Figure 2 plots how the latency penalty increases with the number of observed writings.

The system's overall speed factor is computed as:

$$speed = (1 - \text{median}\{penalty(k_u) : u \in U, d_u = g_u = 1\}) \tag{4}$$

speed equals 1 for a system whose true positives are detected right at the first writing. A slow system, which detects true positives after hundreds of writings, will be assigned a speed score near 0.

Finally, the *latency-weighted* F score is simply:

$$F_{latency} = F \cdot speed \tag{5}$$

---

[13] Again, in eRisk we adopted Sadeque et al.'s proposal but we estimate latency only over the true positives.

[14] In the evaluation we set p to 0.0078, a setting obtained from the eRisk 2017 collection.

Since 2019 user's data was processed by the participants in a post by post basis (i.e. we avoided a chunk-based release of data). Under these conditions, the evaluation approach has the following properties:

- smooth grow of penalties.
- a perfect system gets $F_{latency} = 1$.
- for each user u the system can opt to stop at any point k_u and, therefore, now we do not have the effect of an imbalanced importance of users.
- $F_{latency}$ is more interpretable than ERDE.

4.2 Ranking-based Evaluation

This section discusses an alternative form of evaluation, which was used as a complement of the evaluation described above. After each release of data (new user post or comment) the participants had to send back the following information (for each user in the collection): (i) a decision for the user (alert/no alert), which was used to compute the decision-based metrics discussed above, and (ii) a score that represents the user's level of risk (estimated from the evidence seen so far). We used these scores to build a ranking of users in decreasing estimation of risk. For each participating system, we therefore have one ranking at each point (i.e., ranking after 1 post or comment, ranking after 2 posts/comments, etc.). This simulates a continuous re-ranking approach based on the evidence seen so far. In a real-life application, this ranking would be presented to an expert user who could take decisions (e.g. by inspecting the rankings). Each ranking can be scored with standard IR metrics, such as P@10 or NDCG. Since 2019, the eRisk reports include the ranking-based performance of the systems after seeing k posts or comments (with varying k).

5 eRisk Task on Automatically Filling a Depression Questionnaire

Besides the early detection tasks described above, the eRisk lab incorporated in 2019 a task on estimating the level of depression from a thread of user submissions. The teams were given the full history of posts and comments written by a number of users (in a single release of data) and the task consisted of filling a standard depression questionnaire based on the evidence found in the history of postings.

The questionnaires were derived from the Beck's Depression Inventory (BDI)[2], which assesses the presence of feelings like pessimism, sadness, loss of energy, etc. for the detection of depression. The questionnaire includes 21 questions (see Figs. 3, 4).

The task aims at exploring the viability of automatically estimating the severity of the multiple symptoms associated with depression. Given the user's history of

```
This questionnaire consists of 21 groups of statements. Please read each group of statements
carefully, and then pick out the one statement in each group that best describes the way you feel.
If several statements in the group seem to apply equally well, choose the highest
number for that group.

1. Sadness
   0. I do not feel sad.
   1. I feel sad much of the time.
   2. I am sad all the time.
   3. I am so sad or unhappy that I can't stand it.

2. Pessimism
   0. I am not discouraged about my future.
   1. I feel more discouraged about my future than I used to be.
   2. I do not expect things to work out for me.
   3. I feel my future is hopeless and will only get worse.

3. Past Failure
   0. I do not feel like a failure.
   1. I have failed more than I should have.
   2. As I look back, I see a lot of failures.
   3. I feel I am a total failure as a person.

4. Loss of Pleasure
   0. I get as much pleasure as I ever did from the things I enjoy.
   1. I don't enjoy things as much as I used to.
   2. I get very little pleasure from the things I used to enjoy.
   3. I can't get any pleasure from the things I used to enjoy.

5. Guilty Feelings
   0. I don't feel particularly guilty.
   1. I feel guilty over many things I have done or should have done.
   2. I feel quite guilty most of the time.
   3. I feel guilty all of the time.

6. Punishment Feelings
   0. I don't feel I am being punished.
   1. I feel I may be punished.
   2. I expect to be punished.
   3. I feel I am being punished.

7. Self-Dislike
   0. I feel the same about myself as ever.
   1. I have lost confidence in myself.
   2. I am disappointed in myself.
   3. I dislike myself.

8. Self-Criticalness
   0. I don't criticize or blame myself more than usual.
   1. I am more critical of myself than I used to be.
   2. I criticize myself for all of my faults.
   3. I blame myself for everything bad that happens.

9. Suicidal Thoughts or Wishes
   0. I don't have any thoughts of killing myself.
   1. I have thoughts of killing myself, but I would not carry them out.
   2. I would like to kill myself.
   3. I would kill myself if I had the chance.

10. Crying
   0. I don't cry anymore than I used to.
   1. I cry more than I used to.
   2. I cry over every little thing.
   3. I feel like crying, but I can't.

11. Agitation
   0. I am no more restless or wound up than usual.
   1. I feel more restless or wound up than usual.
   2. I am so restless or agitated that it's hard to stay still.
   3. I am so restless or agitated that I have to keep moving or doing something.
```

Fig. 3 Beck's depression inventory (part 1)

12. Loss of Interest
0. I have not lost interest in other people or activities.
1. I am less interested in other people or things than before.
2. I have lost most of my interest in other people or things.
3. It's hard to get interested in anything.

13. Indecisiveness
0. I make decisions about as well as ever.
1. I find it more difficult to make decisions than usual.
2. I have much greater difficulty in making decisions than I used to.
3. I have trouble making any decisions.

14. Worthlessness
0. I do not feel I am worthless.
1. I don't consider myself as worthwhile and useful as I used to.
2. I feel more worthless as compared to other people.
3. I feel utterly worthless.

15. Loss of Energy
0. I have as much energy as ever.
1. I have less energy than I used to have.
2. I don't have enough energy to do very much.
3. I don't have enough energy to do anything.

16. Changes in Sleeping Pattern
0. I have not experienced any change in my sleeping pattern.
1a. I sleep somewhat more than usual.
1b. I sleep somewhat less than usual.
2a. I sleep a lot more than usual.
2b. I sleep a Iot less than usual.
3a. I sleep most of the day.
3b. I wake up 1-2 hours early and can't get back to sleep.

17. Irritability
0. I am no more irritable than usual.
1. I am more irritable than usual.
2. I am much more irritable than usual.
3. I am irritable all the time.

18. Changes in Appetite
0. I have not experienced any change in my appetite.
1a. My appetite is somewhat less than usual.
1b. My appetite is somewhat greater than usual.
2a. My appetite is much less than before.
2b. My appetite is much greater than usual.
3a. I have no appetite at all.
3b. I crave food all the time.

19. Concentration Difficulty
0. I can concentrate as well as ever.
1. I can't concentrate as well as usual.
2. It's hard to keep my mind on anything for very long.
3. I find I can't concentrate on anything.

20. Tiredness or Fatigue
0. I am no more tired or fatigued than usual.
1. I get more tired or fatigued more easily than usual.
2. I am too tired or fatigued to do a lot of the things I used to do.
3. I am too tired or fatigued to do most of the things I used to do.

21. Loss of Interest in Sex
0. I have not noticed any recent change in my interest in sex.
1. I am less interested in sex than I used to be.
2. I am much less interested in sex now.
3. I have lost interest in sex completely

Fig. 4 Beck's depression inventory (part 2)

writings, the algorithms had to estimate the user's response to each individual question. We collected questionnaires filled by Social Media users together with their history of posts and comments (we extracted each history of postings right after the user provided us with the filled questionnaire). The questionnaires filled by the users (ground truth) were used to assess the quality of the responses provided by the participating systems.

The participants were given a dataset with several users and they were asked to produce a file with the following structure:

```
username1 answer1 answer2 .... answer21
username2 ....
....
```

Each line has a user identifier and 21 values. These values correspond to the responses to the questions of the depression questionnaire (the possible values are 0, 1a, 1b, 2a, 2b, 3a, 3b -for questions 16 and 18- and 0, 1, 2, 3 -for the rest of the questions-).

5.1 *Evaluation Metrics*

For this innovative task, we considered a number of metrics in order to assess the quality of a questionnaire filled by a system when compared to the real questionnaire filled by the actual Social Media user:

- **Average Hit Rate** (AHR): Hit Rate (HR) averaged over all users. HR is a stringent measure that computes the ratio of cases where the automatic questionnaire has exactly the same answer as the real questionnaire. For example, an automatic questionnaire with 5 matches gets HR equal to 5/21 (because there are 21 questions in the form).
- **Average Closeness Rate** (ACR): Closeness Rate (CR) averaged over all users. CR takes into account that the answers of the depression questionnaire represent an ordinal scale. For example, consider the #17 question:

  ```
  17. Irritability
  0. I am no more irritable than usual.
  1. I am more irritable than usual.
  2. I am much more irritable than usual.
  3. I am irritable all the time.
  ```

  Imagine that the real user answered "0". A system S1 whose answer is "3" should be penalised more than a system S2 whose answer is "1".
  For each question, CR computes the absolute difference (ad) between the real and the automated answer (e.g. ad = 3 and ad = 1 for S1 and S2, respectively) and, next, this absolute difference is transformed into an effectiveness score as follows:

$CR = (mad - ad)/mad$, where mad is the maximum absolute difference, which is equal to the number of possible answers minus one.[15]

- **Average DODL (ADODL)**: Difference between overall depression levels (DODL) averaged over all users. The previous measures assess the systems' ability to answer each question in the form. DODL, instead, does not look at question-level hits or differences but computes the overall depression level (sum of all the answers) for the real and automated questionnaire and, next, the absolute difference ($ad\_overall$) between the real and the automated score is computed.
  Depression levels are integers between 0 and 63 and, thus, DODL is normalised into [0,1] as follows: $DODL = (63 - ad\_overall)/63$.
- **Depression Category Hit Rate (DCHR)**. In the psychological domain, it is customary to associate depression levels with the following categories:

```
minimal depression (depression levels 0-9)
mild depression (depression levels 10-18)
moderate depression (depression levels 19-29)
severe depression (depression levels 30-63)
```

  The last effectiveness measure consists of computing the fraction of cases where the automated questionnaire led to a depression category that is equivalent to the depression category obtained from the real questionnaire.

6 Conclusions

Over the years, the eRisk lab, organised under CLEF, has run up to eight shared-tasks. Six of them were devoted to early detecting signs of risk, where the participants had to analyse a sequence of user's posts and comments in an iterative way. This task involves a tradeoff between making early decisions and making more informed but perhaps late decisions. A second class of task was proposed in 2019, when we introduce an innovative challenge where the participants had to analyse the entire history of user's postings and, next, try to estimate the user's responses to a standard depression questionnaire.

Acknowledgements This work was supported by projects RTI2018-093336-B-C21, RTI2018-093336-B-C22 (Ministerio de Ciencia e Innovación, Agencia Estatal de Investigación & ERDF) and PLEC2021-007662 (MCIN/AEI/10.13039/501100011033, Ministerio de Ciencia e Innovación, Agencia Estatal de Investigación, Plan de Recuperación, Transformación y Resiliencia, Unión Europea-Next GenerationEU). The first author thanks the financial support supplied by the Consellería de Educación, Universidade e Formación Profesional (accreditation 2019-2022 ED431G-

[15] In the two questions (#16 and #18) that have seven possible answers {0, $1a$, $1b$, $2a$, $2b$, $3a$, $3b$} the pairs ($1a$, $1b$), ($2a$, $2b$), ($3a$, $3b$) are considered equivalent because they reflect the same depression level. As a consequence, the difference between $3b$ and 0 is equal to 3 (and the difference between $1a$ and $1b$ is equal to 0).

2019/04, ED431C 2018/29) and the European Regional Development Fund, which acknowledges the CiTIUS-Research Center in Intelligent Technologies of the University of Santiago de Compostela as a Research Center of the Galician University System. The third author thanks the financial support supplied by the Consellería de Educación, Universidade e Formación Profesional (accreditation 2019-2022 ED431G/01, ED431B 2019/03) and the European Regional Development Fund, which acknowledges the CITIC Research Center in ICT of the University of A Coruña as a Research Center of the Galician University System.

References

1. Abbasi, A., & Chen, H. (2005). Applying authorship analysis to extremist-group web forum messages. *IEEE Intelligent Systems,* 67–75.
2. Beck, A. T., Ward, C. H., Mendelson, M., Mock, J., & Erbaugh, J. (1961). An inventory for measuring depression. *JAMA Psychiatry 4,*(06), 561–571.
3. Bucci, W., & Freedman, N. (1981). The language of depression. *Bulletin of the Menninger Clinic, 45*(4), 334–358.
4. Choudhury, M. D., Counts, S., & Horvitz, E. (2013). Social media as a measurement tool of depression in populations. In H. C. Davis, H. Halpin, A. Pentland, M. Bernstein, & L. A. Adamic (Eds.), *WebSci* (pp. 47–56). ACM.
5. Choudhury, M. D., Gamon, M., Counts, S., & Horvitz, E. (2013). Predicting depression via social media. In E. Kiciman, N. B. Ellison, B. Hogan, P. Resnick, & I. Soboroff (Eds.), *ICWSM.* The AAAI Press.
6. Coppersmith, G., Dredze, M., & Harman, C. (2014). Quantifying mental health signals in Twitter. In *ACL Workshop on Computational Linguistics and Clinical Psychology.*
7. Inches, G., & Crestani, F. (2012). Overview of the international sexual predator identification competition at pan-2012. In P. Forner, J. Karlgren, and C. Womser-Hacker (Eds.), *CLEF (Online Working Notes/Labs/Workshop), CEUR Workshop Proceedings*, (Vol. 1178). CEUR-WS.org.
8. Losada, D. E., & Crestani, F. (2016). A test collection for research on depression and language use. In *Conference Labs of the Evaluation Forum* (pp. 28–39). Springer.
9. Losada, D. E., Crestani, F., & Parapar, J. (2017). eRISK 2017: CLEF lab on early risk prediction on the internet: Experimental foundations. In *Proceedings Conference and Labs of the Evaluation Forum CLEF 2017.* Dublin, Ireland.
10. Losada, D. E., Crestani, F., & Parapar, J. (2018). Overview of eRisk—Early risk prediction on the internet. In *Experimental IR Meets Multilinguality, Multimodality, and Interaction. Proceedings of the Ninth International Conference of the CLEF Association (CLEF 2018).* Avignon, France.
11. Losada, D. E., Crestani, F., & Parapar, J. (2019). Overview of eRisk 2019—Early risk prediction on the internet. In *Experimental IR Meets Multilinguality, Multimodality, and Interaction. Proceedings of the Ninth International Conference of the CLEF Association (CLEF 2019).* Lugano, Switzerland.
12. Losada, D. E., Crestani, F., & Parapar, J. (2020). Overview of eRisk 2020—Early risk prediction on the internet. In *Experimental IR Meets Multilinguality, Multimodality, and Interaction. Proceedings of the Ninth International Conference of the CLEF Association (CLEF 2020).* Thessaloniki, Greece.
13. Otero, D. (2020). Beaver: Efficiently building test collections for novel tasks. In I. Cantador, M. Chevalier, M. Melucci, & J. Mothe (Eds.), *Proceedings of the Joint Conference of the Information Retrieval Communities in Europe.* CIRCLE '20, CEUR-WS.org.
14. Otero, D., Parapar, J., & Barreiro, A. (2021). The wisdom of the rankers: A cost-effective method for building pooled test collections without participant systems. In *Proceedings of the 36th Annual ACM Symposium on Applied Computing.* New York, NY, USA: SAC '21, Association for Computing Machinery.

15. Park, M., McDonald, D. W., & Cha, M. (2013). Perception differences between the depressed and non-depressed users in Twitter. In E. Kiciman, N. B. Ellison, B. Hogan, P. Resnick, & I. Soboroff (Eds.), *ICWSM*. The AAAI Press.
16. Paul, M. J., & Dredze, M. (2011). You are what you tweet: Analyzing Twitter for public health. In L. A. Adamic, R. A. Baeza-Yates, & S. Counts (Eds.), *ICWSM*. The AAAI Press.
17. Pennebaker, J. W. (2011). *The secret life of pronouns: What our words say about us*. New York: Bloomsbury Press.
18. Pennebaker, J. W., Mehl, M. R., & Niederhoffer, K. G. (2003). Psychological aspects of natural language use: Our words, our selves. *Annual Review of Psychology, 54*(1), 547–577.
19. Rissola, E., Losada, D. E., & Fabio, C. (2021). A survey of computational methods for online mental state assessment on social media. *ACM Transactions on Computing for Healthcare, 2*, 2.
20. Sadeque, F., Xu, D., & Bethard, S. (2018). Measuring the latency of depression detection in social media. In *WSDM* (pp. 495–503). ACM.
21. Skaik, R., & Inkpen, D. (2020). Using social media for mental health surveillance: A review. *ACM Computing Surveys, 53,* 6 Dec.
22. Trotzek, M., Koitka, S., & Friedrich, C. M. (2018). Utilizing neural networks and linguistic metadata for early detection of depression indications in text sequences. arxiv:1804.07000.

A Survey of the First Five Years of eRisk: Findings and Conclusions

Esteban A. Ríssola, Javier Parapar, David E. Losada, and Fabio Crestani

Abstract Early risk detection is a challenging task in which multiple objectives are involved. For this task, getting timely predictions with a reasonable confidence level becomes critical. Over the last five years, eRisk shared-task campaigns have focused on stimulating research in extracting evidences of different types of risk from Internet data (e.g., diagnosis of a mental disorder), fostering the development of early risk detection systems (ERDS). In this chapter, we present an overview of the key aspects and stages involved in the design and development of ERDS. Despite the heterogeneity observed, common elements can be identified from the wealth of systems submitted since eRisk's outset. In particular, we review and summarise what has been learnt from each team contribution, specially focusing on how they built their systems to tackle different early detection tasks. This chapter concludes with several findings and lessons that have been discovered and learnt along the way.

E. A. Ríssola (✉) · F. Crestani
Università della Svizzera italiana (USI), Lugano, Switzerland
e-mail: esteban.andres.rissola@usi.ch

F. Crestani
e-mail: fabio.crestani@usi.ch

J. Parapar
Centro de Investigación en Tecnoloxías da Información e as Comunicacións (CITIC), Universidade da Coruña, A Coruña, Spain
e-mail: javierparapar@udc.es

D. E. Losada
Centro Singular de Investigación en Tecnoloxías Intelixentes (CiTIUS), Universidade de Santiago de Compostela, Santiago de Compostela, Spain
e-mail: david.losada@usc.es

F. Crestani et al. (eds.), *Early Detection of Mental Health Disorders by Social Media Monitoring*, Studies in Computational Intelligence 1018,
https://doi.org/10.1007/978-3-031-04431-1_3

1 Introduction

As it was introduced in chapter "The Challenge of Early Risk Prediction on the Internet", research on language and psychology has shown that various useful cues about individuals' mental state (as well as personality, social and emotional conditions) can be discovered by examining the patterns of their language use [17]. As a matter of fact, language attributes could act as indicators of the current mental state [61, 71], personality [52, 72] and even personal values [12]. The main reason, as argued by Pennebaker et al. [58], is because such latent mental-related variables are encoded in the words that individuals use to communicate. Moreover, language use is relatively reliable over time, consistent, and varies considerably between individuals [11].

The mental and behavioural health domain has witnessed an increasing research interest in the identification of mental state alterations through the exploitation of online digital traces. This interest is a result of the intensive publication activity of social media users, who often share online their thoughts and disclose their feelings and moods. On the top of this, the constraints dictated by reality, such as cost and time, make the efficient process of personal diagnosis unfeasible. Initiatives such as the Strategic Workshop on Information Retrieval in Lorne [21] (SWIRL) are already proposing the application of principles of core Information Retrieval for the development of decision-making systems applied to fields that years back were not easy to conceive or imagine. In particular, they highlight the potential for cross-disciplinary collaboration and impact with a number of scientific fields, including psychology. In this respect, the Early Risk Prediction on the Internet (eRisk) [38–41], as well as the Computational Linguistics and Clinical Psychology (CLPsych) [18, 87] experimental frameworks were the first to propose benchmarks to bring together many researchers to address the automatic detection of mental disorders in online social media. This type of initiatives often contribute to establishing solid foundations, common standards, and a thorough understanding of problems and required data for experimentation.

Over the last five years, eRisk shared-task campaigns have focused on stimulating research in extracting evidences of different types of risk from Internet data (e.g., diagnosis of a mental disorder), mostly fostering the development of early risk detection systems (ERDS). Participants of the campaigns are asked to sequentially process pieces of evidence following the chronological order in which the textual records were created. The main aim is to identify, as soon as possible, early evidences of a mental disorder, such as depression or anxiety. Early detection of a mental disorders can be thought as a binary classification task, given that the ultimate goal is to classify the individuals as positive cases or not (i.e., *at-risk* or not). However, in this scenario an essential feature is the underlying compromise that emerges from making *timely* and *correct* decisions. In other words, when a system receives a piece of data it can either emit a decision or choose to wait for the next piece of evidence in order to take a *more informed* decision. If the system opts to wait then it gets a penalty for its delayed decision. This delay is measured by counting the quantity of textual pieces processed before providing the final answer. In this respect, the eRisk initiative has been the first of its kind to go beyond a traditional binary classification task promoting a benchmark exercise with such characteristics.

The remainder of this chapter is organised as follows. Section 2 introduces the key aspects and stages involved in the design and development of ERDS, particularly focusing on the way participating teams built their systems to tackle different early detection tasks. In 2019, the eRisk lab introduced a novel and complementary task aimed at exploring the feasibility of automatically estimating the severity of multiple symptoms associated with depression. Section 3 provides a overview of the methods and techniques proposed to address this task. Section 4 summarises the several findings and the handful of lessons learnt since the inception of eRisk shared-tasks. Finally, Sect. 5 concludes the chapter.

2 Early Risk Detection Systems Design

Unlike traditional risk-assessment and decision-making applications, a key requirement in the design of ERDS is that, besides the correctness of the decisions, the delays should be also taken into account. Thus, the construction of effective ERDS represents a challenging endeavour. Developer of ERDS need to find the most effective and efficient way to represent and encode the information present in users' posts, taking into account *what* they write about, *how* they write it and, at the same time, keep track of the changes that these variables exhibit over time to spot even subtle and/or sudden variations.

In the following, we present an overview of the main stages involved in the development of ERDS for different tasks, such as the early detection of depression. We particularly focus on the methods and techniques proposed and applied during the last five editions of eRisk. First, we focus on the feature extraction process. The outcomes of this step are the various attributes, know as *features*, which encode several properties and characteristics of the users and their posts. In a subsequent stage, the derived representations are integrated with an assessment technology, or a combination of them, to develop the final assessment system. Since taking timely decisions is equally important as their correctness, we also outline the various strategies that participants included in their systems' design to deal with this trade-off.

2.1 Feature Extraction

There are several ways to encode the information contained in users' posts. For instance, one could take into account quantitative elements of the text, such as the frequency of specific words, or consider other aspects related to the level of engagement that users exhibit in the social media platform, such as the average post length. The computed features and their combination play a very important role in the development of ERDS. In most of the cases, the feature extraction stage involves strategies that were previously shown to be effective in other domains or text classification tasks, such as sentiment analysis. It should be noted that, although related, such domains were not focused on assessing the mental state condition of the users. Subsequently, the generated features are used to train standard machine learning algorithms, given hand-labelled data, or integrated with less sophisticated ruled-based approaches to conduct the assessment. Feature extraction is not a trivial task and a thorough analysis would be required to determine the most useful features for each mental disorder as shown in [70].

Open-Vocabulary: A simple yet effective way to encode the textual content of a document as a vector is known as *Bag-of-Words* (BoW). The basic idea is to focus only on the occurrence and frequency of words in the document, without considering other syntactic attributes, such as their part-of-speech. Thus, any given document can be encoded as a fixed-length vector whose length is equal to the number of terms in the vocabulary. The vocabulary contains the unique set of words found in a collection of documents or as it happens in this case, social media posts. Each position in that vector provides information about the occurrence of a given term in the documents. Such value could simply denote the presence of the term (binary), the number of times that the term is repeated (frequency) or it can represent a more sophisticated term-weighting scheme, such as TF-IDF [20] or Exponential Reward of Personal Information (EXPEI) [54, 55].

Several participants of eRisk have applied BoW to transform users posts into vectorial representations in 2017 [5, 27, 79], 2018 [14, 37, 47, 55, 65, 80, 85], 2019 [23, 51, 54, 66, 77] and 2020 [8, 78]. Most of them extracted single terms (*unigrams*) and sequences of contiguous words, known as *n*-grams (e.g., bigrams, trigrams) to encode textual contents. Usually, the size of the vocabulary can easily reach the order of several thousands of terms [20]. For this reason, feature selection techniques are applied to discard potentially irrelevant and noisy terms, and therefore reduce the feature space favouring the learning process. While a few participants considered filtering out terms below a certain frequency threshold [47, 65, 68], others utilised different metrics to quantify the amount of information that a term can provide, such as *Mutual Information* (MI) [27, 51], *chi-square* (χ^2) [7, 56] or *Discriminative Personal Purity* (DPP) [54, 55]. In this way, only the top-k most discriminating terms are kept.

Villegas et al. [83] introduced a novel document representation approach named *Temporal Variation of Terms* [25] (TVT). This method extended Concise Semantic Analysis [36] (CSA) by defining concepts that capture the temporal aspects in early risk detection tasks. Such method accounts for the variations in the vocabulary at different sequential stages of the users' chronology of posts. CSA is a semantic analysis technique that overcomes certain shortcomings of BoW representations. It models words and documents in a *compact* space of concepts, usually composed of 100 elements. A small and generic set of concepts is derived from a set of category labels defined with human intervention. The idea behind TVT was that the *partial* user history, observed in successive batches of posts, represented *temporal* concepts that should be considered when building the concept space. In particular, the evolution of the word usage through the different sequential stages may reveal relevant information for the task at hand. Funez et al. [28] proposed an improvement of the TVT document representation technique called *Flexible Temporal Variation of terms (FTVT)*. A distinctive feature of TVT was that it provided a convenient way to deal with the unbalance of the minority class. Instead, FTVT introduced a more flexible strategy by allowing to vary the number of batches of posts that enrich the positive class and were used to build the representation. This extension emerged from the necessity to tailor a system depending on the urgency level required, i.e., the speed of the detection.

Aragón [7, 8] presented an innovative document representation method combining information extracted from emotions lexicons and words embeddings called *Bag of Sub-Emotions (BoSE)* [6]. This approach is based on a set of automatically-derived fine-grained emotions used to model the emotional profile of users. Each coarse or basic emotion, such as "anger" or "joy", is represented by several groups of semantically related words, which clustered together, are named "sub-emotions". In this way, users are represented with a histogram of fine-grained emotions (i.e., a frequency distribution) obtained by measuring the similarity between each sub-emotion (centroid of the corresponding cluster) and the text they have written. These representations provide a more flexible and detailed representation of users' textual records providing more interpretable outcomes.

Distributional Word Vectors: An alternative way to generate a fixed-length feature representation from users posts is to consider the semantic relationships between the words in them. Meaning can be understood as emerging from mutual dependencies of words within the language. Semantically related words co-occur in texts with coherent topics at a higher frequency than unrelated words. Using this property, the similarity between two words can be quantitatively measured by the frequency of their co-occurrence.

LSA [22], word2vec [48], GloVe [59], fastText [10, 34] and Random Indexing [35] are associative models that capture the meaning of words by means of linear representations in a high-dimensional semantic space, known as *word embeddings* (WE). The semantic content of a word is encoded as a vector and this vectorial representation can be used to estimate how *similar* other words are. Such natural language representation are known to be *context-free* since they generate a single WE representation for each word in the vocabulary. Because words mean different things in different contexts, such methods require that word representations capture *all* of the possibilities. It should be noted that, although convenient, this makes some assumptions about language that do not fit with reality. Various systems incorporated the used of context-free word embeddings as features to identify different mental disorders in 2017 [79], 2018 [14, 56, 63, 64, 80], 2019 [23, 26, 50, 51, 68] and 2020 [2, 31, 78, 81].

Conversely, in *contextual* representations different WE are generated for each word in the vocabulary based on the words in its nearby context, e.g., in a sentence. Each WE is specific to the token in its particular context, accounting in this way for the various meanings (or *senses*) that a particular word might have. BERT [24],

ELMo [60] and UMLFit [32], are just a few examples of methods (and probably the most popular ones) used to generate contextual language representations. Several eRisk participants have incorporated such representations to design their ERDS [1, 2, 26, 45, 50, 62, 81].

Lexicons: A common method for linking language with psychological variables involves counting words belonging to manually-created categories of language [16–18]. This method is known as "closed-vocabulary" analysis [74]. In this case, a document is represented by the frequency, possibly normalised, of the words that comprise each particular lexicon. Such dictionaries are usually manually constructed by psychologists covering various psychologically meaningful categories which are useful to analyse the linguistic style patterns of an individual's way of writing. Probably one of the most extensively used lexica is the *Linguistic Inquiry and Word Count* [57, 76] (LIWC),[1] which provides mental health practitioners with a tool for gathering quantitative data regarding the mental state of patients from their writing style. Moreover, these lexica are usually extended with other ad-hoc lexica [4, 16, 43, 53] built for specific tasks, such as depression detection or suicide risk assessment. In essence, they consist of words closely associated with texts written by individuals sharing their experience on mental disorders or its symptoms in online settings and also include words related to names of medications. In particular, LIWC [65, 80, 81], the Unified Medical Language System (UMLS) Metathesaurus[2] [23, 56, 73], Non-Suicidal Self-Injury (NSSI) [3], Valence Aware Dictionary and sEntiment Reasoner [33] (VADER) [2] and NRC Word-Emotion Association Lexicon [49] (EmoLex) [81] dictionaries have been utilised by eRisk participants to build their systems.

Social Engagement and Posting Behaviour: These set of features intend to profile certain attributes of users' posts, such as the length or the time they were created, as well as their level of participation in the social media platform. As stated by Coppersmith et al. [19] such attributes provide a proxy, although imperfect, for significant findings in the mental health literature which may manifest and be measured on social media. Moreover, on some occasions they could motivate new inquiries into behavioural traits as quantified on social media [67]. This category of features includes the computation of parameters such as:

- Textual spreading [3, 14, 44, 80]: amount of textual information provided by the users in their posts, such as the length.
- Time gap [2, 14]: time between two consecutive posts
- Time span [14, 27]: profile of the moments (e.g., hour or day of the week) when users published their posts.
- Posting Frequency [5].
- Average/median number of words per post [44, 64, 65].

[1] See: http://liwc.wpengine.com/.

[2] See: https://www.nlm.nih.gov/research/umls/knowledge_sources/metathesaurus/.

Writing Style: Many words such as pronouns, articles and prepositions somehow reveal people's emotional state, personality, thinking style and connection with others individuals [17]. Much of these attributes are used to quantify the importance of personal phrases (i.e., sentences with a first person pronoun) to model the profiles of users suffering from a mental disorder. More specifically, they assumed that the words used in self-reference statements might disclose the individual's social and psychological states and, thus, they might be useful proxies to identify alterations in behaviours and mental states

In particular, these attributes attempt to capture the writing style of the users and are used to quantify specific stylistic patterns that could differentiate positive instances of a mental disorder from control individuals. This set includes part-of-speech (PoS), verbs tense analysis, function words,[3] use of negation words, punctuation and measures of text readability and complexity [3, 5, 44, 64, 79, 81].

2.2 *Assessment Technologies*

The successive stage after deriving different features involves their integration with some kind of predictive technology to develop the final ERDS. Recall that the ultimate goal of risk-assessment and decision-making applications is to aid and facilitate health practitioners daily labour. Therefore, such a system should be able to effectively determine at early stages whether an individual is likely to develop (or has already developed) a mental disorder. The various types of features previously outlined provide a way to encode the latent information associated with the mental state of the individuals such that a decision-making algorithm could *learn* or *leverage* the patterns present in the data to conduct the assessment. In this case, the outcome of such assessment is a binary variable stating, usually with a certain level confidence, whether the individual is suffering from a specific mental disorder or not. Most of the assessment technologies utilised by eRisk participants are based on standard supervised learning algorithms without any modification and, generally, with their parameters optimised for the task. Meanwhile, other participants proposed less sophisticated yet effective ruled-based approaches to conduct the assessment.

Supervised Learning Approaches: The majority of the approaches that deal with the early detection of signs of mental disorders on social media use a standard prediction algorithm from the field of machine learning, which is usually trained on various combinations of features by utilising hand-labelled examples to learn meaningful patterns and optimise their parameters. The great success of such algorithms lies in their ability to learn latent nuances in the input data. Subsequently, the outcome and generalisation ability of the prediction algorithm is evaluated using a set of unseen instances. Although there is not a general consensus on the best prediction algorithm (or combination of them) for each task, participants have utilised a variety statistical

[3] A *function word* is a word whose purpose is to contribute to the syntax rather than to the meaning of the sentence.

learning algorithms including Naïve Bayes (NB), Support Vector Machines (SVM), Logistic/Linear Regression (LR), Random Forest (RF), Ada Boost (AB) and *K*-nearest Neighbours (KNN). Furthermore, individual prediction algorithms can be combined into *ensembles* to produce gains in performance. In such cases, the final output of the ensemble can be, for instance, calculated as an unweighted mean of each individual member.

More recently, the emergence of *deep learning*, one of the fastest-growing fields of machine learning, has influenced and changed the way in which participants design their ERDS. As a matter of fact, during the first eRisk editions it was hard to find teams that utilised deep learning approaches to develop their systems. However, as deep learning models became more popular and accessible showing their potential on several related task, they slowly started to permeate into ERDS design, to the point that in late editions of eRisk most of the systems presented were based on some deep learning architecture.

The main difference with the previously outlined statistical learning methods is that deep learning approaches use neural networks, usually with a *deep* or large number of hidden layers, to learn several levels of abstraction. While a few teams applied simple network architectures, such as Multilayer Perceptron (MLP), others adopted more complex architectures tailored for sequential data, such as Long Short-Term Memory (LSTM) [30] and Gated Recurrent Unit (GRU) [15], or other successful methods in the field image recognition, such as Convolutional Neural Network (CNN) [29]. It should be noted that the learning algorithms of these deep learning architectures rely on massive sets of hand-labelled training data, which in some occasions might prevent their application as it not always possible to count on such large datasets. Moreover, their complex design and functioning make usually hard to understand and interpret the rational behind their outcomes. In spite of their competitive performance, for the clinical practice this is a very sensitive issue that might hinder their application in real-life settings.

Table 1 provides a summary of the supervised learning algorithms utilised by the participants over the various eRisk editions.

Ruled-Based Approaches: Although less sophisticated, ruled-based approaches are more general and less prone to overfitting in comparison with other complex supervised learning-based solutions.

Funez et al. [28] proposed a rule-based approach called *Sequential Incremental Classification (SIC)*. This strategy consists of incrementally reading and estimating the evidence that words provide for positive and control classes, and identifying users at-risk as soon as the cumulative signs of the positive category exceeds the cumulative signs of the control one. During the training stage, a dictionary of words is built for each category where the frequency of each word is collected. At the test stage, weights for the user's words are accumulated based on their frequencies in the different categories of the dictionary created. Finally, all the weights for a particular user are added per category. This weight represents the extent to which a particular word is assumed to belong exclusively to a specific category. Since there were two classes, a user was classified to be at-risk when the cumulative sum

Table 1 Summary of the supervised learning approaches utilised by the participants over the various eRisk editions

Category	Assessment technology	2017	2018	2019	2020
Statistical learning	Naïve Bayes	[27, 73, 83]	[28]	[77]	–
	Support vector machines	[73]	[28, 37, 55, 56]	[7, 23, 50, 51, 54, 66, 77]	[3, 31, 78]
	Logistic/linear regression	[79]	[28, 56, 64, 65, 80]	[26, 51]	–
	Random forest	[5, 44, 83]	[14, 56, 63–65]	[62]	–
	Ada boost	–	[56]	–	[78]
	K-nearest neighbours	[82]	–	–	–
	Ensemble	[5, 79]	[64, 80]	[50, 51]	[2, 31, 81]
Deep learning	Multilayer perceptron	–	[47, 63]	[26, 62]	–
	Long short-term memory	[79]	[37, 56]	[26, 50, 62, 66, 68]	[2, 31, 81]
	Gated recurrent unit	[73]	–	[50, 68]	–
	Convolutional neural network	–	[37, 80, 85]	[50, 51, 68]	[2, 31, 81]

of weights for the positive category exceeded the cumulative sum for the control category. Furthermore, Burdisso et al. [13] extended and generalised this approach improving its performance on early risk detection tasks and showing its flexibility and interpretability potential for the assessment of different mental disorders.

Ragheb et al. [63] developed a two-step procedure in order to model the *temporal mood variation* of users. They first built a time series encoding user mood variation over batches of posts and attempted to estimate how positive or negative a batch was by using the distributed representation obtained from the set of posts corresponding to each class. More specifically, they computed the probability that a posts belonged to a certain class given a distributed representation using Bayes rule. By normalising the count of positive (e.g., depressed) and negative sentences found in a user's posts, they derived a ten-point time series. Finally, the moving average of the time series was computed and used to determine the class of the user.

2.3 Decision Policy

As it was outlined at the beginning of this chapter, producing timely alerts is as important as their accuracy. This is a key feature that differentiates traditional risk-assessment and decision-making applications from ERDS. Once that features have been extracted and integrated with an assessment technology, the final step in the design of ERDS involves the definition of a decision policy. Although these stages seem independent from each other, they are tightly coupled. In fact, it is this relation which greatly influences how accurately a system will perform in terms of speed and correctness.

ERDS designers need to adopt a criterion, or series of them, about the moment in which the system will take the decision of whether to emit an alert or wait to observe and collect more evidences from a user. Usually, this criterion is implemented as a *threshold* based on the confidence score of the prediction produced by the system and the quantity of posts processed. Such threshold might be static, according to the performance fluctuations and tuning observed during the development and validation steps of the ERDS, or dynamic, in which case it could change and become more flexible as delay penalties grow. For instance, Trotzek et al. [79, 80], whose systems were among of the top-performing ones in the 2017 and 2018 depression assessment tasks, defined a decision policy comprised of several thresholds based on the output probability of the system and the number of posts written by each user. For example, one of their ERDS would label a user as depressed when the system's output probability was larger than 0.6 with at least 20 posts, 0.7 with at least 10 posts, and all probabilities above 0.9 without considering the number of posts. Given that the various system configurations they proposed were highly dependent on the number of posts used at the training step, accounting for this variable in the threshold's definition was important to avoid generating too many false positives. However, in light of the performance achieved in 2017 edition and the changes on the systems configuration, in 2018 the authors decided to adopt a simpler approach and defined a single prediction threshold. Interestingly, the number of posts processed per user was not considered anymore as they observed that the systems developed were less prone to produce many false positives after processing only few posts.

Conversely, a few participants followed a more dynamic approach, such as Cacheda et al. [14] and Ramiandrisoa et al. [64] who utilised a threshold computed on the basis of a decreasing step function that depended on the number of chunks processed. As more chunks were processed, less stringent the threshold became. Meanwhile others such as Ortega-Mendoza et al. [55] followed a criterion to emit alerts based on the accumulation of evidences. An alert was submitted only if the user was classified as positive in both the current and previous chunks.

It should be noted that the modification in the experimental design and evaluation framework introduced from 2019 influenced and changed the way in which the participating teams define and execute their decision policy. Although the systems have more flexibility to decide when to trigger alerts, as test data is released item-by-item instead of chunks, concerns such as the number of false positives need still to be considered. In this sense, the task became more similar to a stream processing problem. For instance, Ragheb et al. [62] and Ageitos et al. [3] processed the incoming posts with a moving window of size N. In order to make a decision after observing a post at time t, the system processed all the user's posts starting from $(t - N - 1)$. This provided more information on the context of a post and reduced the effect of noisy and irrelevant ones. In a similar way, given a growing list of posts, Martínez-Castaño [45]'s systems took into account the average probability of the posts observed so far in the stream for each user as well as the minimum and maximum number of posts that the system should processed before making a decision.

Overall, most of the participating teams defined thresholds that were equally stringent or flexible for every user. However, there are users whose signs make their probability of being affected by a mental disorder very close to the threshold but do not surpass it until a breaking point. This observation suggest that performance could be enhanced if thresholds are defined on a user-dependent basis, to capture the very subjective behaviour of each user. For instance, users with similar characteristics could be grouped in order to create different *stereotypes* or *profiles*. In this way, each group of users would have its own threshold. When new users arrive they would be associated with the group that better suits their characteristics and the corresponding thresholds would be selected. As discussed later in Sect. 4, finding an appropriate trade-off between accuracy and speed, although feasible, is a challenging endeavour as multiple objectives need to be optimised.

3 Measuring the Severity of the Signs of Depression

From 2019, a novel and equally challenging exercise extended eRisk's suite of shared-tasks: measuring the severity of the signs of depression. This task aims at exploring the feasibility of automatically estimating the severity of multiple symptoms associated with depression, as measured by the Beck's Depression Inventory [9] questionnaire (BDI). In essence, the BDI is a self-report rating inventory for measuring characteristic attitudes and symptoms of depression. Through a set of 21 multiple-choice questions it gauges the presence and intensity of feelings like sadness, hopelessness, self-dislike, social withdrawal, and loss of energy. Participants were given users' history of posts, and had to design algorithms which could extract useful evidence related to depression in order to estimate users' response to each individual BDI item. Further details about this task are given in Sect. 5 of chapter "The Challenge of Early Risk Prediction on the Internet".

The first execution of the task did not count with any training data release, and for this reason most of the participating teams proposed various ruled-based solutions. Similar to the design and development of ERDS, at a first stage a set of features which attempt to capture evidences of the BDI items from users' posts are extracted. Based on the intensity and variation of these attributes, for instance observing the resulting features distribution, participants manually defined various thresholds to determine which option should be selected for each item in the questionnaire.

There were participants who defined a set of hand-crafted features [1, 69, 77] mostly associated with behavioural and psycholinguistics cues that are usually correlated with with depressive states, such as word polarities, LIWC psychometric attributes, usage of absolutist, self-reflective, and antidepressant words. Meanwhile others decided to exploit the semantic similarity patterns between the textual content of the posts and the items through the utilisation of WE [1, 69]. In addition, Abed-Esfahani et al. [1] and Rijen et al. [69] also leveraged external data to provide some sort training to their systems. Similarly, Burdisso et al. [13] re-utilised the system developed for different early risk detection tasks and trained it with the eRisk 2018 depression dataset. By taking advantage of the system's prediction scores they transformed its output from a 2-dimensional vector into a BDI depression level, ranging from 0 to 63. The system compiled the questionnaire utilising the estimated depression level and considering textual evidences found in the posts, mainly through regular expressions manually defined for each item, or randomly choosing an option.

In 2020, the participating teams could use the data from 2019 to train and fine-tune their systems. As a result, most of the systems submitted were not built upon ruled-based approaches anymore but supervised learning ones. In particular, there were participants who approached the problem as a multi-class classification task [45, 81]. Hence, they trained one classifier for each individual BDI item, where each item can be assigned one of 4-6 labels depending on the item. However, in light of the effectiveness achieved, specially in terms of DCHR, the authors noted that it might be more appropriate to jointly predict the results of all items and the final depression category. The main reason is because the items will likely have a high correlation between the answers, and thus the information for inferring the answer for one item may be useful for inferring others when considered together. Moreover, the teams leveraged contextual language representations, such as BERT, to capture the latent semantic patterns in users' sentences with regard to each item option. Similarly, another team considered topic models and stylometry features to model the problem as an authorship attribution task [46]. Due to the reduced size of the training data the prediction algorithms chosen were mostly statistical learning methods [78, 81], such as SVM and LR. Only one team attempted, although not with a successful outcome, to tackle the problem utilising deep learning architectures [42], such as CNN and LSTM.

Finally, Table 2 shows the top-performing systems for 2019 and 2020 editions according to the evaluation metrics assessed. Overall, we observe that the task is feasible, although, of a great complexity. The effectiveness achieved by the different systems indicates that the BDI questionnaire could be automatically estimated based on the evidence available on social media. However, we are still far from a really effective depression screening tool. For instance, in 2019 UNSLC provided evidence that it is possible to obtain more than 40% of the questionnaire answers right (AHR). Moreover, the ACR (distance-based variant of AHR) of this system was the second highest, with a closed margin to the first one, and even outperforming a random baseline algorithm. However, none of the submitted systems was able to surpass the ACR achieved by an all 1s baseline algorithm. It should be noted that this metric penalises large distances between the correct answer and the answers

Table 2 Top-performing systems for the task of measuring the severity of the signs of depression

		AHR (%)	*ACR* (%)	*ADODL* (%)	*DCHR* (%)
2019	UNSLC	**41.43**	69.13	78.02	40.00
	UNSLE	40.71	**71.27**	80.48	35.00
	CAMH_GPT_ nearest_unsupervised	23.81	57.06	**81.03**	**45.00**
2020	BioInfo@UAVR	**38.30**	69.21	76.01	30.00
	iLab run 2	37.07	**69.41**	81.70	27.14
	prhlt_svm_features	34.56	67.44	80.63	**35.71**
	relai_lda_user	36.39	68.32	**83.15**	34.29

estimated by a system. Therefore, it tends to favour *conservative* answers. ADODL and, in particular, DHCR exhibited that the systems developed were not successful at estimating the overall users' depression level. The top-performing system, CAMH_GPT_nearest_unsupervised, accurately predicted the right depression category for only 45% of the individuals. Interestingly, despite that in 2020 participants could use the training data from 2019, the systems tended to perform worse. In fact, a higher score is observed only for ADODL. Even though there is still a lot of room for improvement, these effectiveness figures are encouraging as they demonstrate that for the time being such tools could be used at least to raise awareness.

4 Findings and Lessons

The various shared-tasks conducted over the years have attracted an increasing number of participants as it is observed in Table 3. One of the most interesting findings, and possibly the most significant one, that the last five years of eRisk has left is that the tasks are feasible. Although challenging, identifying early traces of mental disorders and track their evolution by leveraging user-generated content, in particular textual records, is possible. Interestingly, we could not find a single combination of features, assessment technologies and decision policy which yields the best performance for every situation. Several feature extraction methods (linguistic, syntactic, dictionary-based, word embeddings, among others), assessment technologies (LR, NB, RF, SVM, LSTM, CNN, GRU, just to name a few) and decision policies were combined to build ERDS with different particularities and tailored for the assessment of a variety of mental disorders. Table 4 summarises the characteristics of the top-performing ERDS for each task according to the performance metrics included in the eRisk evaluation framework (see also Tables 5, 6 and 7). Despite observing such heterogeneity, common elements can be identified from the wealth of systems submitted over the various editions and a handful of lessons have been learnt along the way.

Table 3 Summary of eRisk shared-tasks campaign participation

	2017	2018		2019			2020	
	Depression	Depression	Anorexia	Anorexia	Self-Harm	BDI	Self-Harm	BDI
Teams	9	11	9	14	8	8	12	5
Submissions	30	45	35	54	33	33	56	17

Table 4 Summary of the top-performing ERDS according to the performance metrics included in the eRisk evaluation framework (alphabetically ordered)

ERDS	Features	Assessment technologies
CLac [50]	Open Vocabulary (BoW, WE/ELMo-GloVe)	CNN, LSTM, GRU, Ensemble, SVM
FHDO [79]	Open Vocabulary (BoW, WE/LSA-W2V), Lexicon-based, Syntactic Structure	LSTM, LR(Ensemble)
FHDO-BCSG [80]	Open Vocabulary (BoW, WE/GloVe), Lexicon-Based (LIWC), Syntactic Structure	CNN, LR (Ensemble)
iLab [45]	Open Vocabulary (WE/BERT)	BERT-based classifiers
LTL-INOAE [54]	Open Vocabulary (BoW/EXPEI-DPP)	SVM
lirmm [63]	Open Vocabulary (WE/ULMFit)	MLP, RF, LSTM
RKMVERIC [56]	Open Vocabulary (BoW, WE/GloVe-fastText), Lexicon-based (UMLS)	SVM, LR, RF, AB, LSTM
UArizona [73]	Lexicon-based (UMLS)	NB, SVM, GRU
UDC [14]	Open Vocabulary (BoW, WE/LSA), Social Engagement and Writing Behaviour	RF
UNSL [13, 28, 83]	Open Vocabulary (TVT,FTVT)	NB, RF, SVM, LR, SIC

4.1 A Challenging Trade-Off

The initial editions of eRisk (2017/2018) showed that, overall, most of the participants focused on the effectiveness of their estimates rather than on the trade-off between effectiveness and delay (i.e., speed of detection). This issue can be observed by analysing the number of users posts processed by each participating system. In general, the majority of the systems were rather conservative and waited to process hundreds of posts (actually, in most cases the number approaches to a thousand) per user before taking a decision.

Table 5 Top-performing systems in depression early detection task according to the performance metrics included in the eRisk evaluation framework

	ERDS	$ERDE_5$ (%)	$ERDE_{50}$ (%)	F1	P	R
2017	FHDOB	**12.70**	10.39	0.55	**0.69**	0.46
	UNSLA	13.66	**9.68**	0.59	0.48	0.79
	FHDOA	12.82	9.69	**0.64**	0.61	0.67
	UArizonaC	17.93	12.74	0.34	0.21	**0.92**
2018	UNSLA	**8.78**	7.39	0.38	0.48	0.32
	FHDO-BCSGB	9.50	**6.44**	**0.64**	0.64	0.65
	RKMVERIC	9.81	9.08	0.48	**0.67**	0.38
	UDCB	15.79	11.95	0.18	0.10	**0.95**

Table 6 Top-performing systems in anorexia early detection task according to the performance metrics included in the eRisk evaluation framework

	ERDS	$ERDE_5$ (%)	$ERDE_{50}$ (%)	F1	P	R	$F_{latency}$
2018	UNSLB	**11.40**	7.82	0.61	0.75	0.51	–
	FHDO-BCSGD	12.15	**5.96**	0.81	0.75	**0.88**	–
	FHDO-BCSGE	11.98	6.61	**0.85**	0.87	0.83	–
	UNSLD	12.93	9.85	0.79	0.91	**0.71**	–
2019	UNSL0	**5.54**	3.92	0.55	0.42	0.78	0.55
	UNSL4	6.14	**2.97**	0.47	0.31	0.92	0.46
	CLaC4	6.25	3.43	**0.71**	0.64	0.79	**0.69**
	lirmm1	9.10	5.51	0.68	**0.77**	0.60	0.62
	Fazl2	17.11	11.22	0.16	0.09	**1.00**	0.14

As a result, many of the models with high F-score usually performed poorly in terms of $ERDE_5$. Recall from chapter "The Challenge of Early Risk Prediction on the Internet" that ERDE is an error measure that introduces a penalty for late correct alerts (true positives). In particular, $ERDE_5$ is extremely stringent with delays (after 5 writings, penalties grow quickly), and thus, there is very little room for mistakes. Its goal is to encourage the design of systems that provide few but quick and correct decisions. Although, finding an equilibrium in such delicate balance represents a challenging endeavour. Instead, for $ERDE_{50}$ delays penalties are smoother, and therefore the participating teams were able to reach a better comprise between speed and effectiveness. For instance, as it is shown in Table 5, FHDO-BCSGB

Table 7 Top-performing systems in Self-harm early detection task according to the performance metrics included in the eRisk evaluation framework

	ERDS	$ERDE_5$ (%)	$ERDE_{50}$ (%)	F1	P	R	$F_{latency}$
2019	UNSL4	**8.21**	**4.93**	0.46	0.31	0.88	0.45
	UNSL0	9.01	7.31	**0.52**	**0.71**	0.41	**0.52**
	LTL-INAOE0	12.53	10.60	0.22	0.12	**1.00**	0.22
2020	iLab2	**13.40**	11.80	0.59	0.54	0.65	0.59
	iLab3	28.7	**7.10**	0.69	0.56	0.89	0.57
	iLab4	25.50	25.50	**0.75**	0.83	0.69	0.48
	iLab1	24.80	14.90	0.56	**0.91**	0.40	0.54
	SSN_NLP1	20.50	15.80	0.44	0.28	**1.00**	0.44
	iLab0	25.20	11.10	0.68	0.83	0.58	**0.66**

achieved the lowest $ERDE_{50}$ as well as the highest $F1$ in the 2018 depression task. This shows that, although complex, finding a reasonable compromise is feasible. A similar situation is observed for the case of FHDO-BCSGD in the 2018 Anorexia task (Table 5). It should be noted that there was a marked improvement in terms of ERDE between the depression early detection tasks of 2017 and 2018. However, there were not substantial improvements in the rest of the effectiveness metrics assessed.

It should be noted that the introduction of complementary evaluation measures, like latency-weighted $F1$, as well as the change in the experimental design (from a chunk-based release of data to an item-by-item one) in the latest eRisk's editions (2019/2020) provided a finer-grained lens to better analyse how the participating systems were addressing this challenging trade-off. Overall, the fact that participants had the opportunity to stop and emit an alert at any point of users' chronology showed that with a few dozens of posts it is possible to achieved a reasonably high effectiveness without considerably compromising the speed.

In 2019 (Table 7) CLaC4 yielded an effectiveness of around 70% based on a median of 7 user writings processed for the true positives identified. As it was concluded previously, a reasonable compromise between effectiveness and delay is feasible. It is worth noting that there were systems which emitted quicker decisions ($latency_{TP}$ and $speed$ equal to 1) but the associated effectiveness was rather poor (e.g., $F1$ of 0.37). Such outcome is expected as decisions based on a single post are likely to be premature. On the other extreme, there were systems which achieved a perfect recall (as Fazl2 in Table 7) but perform poorly in the rest of the metrics assessed. The utilisation of such systems in a real-life scenario is rather questionable. Other participants like lirmm1 in Table 7 decided to prioritise the precision of their estimates. This ERDS looks also quite promising as its true positive decisions were fast (around 20 post processed per user) achieving a satisfactory comprise. A similar situation was observed in 2020 edition as Table 7 shows. Although, we note that despite the good performance achieved in terms of $F1$ and its latency-weighted variant, overall, recall was lower than in previous years. This could be associated with the fact that detecting early traces of self-harm might be more complex than it is for depression or anorexia. Finally, iLab2 and iLab3 achieved the the lowest $ERDE_5$ and $ERDE_{50}$, respectively, showing a good compromise between accuracy and delay. Moreover, the latency of the true positive was 2 and 45, respectively.

4.2 *Experimental Design and Evaluation Framework*

It is clear that the experimental design and evaluation framework influence the way in which eRisk participants designed their systems. Initially, at the test stage, each system received a weekly chunk of data that contained the 10% of every user collection of posts (*chunk-based* released of data). For instance, a user with 1580 posts has 158 posts per chunk and such a large number of texts imposes a large ERDE penalty. However, a system might not need such a large number of posts to determine whether a user is at-risk or not. Moreover, the contribution of each user to the performance evaluation had a large variance. While there are users with only 10 posts, others have more than a thousand. For this reason, the evaluation framework changed from 2019 so that systems received a single post at a time from each user in the dataset (*item-by-item* release of data). This gave the participants the alternative to stop at any given point in the stream and the subsequent ERDE penalties ranged over the full extent of users' collection of posts. In fact, this simulates a real-life scenario where health practitioners analyse social media posts as they are published. Interestingly, this modification revealed that various systems incorporated some form of offline processing as there were cases in which they took several days to run the whole assessment process. This is an interesting point to consider given that in a real-life scenario, time is also an essential variable. Moreover, it would be interesting to think how different ERDS would perform or should be designed to incorporate real-time processing.

Early risk detection is challenging because multiple objectives are involved (ERDE, Precision, Recall, Latency). For this task, getting timely predictions with a reasonable confidence level becomes critical. In this regard, the final goal of a competitive system would be to minimise ERDE and maximise the F-score. However, finding a proper balance between them is far from trivial. Making rushed decisions might lead to a high rate of false alarms (FP), diminishing the precision and consequently, affecting the overall F-score. A first simple solution to mitigate this effect would be to observe more documents before annotating a user. Nevertheless, by doing so, ERDE would start to increase.

Bearing this in mind, it becomes essential to understand the practical implications of using ERDS systems in the clinical practice. For instance, consider the difference that $ERDE_5$ and $ERDE_{50}$ could have in a real-life scenario. A mental health agency might decide to set the penalty costs on the consequences of late detection. This leads to a natural trade-off depending on whether the goal is to be more conservative and raise a handful of timely alerts or to maximise the recall at the cost of issuing false alarms. To illustrate this point, Tables 5, 6 and 7 present the top-performing ERDS considering the performance metrics assessed in each corresponding eRisk edition and task. It is worth noting that, in most of the cases, none of the systems overlap. Different system configurations achieve the highest effectiveness at each metric. Even though the metrics are correlated, each measure captures a particular aspect of the problem (e.g., speed) and altogether provide an integral evaluation of the system.

Figure 1 depicts the performance figures achieved by averaging the contribution of the participating systems in each task. In this way, one could observe whether the understanding of the challenges addressed has improved over the years and how such improvement impacted on the performance. A first glance reveals that the highest performance across the different metrics has been achieved for self-harm task in 2020. While depression task in 2018 was the lowest one in terms of ERDE. It should be noted that comparisons are not completely fair as the experimental design and evaluation framework changed from 2019. Therefore, metrics like ERDE were previously computed over the posts in a chunk, instead of the actual number of posts processed by a system to emit an alert. Self-harm scores in 2019 are quite low in comparison with the rest of the tasks. As it is discussed later, this could be due to the lack of training data. Overall, systems fare modestly at detecting individuals at-risk as an average recall close to 60% is achieved for all the tasks.

Finally, we note that systems tend to perform better at detecting non-risk users. Given the imbalanced nature of the task such outcome is expected. In addition, these users usually do not engage in conversations related to any of the mental disorders under analysis, allowing systems to better differentiate them from at-risk cases. Interestingly, we found that in 2017/2018 depression tasks there was not a single at-risk user which could be identified by all the submitted systems. However, every one of them was detected by at least one system. A similar, although slightly better situation, is observed in 2018 anorexia task. Moreover, in both cases a considerable number of users are only detected by less than a half of the systems. This poses several interesting questions regarding the attributes that such individuals have and what makes them so difficult to spot. Is it related to the way they express? Is the amount of textual information available enough to identify consistent and significant signals? Are the systems properly capturing the nuances of the linguistic patterns that differentiate them from control individuals? All this reinforces the argument that not all the features are able to capture every signal with the same strength. Furthermore, different portions of the population of users at-risk might not evidence overlapping signals.

4.3 Signals Crossover

Another important finding that deserves attention, and which possibly opens new avenues for further research is related to the ways in which different disorders manifest through users' writing. Specially, whether a system that exhibit competitive

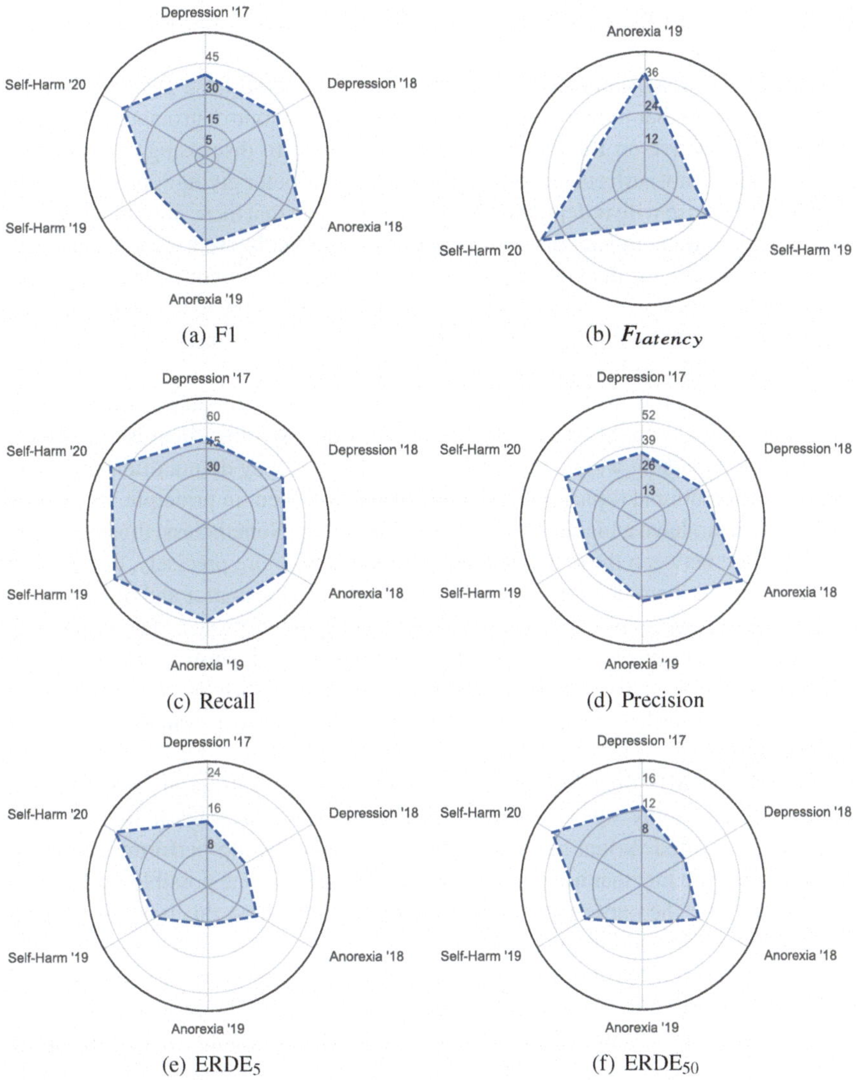

Fig. 1 Average performance for each task according to the performance metrics included in the eRisk evaluation framework. All the values are expressed as percentages

performance figures for a particular task could perform equally well for a different but related one. The performance of the same systems in eRisk 2018 depression and anorexia tasks revealed very different outcomes. For instance, while the lowest $ERDE_{50}$ achieved for anorexia was 5.96%, the lowest error for depression was 9.68% (Tables 5 and 6). Remarkably, the most effective system yielded an F1 of 0.85 for anorexia, while the top-performing system for depression reached a score of 0.64 (Tables 5 and 6).

One possible reason could be the proportion of potential false positives in each collection. Recall that to build more realistic collections control groups contain also users who are active on Reddit's communities devoted to discussing about mental disorders but are not suffering from any of them (e.g., a doctor giving support to others or a husband whose wife is depressed or anorexic). Given that these individuals would often write about the mental disorder in question, and likely use a style that suggest they are affected by the disorder although they are not, could potentially lead systems to label them as positives cases (false positives). It could be the case that the number of such users might be lower for anorexia than for depression and for this reason we observe such differences in terms of performance.

Another reasonable explanation could be that they way individuals suffering from anorexia expressed might be extremely biased towards writing about issues related to eating habits, losing weight and body image. Thus, if they do not often engage in general conversational topics (i.e., anorexia unrelated) then, in principle, this would allow systems to have a higher chance of spotting them. Nonetheless, this highlights the difference between these two mental disorders and, more precisely, the features that characterise them. Ríssola et al. [70] shed light on this matter and highlight the importance of steering research towards building new metrics that can correlate with a disease before traditional symptoms arise and which clinicians can use as leading indicators of traditional later-onset symptoms. Moreover, this also poses a broader question related to the adaptability of the approaches to other domains and social media sources.

Similarly, on 2019 the effectiveness scores observed for self-harm early detection task were considerably lower than those achieved for the anorexia task. Both, $F1$ and its latency-weighted variant hardly exceed 50% for the the top-performing systems (see Table 7). The fact that no training data was provided is one possible explanation of this outcome. The participating teams attempted to address this issue by training their models with external datasets related to the task. For instance, based on the assumption that self-harm ideation is often related to depression, Trifan et al. [77] utilised the Reddit Self-reported Depression Diagnosis (RSDD) [86], a large corpus utilised for the assessment of depression on social media, as training data. In a similar way, Abed-Esfahani et al. [1] employed the University of Maryland (UMD) Reddit Suicidality Dataset [75], a dataset developed for the assessment of suicide risk from online posting, to fine-tune their systems. Other participants, as Naderi et al. [51] and Burdisso et al. [13] leveraged various collections of Reddit posts and tweets related to self-harm. Although innovative, this strategy did not worked as expected given that the performance achieved by the different ERDS was still low. In addition, users' chronology was entirely comprised of posts written before they entered the Reddit self-harm community. Hence, signals related to this disorder might not be that explicit, making them harder to detect in comparison with other disorders included the datasets such as depression.

An interesting lesson to take here is that, overall, designing and implementing ERDS that can equally perform for different early detection tasks is still a complex endeavour. Despite that there might be overlapping features associated with the identification of different disorders, such as self-harm and depression, the way individuals express has subtle variations depending on the disorder under analysis [70]. Although these nuances in the data allow systems to effectively discover positive cases, they prevent them to be applicable for detecting other disorders than the one they were meant to identify. Furthermore, it could happen that an individual is suffering from more than one disorder at the same time, although has been diagnosed with one. This situation is commonly known as *comorbidity*. For instance, according to the DSM, a Major Depressive Disorder is a very common comorbid disorder, and it frequently coexists with other disorders, such as PTSD. This issue highlights the fact that computational tools should not be expected to serve as standalone diagnostic instruments but as unobtrusive mechanisms for early identification of potential mental problems.

5 Conclusions

Recall from the introduction of this chapter that the main motivation behind eRisk shared-task campaigns is to foster the development of risk-assessment and decision-making technologies, in particular ERDS. The ultimate goal of these language-based technologies is to aid and facilitate health practitioners daily labour. Over these years, we have learned that the interaction between mental disorders and language use is challenging and, overall, the effectiveness of most participating systems is modest. For instance, most tasks had levels of performance (e.g., in terms of $F1$) below 70%. This suggests that this kind of early prediction tasks require further research and solutions proposed so far still have much room for improvement.

In a real-life setting, one would have to decide which metrics to focus when optimising the various parameters of a specific system. This decision could be taken with the assistance and advice of professionals in the health domain. For instance, under certain circumstances, producing a considerable amount of false alarms can be tolerated at the benefit of quickly discovering true cases. This could help to prevent further consequences (*e.g*, suicide). Moreover, achieving an effective performance is equally relevant as being able to track the onset and development of a mental disorder. For this reason, a system could be more useful if it provides a way of understanding the explanatory factors that lead to such disorder. As argued by Walsh et al. [84], this issue, along with other factors, might prevent most of the risk-assessment and decision-making technologies to ever been used in the clinical practise.

To date, the judgement and expertise of a mental health practitioner has no technological substitute. However, new solutions involving the use of language technologies should be considered at least for a preliminary screening process and to raise awareness. There is a real possibility of leveraging social media data to assist clinicians (and other relevant stakeholders) in screening individuals or communities "at-risk". Large-scale early screening utilising low-cost unobtrusive mechanisms could be offered to mental health agencies to proactively identify individuals that should be closely followed by a health professional anticipating further consequences.

These five years of eRisk have been more than a proof-of-concept to support and strengthen this argument. As it is discussed throughout the book, language technologies have a great potential to identify and exploit latent linguistic nuances encoded in users' textual records that correlate with mental disorders, like depression, anorexia or suicide behaviour. Thus, they can provide practitioners with a holistic and comprehensive way to assess the individual.

Acknowledgements This work was supported by projects RTI2018-093336-B-C21, RTI2018-093336-B-C22 (Ministerio de Ciencia e Innovación, Agencia Estatal de Investigación & ERDF) and PLEC2021-007662 (MCIN/AEI/10.13039/501100011033, Ministerio de Ciencia e Innovación, Agencia Estatal de Investigación, Plan de Recuperación, Transformación y Resiliencia, Unión Europea-Next GenerationEU). The second author thanks the financial support supplied by the Consellería de Educación, Universidade e Formación Profesional (accreditation 2019-2022 ED431G/01, ED431B 2019/03) and the European Regional Development Fund, which acknowledges the CITIC Research Center in ICT of the University of A Coruña as a Research Center of the Galician University System. The third author thanks the financial support supplied by the Consellería de Educación, Universidade e Formación Profesional (accreditation 2019-2022 ED431G-2019/04, ED431C 2018/29) and the European Regional Development Fund, which acknowledges the CiTIUS-Research Center in Intelligent Technologies of the University of Santiago de Compostela as a Research Center of the Galician University System.

References

1. Abed-Esfahani, P., Howard, D., Maslej, M., Patel, S., Mann, V., Goegan, S., & French, L. (2019). Transfer learning for depression: Early detection and severity prediction from social media postings. In *Working Notes of CLEF 2019 - Conference and Labs of the Evaluation Forum, Lugano, Switzerland, September 9–12* (vol. 2380). *CEUR Workshop Proceedings*, CEUR-WS.org.
2. Achilles, L., Kisselew, M., Schäfer, J., & Kölle, R. (2020). Using surface and semantic features for detecting early signs of self-harm in social media postings. In *Working Notes of CLEF 2020 - Conference and Labs of the Evaluation Forum, Thessaloniki, Greece, September 22–25, 2020* (vol. 2696). *CEUR Workshop Proceedings*, CEUR-WS.org.
3. Ageitos, E. C., Martínez-Romo, J., & Araujo, L. (2020). NLP-UNED at erisk 2020: Self-harm early risk detection with sentiment analysis and linguistic features. In *Working Notes of CLEF 2020 - Conference and Labs of the Evaluation Forum, Thessaloniki, Greece, September 22–25, 2020* (vol. 2696). *CEUR Workshop Proceedings*, CEUR-WS.org.
4. Al-Mosaiwi, M., & Johnstone, T. (2018). In an absolute state: Elevated use of absolutist words is a marker specific to anxiety, depression, and suicidal ideation. *Clinical Psychological Science, 6*(4), 529–542.
5. Almeida, H., Briand, A., & Meurs, M. (2017). Detecting early risk of depression from social media user-generated content. In *Working Notes of CLEF 2017 - Conference and Labs of the Evaluation Forum, Dublin, Ireland, September 11–14, 2017*.
6. Aragón, M. E., López-Monroy, A. P., González-Gurrola, L. C., & Montes-y-Gómez, M. (2019). Detecting depression in social media using fine-grained emotions. In *Proceedings of the 2019 Conference of the North American Chapter of the Association for Computational Linguistics: Human Language Technologies, NAACL-HLT 2019, Minneapolis, USA, June 2-7, 2019* (pp. 1481–1486).
7. Aragón, M. E., López-Monroy, A. P., & Montes-y-Gómez, M. (2019). INAOE-CIMAT at erisk 2019: Detecting signs of anorexia using fine-grained emotions. In *Working Notes of CLEF*

2019 - Conference and Labs of the Evaluation Forum, Lugano, Switzerland, September 9–12, 2019 (vol. 2380). *CEUR Workshop Proceedings*, CEUR-WS.org.
8. Aragón, M. E., López-Monroy, A. P., & Montes-y-Gómez, M. (2020). INAOE-CIMAT at erisk 2020: Detecting signs of self-harm using sub-emotions and words. In *Working Notes of CLEF 2020 - Conference and Labs of the Evaluation Forum, Thessaloniki, Greece, September 22–25, 2020* (vol. 2696). *CEUR Workshop Proceedings*, CEUR-WS.org.
9. Beck, A. T., Steer, R. A., & Carbin, M. G. (1988). Psychometric properties of the beck depression inventory: Twenty-five years of evaluation. *Clinical Psychology Review, 8*(1), 77–100.
10. Bojanowski, P., Grave, E., Joulin, A., & Mikolov, T. (2017). Enriching word vectors with subword information. *Transactions of the Association for Computational Linguistics, 5*, 135–146.
11. Boyd, R. L., & Pennebaker, J. W. (2017). Language-based personality: a new approach to personality in a digital world. *Current Opinion in Behavioral Sciences, 18,* 63–68. Big data in the behavioural sciences.
12. Boyd, R. L., Wilson, S. R., Pennebaker, J. W., Kosinski, M., Stillwell, D. J., & Mihalcea, R. (2015). Values in words: Using language to evaluate and understand personal values. In *Proceedings of the Ninth International Conference on Web and Social Media, ICWSM 2015, University of Oxford, Oxford, UK, May 26–29, 2015* (pp. 31–40).
13. Burdisso, S. G., Errecalde, M., & Montes-y-Gómez, M. (2019). UNSL at erisk 2019: A unified approach for anorexia, self-harm and depression detection in social media. In *Working Notes of CLEF 2019 - Conference and Labs of the Evaluation Forum, Lugano, Switzerland, September 9–12, 2019* (vol. 2380). *CEUR Workshop Proceedings*, CEUR-WS.org.
14. Cacheda, F., Iglesias, D. F., Nóvoa, F. J., & Carneiro, V. (2018). Analysis and experiments on early detection of depression. In *Working Notes of CLEF 2018 - Conference and Labs of the Evaluation Forum, Avignon, France, September 10–14, 2018.*
15. Cho, K., van Merrienboer, B., Gülçehre, Ç., Bahdanau, D., Bougares, F., Schwenk, H., & Bengio, Y. (2014). Learning phrase representations using RNN encoder-decoder for statistical machine translation. In *Proceedings of the 2014 Conference on Empirical Methods in Natural Language Processing, EMNLP 2014, October 25–29, 2014, Doha, Qatar, A meeting of SIGDAT, a Special Interest Group of the ACL* (pp. 1724–1734).
16. Choudhury, M. D., Gamon, M., Counts, S., & Horvitz, E. (2013). Predicting depression via social media. In *Proceedings of the Seventh International Conference on Weblogs and Social Media, ICWSM 2013, Cambridge, Massachusetts, USA, July 8–11, 2013.*
17. Chung, C., & Pennebaker, J. (2007). The psychological functions of function words. *Frontiers of social psychology. Social communication.*
18. Coppersmith, G., Dredze, M., Harman, C., Hollingshead, K., & Mitchell, M. (2015). Clpsych 2015 shared task: Depression and PTSD on twitter. In *Proceedings of the 2nd Workshop on Computational Linguistics and Clinical Psychology: From Linguistic Signal to Clinical Reality, CLPsych@NAACL-HLT 2015, June 5, 2015, Denver, Colorado, USA* (pp. 31–39).
19. Coppersmith, G., Harman, C., & Dredze, M. (2014). Measuring post traumatic stress disorder in twitter. In *Proceedings of the 8th International Conference on Weblogs and Social Media, ICWSM 2014.*
20. Croft, B., Metzler, D., & Strohman, T. (2009). *Search Engines: Information Retrieval in Practice* (1st ed.). USA: Addison-Wesley Publishing Company.
21. Culpepper, J. S., Diaz, F., & Smucker, M. D. (2018). Research frontiers in information retrieval: Report from the third strategic workshop on information retrieval in lorne (swirl 2018). *SIGIR Forum, 52*(1), 34–90.
22. Deerwester, S., Dumais, S. T., Furnas, G. W., Landauer, T. K., & Harshman, R. (1990). Indexing by latent semantic analysis. *Journal of the American Society for Information Science, 41*, 6.
23. del Arco, F. M. P., López-Úbeda, P., Díaz-Galiano, M. C., López, L. A. U., & Valdivia, M. T. M. (2019). Integrating UMLS for early detection of sings of anorexia. In *Working Notes of CLEF 2019 - Conference and Labs of the Evaluation Forum, Lugano, Switzerland, September 9–12* (vol. 2380). *CEUR Workshop Proceedings*, CEUR-WS.org.

24. Devlin, J., Chang, M., Lee, K., & Toutanova, K. (2018). BERT: pre-training of deep bidirectional transformers for language understanding. *CoRR abs/1810.04805*.
25. Errecalde, M. L., Villegas, M. P., Funez, D. G., Ucelay, M. J. G., & Cagnina, L. C. (2017). Temporal variation of terms as concept space for early risk prediction. In *Working Notes of CLEF 2017 - Conference and Labs of the Evaluation Forum, Dublin, Ireland, September 11–14, 2017*.
26. Fano, E., Karlgren, J., & Nivre, J. (2019). Uppsala university and gavagai at CLEF erisk: Comparing word embedding models. In *Working Notes of CLEF 2019 - Conference and Labs of the Evaluation Forum, Lugano, Switzerland, September 9–12* (vol. 2380). *CEUR Workshop Proceedings*, CEUR-WS.org.
27. Farias-Anzaldua, A. A., Montes-y-Gómez, M., López-Monroy, A. P., & González-Gurrola, L. C. (2017). UACH-INAOE participation at erisk2017. In *Working Notes of CLEF 2017 - Conference and Labs of the Evaluation Forum, Dublin, Ireland, September 11–14, 2017*.
28. Funez, D. G., Ucelay, M. J. G., Villegas, M. P., Burdisso, S., Cagnina, L. C., Montes-y-Gómez, M., & Errecalde, M. (2018). Unsl's participation at erisk 2018 lab. In *Working Notes of CLEF 2018 - Conference and Labs of the Evaluation Forum, Avignon, France, September 10–14, 2018*.
29. Goodfellow, I., Bengio, Y., & Courville, A. (2016). *Deep Learning*. The MIT Press.
30. Hochreiter, S., & Schmidhuber, J. (1997). Long short-term memory. *Neural Computation, 9*(8), 1735–1780. Nov.
31. Hosseinabad, H. B., Ersi, E. F., & Vahedian, A. (2020). Detection of early sign of self-harm on reddit using multi-level machine. In *Working Notes of CLEF 2020 - Conference and Labs of the Evaluation Forum, Thessaloniki, Greece, September 22–25, 2020* (vol. 2696). *CEUR Workshop Proceedings*, CEUR-WS.org.
32. Howard, J., & Ruder, S. (2018). Universal language model fine-tuning for text classification. In *Proceedings of the 56th Annual Meeting of the Association for Computational Linguistics* (Melbourne, Australia, 2018) (pp. 328–339).
33. Hutto, C. J., & Gilbert, E. (2014). Vader: A parsimonious rule-based model for sentiment analysis of social media text. In E. Adar, P. Resnick, M. D. Choudhury, B. Hogan, & A. H. Oh (Eds.), *ICWSM*. The AAAI Press.
34. Joulin, A., Grave, E., Bojanowski, P., & Mikolov, T. (2017). Bag of tricks for efficient text classification. In *Proceedings of the 15th Conference of the European Chapter of the Association for Computational Linguistics: Volume 2, Short Papers* (pp. 427–431). Association for Computational Linguistics.
35. Kanerva, P., Kristoferson, J., & Holst, A. (2000). Random indexing of text samples for latent semantic analysis. In *In Proceedings of the 22nd Annual Conference of the Cognitive Science Society* (pp. 103–6). Erlbaum.
36. Li, Z., Xiong, Z., Zhang, Y., Liu, C., & Li, K. (2011). Fast text categorization using concise semantic analysis. *Pattern Recognition Letters, 32*, 441–448.
37. Liu, N., Zhou, Z., Xin, K., & Ren, F. (2018). TUA1 at erisk 2018. In *Working Notes of CLEF 2018 - Conference and Labs of the Evaluation Forum, Avignon, France, September 10–14, 2018*.
38. Losada, D. E., Crestani, F., & Parapar, J. (2017). eRISK 2017: CLEF lab on Early Risk Prediction on the Internet: Experimental foundations. In G. J. Jones, S. Lawless, J. Gonzalo, L. Kelly, L. Goeuriot, T. Mandl, et al. (Eds.), *Experimental IR Meets Multilinguality, Multimodality, and Interaction* (pp. 346–360). Springer International Publishing.
39. Losada, D. E., Crestani, F., & Parapar, J. (2018). Overview of eRisk: Early Risk Prediction on the Internet. In *Experimental IR Meets Multilinguality, Multimodality, and Interaction - 9th International Conference of the CLEF Association, CLEF 2018, Avignon, France, September 10–14, 2018, Proceedings* (pp. 343–361).
40. Losada, D. E., Crestani, F., & Parapar, J. (2019). Overview of erisk 2019 early risk prediction on the internet. In *Experimental IR Meets Multilinguality, Multimodality, and Interaction - 10th International Conference of the CLEF Association, CLEF 2019, Lugano, Switzerland*, (pp. 340–357).

41. Losada, D. E., Crestani, F., & Parapar, J. (2020). Overview of eRisk 2020: Early Risk Prediction on the Internet. In *Experimental IR Meets Multilinguality, Multimodality, and Interaction Proceedings of the Eleventh International Conference of the CLEF Association (CLEF 2020)*.
42. Madani, A., Boumahdi, F., Boukenaoui, A., Kritli, M. C., & Hentabli, H. (2020). USDB at erisk 2020: Deep learning models to measure the severity of the signs of depression using reddit posts. In *Working Notes of CLEF 2020 - Conference and Labs of the Evaluation Forum, Thessaloniki, Greece, September 22–25, 2020* (vol. 2696). *CEUR Workshop Proceedings*, CEUR-WS.org.
43. Maigrot, C., Bringay, S., & Azé, J. (2017). Concept drift vs suicide: How one can help prevent the other? *International Journal of Computational Linguistics and Applications, 8*, 1. Oct.
44. Malam, I. A., Arziki, M., Bellazrak, M. N., Benamara, F., Kaidi, A. E., Es-Saghir, B., He, Z., Housni, M., Moriceau, V., Mothe, J., & Ramiandrisoa, F. (2017). IRIT at e-risk. In *Working Notes of CLEF 2017 - Conference and Labs of the Evaluation Forum, Dublin, Ireland, September 11–14, 2017*.
45. Martínez-Castaño, R., Htait, A., Azzopardi, L., & Moshfeghi, Y. (2020). Early risk detection of self-harm and depression severity using bert-based transformers. In *Working Notes of CLEF 2020 - Conference and Labs of the Evaluation Forum, Thessaloniki, Greece, September 22–25, 2020* (vol. 2696). *CEUR Workshop Proceedings*, CEUR-WS.org.
46. Maupomé, D., Armstrong, M. D., Belbahar, R. M., Alezot, J., Balassiano, R., Queudot, M., Mosser, S., & Meurs, M. (2020). Early mental health risk assessment through writing styles, topics and neural models. In *Working Notes of CLEF 2020 - Conference and Labs of the Evaluation Forum, Thessaloniki, Greece, September 22–25, 2020* (vol. 2696). *CEUR Workshop Proceedings*, CEUR-WS.org.
47. Maupomé, D., & Meurs, M. (2018). Using topic extraction on social media content for the early detection of depression. In *Working Notes of CLEF 2018 - Conference and Labs of the Evaluation Forum, Avignon, France, September 10–14, 2018*.
48. Mikolov, T., Sutskever, I., Chen, K., Corrado, G., & Dean, J. (2013). Distributed representations of words and phrases and their compositionality. In *Proceedings of the 26th International Conference on Neural Information Processing Systems* (Lake Tahoe, USA, 2013), NIPS'13 (pp. 3111–3119).
49. Mohammad, S., & Turney, P. D. (2013). Crowdsourcing a word-emotion association lexicon. *Computational Intelligence, 29*(3), 436–465.
50. Mohammadi, E., Amini, H., & Kosseim, L. (2019). Quick and (maybe not so) easy detection of anorexia in social media posts. In *Working Notes of CLEF 2019 - Conference and Labs of the Evaluation Forum, Lugano, Switzerland, September 9–12* (vol. 2380). *CEUR Workshop Proceedings*, CEUR-WS.org.
51. Naderi, N., Gobeill, J., Teodoro, D., Pasche, E., & Ruch, P. (2019). A baseline approach for early detection of signs of anorexia and self-harm in reddit posts. In *Working Notes of CLEF 2019 - Conference and Labs of the Evaluation Forum, Lugano, Switzerland, September 9–12* (vol. 2380). *CEUR Workshop Proceedings*, CEUR-WS.org.
52. Neuman, Y. (2016). *Computational personality analysis: Introduction, practical applications and novel directions*. Springer.
53. Neuman, Y., Cohen, Y., Assaf, D., & Kedma, G. (2012). Proactive screening for depression through metaphorical and automatic text analysis. *Artificial Intelligence in Medicine, 56*(1), 19–25.
54. Ortega-Mendoza, R. M., Farías, D. I. H., & Montes-y-Gómez, M. (2019). Ltl-inaoe's participation at erisk 2019: Detecting anorexia in social media through shared personal information. In *Working Notes of CLEF 2019 - Conference and Labs of the Evaluation Forum, Lugano, Switzerland, September 9–12* (vol. 2380). *CEUR Workshop Proceedings*, CEUR-WS.org.
55. Ortega-Mendoza, R. M., López-Monroy, A. P., Franco-Arcega, A., & Montes-y-Gómez, M. (2018). PEIMEX at erisk2018: Emphasizing personal information for depression and anorexia detection. In *Working Notes of CLEF 2018 - Conference and Labs of the Evaluation Forum, Avignon, France, September 10–14, 2018*.
56. Paul, S., Jandhyala, S. K., & Basu, T. (2018). Early detection of signs of anorexia and depression over social media using effective machine learning frameworks. In *Working Notes of CLEF*

2018 - Conference and Labs of the Evaluation Forum, Avignon, France, September 10–14, 2018.
57. Pennebaker, J. W., Chung, C. K., Ireland, M., Gonzales, A., & Booth, R. J. (2015). The development and psychometric properties of liwc2015. Ut faculty/researcher works.
58. Pennebaker, J. W., Mehl, M. R., & Niederhoffer, K. G. (2003). Psychological aspects of natural language use: Our words, our selves. *Annual Review of Psychology, 54*, 1.
59. Pennington, J., Socher, R., & Manning, C. D. (2014). Glove: Global vectors for word representation. In *Proceedings of the 2014 Conference on Empirical Methods in Natural Language Processing, EMNLP 2014, October 25–29, 2014, Doha, Qatar, A meeting of SIGDAT, a Special Interest Group of the ACL* (pp. 1532–1543).
60. Peters, M., Neumann, M., Iyyer, M., Gardner, M., Clark, C., Lee, K., & Zettlemoyer, L. (2018) Deep contextualized word representations. In *Proceedings of the 2018 Conference of the North American Chapter of the Association for Computational Linguistics: Human Language Technologies* (pp. 2227–2237).
61. Preoţiuc-Pietro, D., Eichstaedt, J., Park, G., Sap, M., Smith, L., Tobolsky, V., Schwartz, H. A., & Ungar, L. (2015). The role of personality, age and gender in tweeting about mental illnesses. In *Proceedings of the 2nd Workshop on Computational Linguistics and Clinical Psychology: From Linguistic Signal to Clinical Reality.*
62. Ragheb, W., Azé, J., Bringay, S., & Servajean, M. (2019). Attentive multi-stage learning for early risk detection of signs of anorexia and self-harm on social media. In *Working Notes of CLEF 2019 - Conference and Labs of the Evaluation Forum, Lugano, Switzerland, September 9–12* (vol. 2380). *CEUR Workshop Proceedings*, CEUR-WS.org.
63. Ragheb, W., Moulahi, B., Azé, J., Bringay, S., & Servajean, M. (2018). Temporal mood variation: at the CLEF erisk-2018 tasks for early risk detection on the internet. In *Working Notes of CLEF 2018 - Conference and Labs of the Evaluation Forum, Avignon, France, September 10–14, 2018.*
64. Ramiandrisoa, F., Mothe, J., Benamara, F., & Moriceau, V. (2018). IRIT at e-risk 2018. In *Working Notes of CLEF 2018 - Conference and Labs of the Evaluation Forum, Avignon, France, September 10–14, 2018.*
65. Ramírez-Cifuentes, D., & Freire, A. (2018). Upf's participation at the CLEF erisk 2018: Early risk prediction on the internet. In *Working Notes of CLEF 2018 - Conference and Labs of the Evaluation Forum, Avignon, France, September 10–14, 2018.*
66. Ranganathan, A., A, H., Thenmozhi, D., & Aravindan, C. (2019). Early detection of anorexia using RNN-LSTM and SVM classifiers. In *Working Notes of CLEF 2019 - Conference and Labs of the Evaluation Forum, Lugano, Switzerland, September 9–12* (vol. 2380). *CEUR Workshop Proceedings*, CEUR-WS.org.
67. Reece, A. G., & Danforth, C. M. (2017). Instagram photos reveal predictive markers of depression. *EPJ Data Science, 6*(1), 15. Aug.
68. Retamero, P. R. G., & Segura-Bedmar, I. (2019). Early risk prediction by means of deeplearning. In *Working Notes of CLEF 2019 - Conference and Labs of the Evaluation Forum, Lugano, Switzerland, September 9–12* (vol. 2380). *CEUR Workshop Proceedings*, CEUR-WS.org.
69. Rijen, P. V., Teodoro, D., Naderi, N., Mottin, L., Knafou, J., Jeffryes, M., & Ruch, P. (2019). A data-driven approach for measuring the severity of the signs of depression using reddit posts. In *Working Notes of CLEF 2019 - Conference and Labs of the Evaluation Forum, Lugano, Switzerland, September 9–12, 2019* (vol. 2380). *CEUR Workshop Proceedings*, CEUR-WS.org.
70. Ríssola, E. A., Aliannejadi, M., & Crestani, F. (2020). Beyond modelling: Understanding mental disorders in online social media. In *Advances in Information Retrieval - 42nd European Conference on IR Research, ECIR 2020, Lisbon, Portugal, April 14–17* (vol. 12035, pp. 296–310).
71. Ríssola, E. A., Bahrainian, S. A., & Crestani, F. (2019). Anticipating depression based on online social media behaviour. In *Flexible Query Answering Systems - 13th International Conference, FQAS 2019, Amantea, Italy, July 2–5, 2019, Proceedings* (pp. 278–290).
72. Ríssola, E. A., Bahrainian, S. A., & Crestani, F. (2019). Personality recognition in conversations using capsule neural networks. In *2019 IEEE/WIC/ACM International Conference on Web Intelligence, WI 2019, Thessaloniki, Greece, October 14–17, 2019* (pp. 180–187).

73. Sadeque, F., Xu, D., & Bethard, S. (2017). Uarizona at the CLEF erisk 2017 pilot task: Linear and recurrent models for early depression detection. In *Working Notes of CLEF 2017 - Conference and Labs of the Evaluation Forum, Dublin, Ireland, September 11–14, 2017.*
74. Schwartz, H. A., Eichstaedt, J. C., Kern, M. L., Dziurzynski, L., Ramones, S. M., Agrawal, M., et al. (2013). Personality, gender, and age in the language of social media: The open-vocabulary approach. *PLoS ONE, 8*(9), e73791.
75. Shing, H.-C., Nair, S., Zirikly, A., Friedenberg, M., Daumé III, H., & Resnik, P. (2018). Expert, crowdsourced, and machine assessment of suicide risk via online postings. In *Proceedings of the Fifth Workshop on Computational Linguistics and Clinical Psychology: From Keyboard to Clinic* (pp. 25–36).
76. Tausczik, Y. R., & Pennebaker, J. W. (2009). The psychological meaning of words: Liwc and computerized text analysis methods. *Journal of Language and Social Psychology.*
77. Trifan, A., & Oliveira, J. L. (2019). Bioinfo@uavr at erisk 2019: delving into social media texts for the early detection of mental and food disorders. In *Working Notes of CLEF 2019 - Conference and Labs of the Evaluation Forum, Lugano, Switzerland, September 9–12* (vol. 2380). *CEUR Workshop Proceedings*, CEUR-WS.org.
78. Trifan, A., Salgado, P., & Oliveira, J. L. (2020). Bioinfo@uavr at erisk 2020: on the use of psycholinguistics features and machine learning for the classification and quantification of mental diseases. In *Working Notes of CLEF 2020 - Conference and Labs of the Evaluation Forum, Thessaloniki, Greece, September 22–25, 2020* (vol. 2696). *CEUR Workshop Proceedings*, CEUR-WS.org.
79. Trotzek, M., Koitka, S., & Friedrich, C. M. (2017). Linguistic metadata augmented classifiers at the CLEF 2017 task for early detection of depression. In *Working Notes of CLEF 2017 - Conference and Labs of the Evaluation Forum, Dublin, Ireland, September 11–14, 2017.*
80. Trotzek, M., Koitka, S., & Friedrich, C. M. (2018). Word embeddings and linguistic metadata at the CLEF 2018 tasks for early detection of depression and anorexia. In *Working Notes of CLEF 2018 - Conference and Labs of the Evaluation Forum, Avignon, France, September 10–14, 2018.*
81. Uban, A. S., & Rosso, P. (2020). Deep learning architectures and strategies for early detection of self-harm and depression level prediction. In *Working Notes of CLEF 2020 - Conference and Labs of the Evaluation Forum, Thessaloniki, Greece, September 22–25, 2020* (vol. 2696). *CEUR Workshop Proceedings*, CEUR-WS.org.
82. Villatoro-Tello, E., Ramírez-de-la-Rosa, G., & Jiménez-Salazar, H. (2017). Uam's participation at CLEF erisk 2017 task: Towards modelling depressed blogers. In *Working Notes of CLEF 2017 - Conference and Labs of the Evaluation Forum, Dublin, Ireland, September 11–14, 2017.*
83. Villegas, M. P., Funez, D. G., Ucelay, M. J. G., Cagnina, L. C., & Errecalde, M. L. (2017). LIDIC - unsl's participation at erisk 2017: Pilot task on early detection of depression. In *Working Notes of CLEF 2017 - Conference and Labs of the Evaluation Forum, Dublin, Ireland, September 11–14, 2017.*
84. Walsh, C. G., Chaudhry, B., Dua, P., Goodman, K. W., Kaplan, B., Kavuluru, R., Solomonides, A., & Subbian, V. (2020). Stigma, biomarkers, and algorithmic bias: recommendations for precision behavioral health with artificial intelligence. *JAMIA Open.*
85. Wang, Y., Huang, H., Chen, H. (2018). A neural network approach to early risk detection of depression and anorexia on social media text. In *Working Notes of CLEF 2018 - Conference and Labs of the Evaluation Forum, Avignon, France, September 10–14, 2018.*
86. Yates, A., Cohan, A., & Goharian, N. (2017). Depression and self-harm risk assessment in online forums. In *Proceedings of the 2017 Conference on Empirical Methods in Natural Language Processing* (Copenhagen, Denmark, 2017) (pp. 2968–2978).
87. Zirikly, A., Resnik, P., Uzuner, Ö., & Hollingshead, K. (2019). CLPsych 2019 shared task: Predicting the degree of suicide risk in Reddit posts. In *Proceedings of the Sixth Workshop on Computational Linguistics and Clinical Psychology: From Keyboard to Clinic.*

The Best of eRisk

From Bag-of-Words to Transformers: A Deep Dive into the Participation in the eRisk *Early Risk Detection of Depression* Tasks with Classical and New Approaches

Hendrik Damm, Marcel Trotzek, Sven Koitka, Henning Schäfer, Ahmad Idrissi-Yaghir, and Christoph M. Friedrich

Abstract World Health Organization (WHO) describes depression as the leading contributor to global disability and names it a major reason for suicide. Regardless of the prevalence and seriousness of depression, only about 50% of all affected individuals are under professional treatment. Pandemics such as COVID-19 have shown that a global crisis with drastic changes in living conditions can lead to increased symptoms of anxiety and depression, making the demand for early risk detection more relevant than ever. This chapter describes the models and results submitted by the FHDO Biomedical Computer Science Group (BCSG) to the eRisk tasks of 2017 and 2018 on Early Detection of Signs of Depression. After those challenges, some extended models have been developed to see if the results could be improved. These

---

Hendrik Damm Contributed equally to this work.

H. Damm · M. Trotzek (✉) · S. Koitka · H. Schäfer · A. Idrissi-Yaghir · C. M. Friedrich
Department of Computer Science, University of Applied Sciences and Arts Dortmund (FHDO), Emil-Figge-Str. 42, 44227 Dortmund, Germany
e-mail: mtrotzek@stud.fh-dortmund.de

H. Damm
e-mail: dammh@uni-muenster.de

S. Koitka
e-mail: sven.koitka@uk-essen.de

H. Schäfer
e-mail: henning.schaefer@uk-essen.de

A. Idrissi-Yaghir
e-mail: ahmad.idrissi-yaghir@fh-dortmund.de

C. M. Friedrich
e-mail: christoph.friedrich@fh-dortmund.de

H. Damm
Institute of Epidemiology and Social Medicine, University of Münster, Albert-Schweitzer-Campus 1, 48149 Münster, Germany

F. Crestani et al. (eds.), *Early Detection of Mental Health Disorders by Social Media Monitoring*, Studies in Computational Intelligence 1018,
https://doi.org/10.1007/978-3-031-04431-1_4

tests include the use of language models, which will be described in this chapter as well. Besides using hand-crafted features based on linguistic metadata, there were also attempts to use emotions and sentiment lexica for the early risk detection of depression. For experiments with machine learning models, a new word embedding was trained on a large corpus of the same domain as the described task and is evaluated. Finally, different prediction thresholds and ensembles of the developed models are used to explore the possible improvements, and the proposed alternative early detection metrics ($F_{latency}$ and $\text{ERDE}_o^{\%}$) are evaluated.

1 Introduction

More than 300 million people worldwide are suffering from depression, according to data collected by World Health Organization (WHO) [54]. Depression occurs in any age group and any region of the world as well as for any social status [5], which leads to the common statement that depression is often accompanied by paradoxes, caused by a contrast between a patient's self-image and the actual facts. The worst case is that depression can lead to suicide and is therefore declared a major contributor to the nearly 800,000 [54] people who are dying by suicide every year. The WHO lists self-harm as the second leading cause of death in the age group between 15 and 29 [54]. In addition, recent events [23, 60] have shown that the COVID-19 pandemic and its subsequent drastic changes in living conditions can lead to increased symptoms of anxiety, depression, and trauma, making the demand for early risk detection more relevant than ever. Although the severity of depression is well-known, it is estimated that only half of the individuals who have any mental disorder are in professional treatment [3]. Methods that help identify risk cases or already affected individuals automatically can play an important role in future early risk detection of depression.

As several studies have shown (see e.g., [7, 25, 52, 53]), individuals with mental disorders or other stigmatized illnesses are more likely to use internet resources to get informed, connect with others, and share experiences. These results show the importance of research that could assist affected individuals on social media platforms and the internet in general.

S. Koitka
Department of Diagnostic and Interventional Radiology and Neuroradiology, University Hospital Essen, Essen, Germany

Institute for Artificial Intelligence in Medicine, University Hospital Essen, Essen, Germany

H. Schäfer
Institute for Transfusion Medicine, University Hospital Essen, Essen, Germany

C. M. Friedrich
Institute for Medical Informatics Biometry and Epidemiology (IMIBE), University Hospital Essen, Essen, Germany

As more and more data has become available for research due to the popularity of social media platforms, completely new research possibilities have emerged, for example, in the field of text classification. Extracting information about a person's mental status from a spoken and written text is already a well-studied area (see e.g., [64, 70, 79]) that has also been applied to text classification based on social media in several works (see e.g., [17, 27, 31, 51]). The work presented in this chapter focuses on a twofold medical text classification task. The first aspect of this task is detecting depression indications in written texts, which is done based on various standard machine learning methods, neural networks, and a set of linguistic metadata features. The second aspect is the early detection of such indications using as few texts as possible. Furthermore, this work contributes to the discussion about early detection tasks in general by giving detailed insights into a current metric for such a task and proposing an alternative. Finally, it has been tested if the Transformer Architecture [77] is applicable to the task of early risk detection. All this work is based on the shared task about the early detection of depression as part of the eRisk workshop at the Conference and Labs of the Evaluation Forum (CLEF) in 2017 [41] and 2018 [42] as well as related work to those tasks. This chapter summarizes all the work done in the following submissions and publications:

- Participation of FHDO Biomedical Computer Science Group (BCSG) at the Conference and Labs of the Evaluation Forum (CLEF) 2017 eRisk task [72].
- Related work to the eRisk 2017 task, based on Linguistic Metadata Augmented Classifiers [71].
- IEEE Publication for detection of depression using machine learning models based on messages on a social platform. In particular, a convolutional neural network based on different word embeddings [74].
- Participation of FHDO Biomedical Computer Science Group (BCSG) at the Conference and Labs of the Evaluation Forum (CLEF) 2018 eRisk task [73].

In the remainder of this chapter, Sect. 2 provides a short overview of the tasks, which form the basis of this work (detailed information can be found in chapter "The Challenge of Early Risk Prediction on the Internet"). Section 3 describes the evaluation criteria for the task and proposes alternatives. Section 4 details all features and architectures used for the proposed models, which are displayed in Sect. 5. In Sect. 6 the obtained results are reported and discussed afterwards in Sect. 7. Finally, Sect. 8 presents the overall conclusion for this chapter.

2 eRisk 2017/2018 Task for Early Detection of Depression

2.1 Overview

The eRisk 2017 Task for Early Detection of Depression [41] was the pilot task for early detection of depression followed by the eRisk 2018 Task for Early Detection of Depression [42]. The following sections describe the participation of the BCSG in those tasks. For the 2017 task, the BCSG submitted models from four different approaches and an additional fifth [72] optimized variation as a late submission. For the 2018 task, the BCSG again submitted four different models and a late fusion ensemble [73] of three of them. These models and the findings concerning the datasets are described in this chapter and an outlook on possible improvements and future research is given. The work described in this chapter also includes further research based on the same datasets, as well as ongoing work. Furthermore, the tasks were extended with a newly proposed metric and the generated results with that metric were examined.

2.2 Datasets

The dataset presented in the CLEF 2017 eRisk pilot task consists of text contents written by users of Reddit,[1] which is a communication platform widely used for creating communities, called *subReddits*, that cover all kinds of topics.[2]

The given dataset for the 2017 task contains all three kinds of content written by 887 users resulting in 10 to 2,000 documents per user. Table 1 gives a summary of some basic characteristics of the training and test split. The task's goal is to classify which of these users show indications of depression by reading as few of their posts as possible in chronological order. Each document contains a timestamp of publication, the title, and the text content, while the title or text can be empty. Overall, there are 91 documents with both an empty title and text. The URL or image of link entries is not provided in the dataset. The number of unique *n*-grams, shown in Table 1, contains all tokens with more than one alphabetical character (and the word "I") that occur at least in two documents, also including numbers, emoticons, and words that contain hyphens or apostrophes.

Similar to the task in 2017, the 2018 dataset consists of messages obtained from the subReddit `/r/depression`. The training data of the 2018 task is a combination of the training and test data of the previous task in 2017. For the 2018 task, there were exceptions of the general rule of 10% of the user's messages being provided in each chunk because three depression test users (subject5161, subject5301, and subject8719) did not have any messages in the final week, resulting in only nine messages of these users. Table 2 displays the main characteristics of the dataset. The average amount of characters and unigrams per document was calculated based on a concatenation of the *text* and *title* field.

[1] https://www.Reddit.com, accessed on 2021-01-04.

[2] https://Redditblog.com/2014/07/30/how-Reddit-works-2/, accessed on 2021-01-04.

Table 1 Characteristics of the 2017 training and test datasets

	Training	Test
Users	486	401
Depressed/Non-depressed	83/403	52/349
Documents	295,023	236,371
Comments (empty title)	198,731	168,708
Links/One-liners (empty text)	84,288	57,561
Empty documents	46	45
Avg. documents per user	607.04	589.45
Avg. characters per document (title + text)	172.19	182.29
Avg. unigrams per document (title + text)	29.80	32.27
Unique unigrams	73,501	69,587
Unique bigrams	606,608	526,380
Unique trigrams	778,694	673,048

Table 2 Characteristics of the 2018 training and test datasets

	Training	Test
Users	887	820
Depressed/Non-depressed	135/752	79/741
Documents	531,394	544,447
Comments (empty title)	367,439	366,845
Links/One-liners (empty text)	141,849	147,197
Empty documents	91	219
Avg. documents per user	599.09	663.96
Avg. characters per document (title + text)	174.54	197.47
Avg. unigrams per document (title + text)	30.83	34.53
Unique unigrams	85,558	94,569
Unique bigrams	859,148	956,268
Unique trigrams	1,177,839	1,309,493

3 Evaluation Criteria and Concerns About ERDE Score

Before examining the results of the models in the tasks described in Sect. 5, it is necessary to analyze the utilized *Early Risk Detection Error* ($ERDE_o$) metric used to assess early detection systems. The given dataset was explicitly published for early risk detection of depression within the task. To measure this criterion, the data was

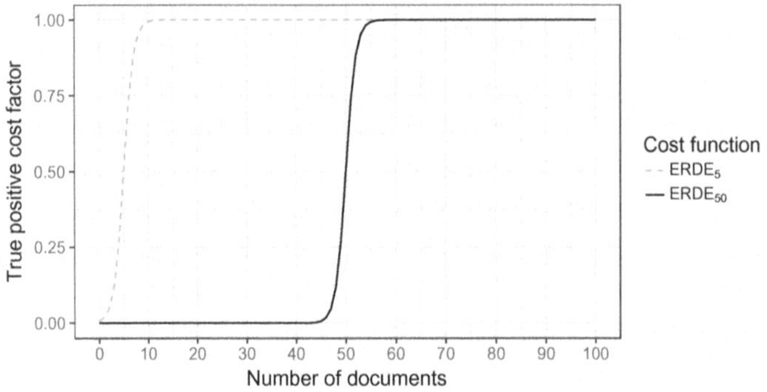

Fig. 1 Plot of the true positive cost factor $lc_o(k)$ for ERDE_5 and ERDE_{50}. License: Creative Commons CC-BY Trotzek et al. [74]

also split into ten chunks by the organizers, containing 10% of each user's messages in chronological order.

The concept of the ERDE_o metric will only be briefly addressed in this Section. The details can be found in chapter "The Challenge of Early Risk Prediction on the Internet" (Sect. 4).

Since the results given for the baseline experiments in the original paper [40] were obtained by using systems that could submit a prediction after reading each message per user separately, they cannot be compared to results of the actual eRisk task that required to read a whole chunk of between 1 and 200 messages per user. As Fig. 1 illustrates, this means that depressed users with about ten and more (for ERDE_5) or about 55 and more (for ERDE_{50}) messages per chunk basically cannot be predicted correctly because the cost would be very close to c_{fn}.

Table 3 shows the ERDE_o scores of perfect predictions ($F_1 = 1.0$) submitted after reading n chunks with no predictions submitted in the chunks before this one. It also includes the corresponding scores obtained from $\text{ERDE}_o^{\%}$ described at the end of this section. The scores obtained for $n = 1$ are the best possible ERDE_o scores for this task in 2017, while $n = 10$ gives the best possible scores for a system that has read all messages. Only predicting the 18 depressed users with less than ten messages per chunk as early as possible and predicting every other user as negative, results in an F_1-Score of 0.51 (1.0 precision and 0.35 recall) but still obtains an ERDE_5 score of 10.61% and ERDE_{50} of 8.48%. The additional F_1-Score is therefore especially important to evaluate systems in the general task of depression detection. To achieve better ERDE_o scores, systems not only have to be optimized for this task but also need optimized prediction thresholds to make early predictions without too many false positives or false negatives. This twofold optimization makes this task especially challenging.

Related experiments described in this chapter are based on the same training and test data from the eRisk 2017 and 2018 tasks which are also processed by evaluating the same chunks of test data in chronological order. This ensures that the results are directly comparable to those of the pilot task.

Table 3 Scores for perfect predictions of the eRisk 2017 test data after reading n chunks according to the original ERDE_o and the newly proposed $\text{ERDE}_o^{\%}$ Score

n	ERDE_5	ERDE_{50}	$\text{ERDE}_{20}^{\%}$	$\text{ERDE}_{50}^{\%}$
1	10.60	3.74	0.00	0.00
2	12.00	5.37	6.48	0.00
5	12.85	8.47	12.97	6.48
10	12.97	10.48	12.97	12.97

Nevertheless, a detailed look at the ERDE_o function shows that there is a need to modify this function especially for future works with data in chunks. The first modification of ERDE has been proposed by [43] and in addition to making the score usable for multi-class problems, it mainly consists of an altered cost function defined now as:

$$lc_o(k) = \frac{k}{o}, \tag{1}$$

where o is no longer used to parameterize the cost but equals the number of documents per user and k is the number of documents already read for this user. This ensures that the cost is based on the proportion of read documents instead of a fixed number. Still, there is no way to parameterize this function and it immediately grows linearly, without any possibility to predict a subject correctly with a cost of zero.

Therefore, a modification of the original sigmoid cost function was proposed [74]:

$$lc_o(p) = 1 - \frac{1}{1 + e^{p-o}} \tag{2}$$

$$p = \frac{100 \cdot k}{n_d}, \tag{3}$$

where n_d is the total number of documents per user and k still equals the number of documents already read per user. The cost can still be parameterized by using $o \in [0, 100]$ to make the cost grow around the point where o percent of data has been read. This results in a more intuitive cost that grows equally for all users independent of their number of messages. The newly proposed error function based on $lc_o(p)$ is denoted as $\text{ERDE}_o^{\%}$ and is evaluated for some of the models. Table 3 shows how this score compares to the original one for perfect predictions on the eRisk 2017 test data. Since at least 10% of the messages per user have to be read and $o = 18$ is the minimum natural value to achieve an error of 0.00%, results are shown for $\text{ERDE}_{20}^{\%}$ instead of $\text{ERDE}_5^{\%}$.

Based on similar findings, an alternative score for early detection systems, namely $F_{latency}$, was recently proposed by another participating team of eRisk 2017 [66]. This metric incorporates the standard F_1-Score measure and uses a cost factor based on the latency of the classification, which is defined as the median number of messages

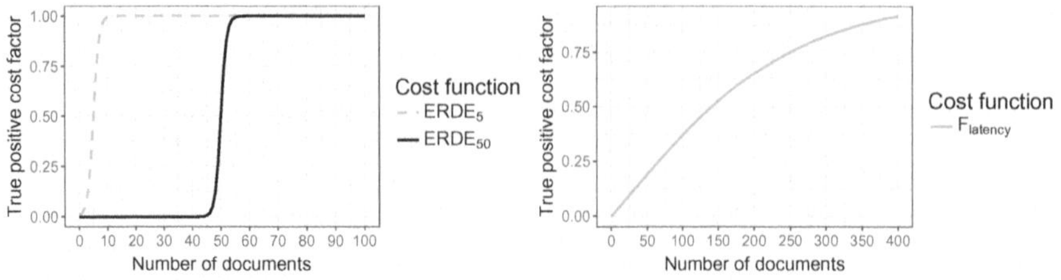

Fig. 2 Plot of the true positive cost functions used for $ERDE_5$ and $ERDE_{50}$ (left) as well as for $F_{latency}$ with $p = 0.0078$ (right). License: Creative Commons CC-BY Trotzek et al. [74]

read before predicting a user depressed. Based on this, they define their cost function $P_{latency}$ and the corresponding score $F_{latency}$ as [66, p. 497]:

$$P_{latency}(u, sys) = -1 + \frac{2}{1 + e^{-p \cdot (time(u,sys)-1)}} \tag{4}$$

$$F_{latency}(U, sys) = F_1(U, sys) \cdot \left(1 - \underset{u \in U \wedge ref(u)=+}{\text{median}} P_{latency}(u, sys)\right), \tag{5}$$

with $time(u, sys)$ denoting the number of documents seen for user u by system sys, the free parameter p to modify how the cost grows, the standard F_1-Score $F_1(U, sys)$ calculated over all users in the dataset U, and $ref(u) = +$ referring to a user with a positive (depressed) label. In addition to the true positive cost function of $ERDE_o$, Fig. 2 also displays a plot of the cost function used for $F_{latency}$. It shows $P_{latency}$ with $p = 0.0078$ as proposed in the paper, which results in a cost of 0.5 for the median number of posts per user (142 for eRisk 2017). This results in a less rapid growth of the cost function, fewer parameters as there are no fixed cost values to define, and already incorporates F_1-Score, which makes this score more meaningful alone. Still, the cost is based on the absolute number of read documents, which leads to the same problem as discussed above for chunk-based shared task scenarios.

4 Features and Architectures Used for Depression Detection

This section gives an overview of the features and architectures used for the eRisk tasks and related work. This includes the creation of Hand-crafted User Features in Sect. 4.1. Next up, additional Linguistic Metadata features based on Linguistic Inquiry and Word Count (LIWC) [70] are presented. The use of emotions and sentiment lexica for early risk detection is examined in Sect. 4.6. The succeeding Sects. 4.7 and 4.8 give a deep analysis on Neural word embeddings. Finally, Sect. 4.9 explains a new approach to the eRisk tasks using language models.

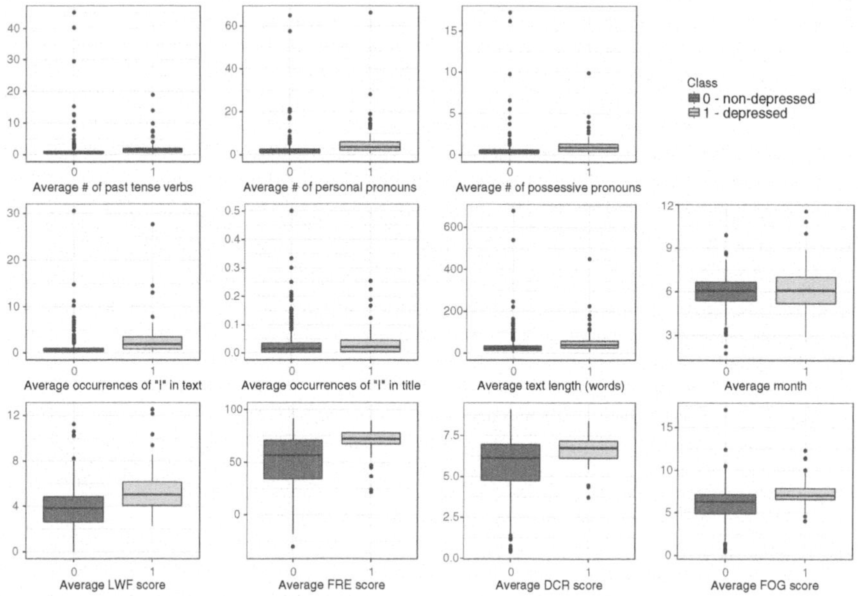

Fig. 3 Boxplots of text features for both classes per user in the eRisk 2017 training dataset. License: Reproduced with authors approval from [72]

4.1 Hand-Crafted User Features

For the eRisk tasks, and specifically for the topic of detecting early depression risk, a set of hand-crafted features for user-level linguistic metadata was created. These were used in several models described in Sect. 5. Various text statistics were computed and compared between depressed and non-depressed users in the given datasets. All text-based features were computed based on concatenation of the *text* and *title* field of each post. The most promising features are shown in Fig. 3 as boxplots for each class. These boxplots represent data from the 2017 task only, and all features were calculated as averages across all texts from the same user. In addition to counts of personal and possessive pronouns, past tense verbs, and especially the word *I*, four standard measures of text readability were calculated for the text content, namely *Gunning Fog Index* (FOG) [26], Flesch Reading Ease (FRE) [21], Linsear Write Formula (LWF)[3] [14], and New Dale-Chall Readability (DCR) [12, 16]. Interestingly, FOG, LWF, and DCR compute higher complexity for texts by depressed users (with scores based on years of schooling in the United States), while FRE also computes a higher score, corresponding to lower complexity in this case. Details on readability are described in Sect. 4.2.

Based on the hypothesis that depressive symptoms may increase during the winter months, the average number of times a user posted in each month were included.

[3] Originally developed by the U.S. Air Force, with no available references.

However, this is difficult to observe in the given datasets because the age of the available texts depends on how often a user posted. This is due to the restriction to the last 2000 writings per user. Therefore, users with many and frequent writings tend to have more samples from early summer 2015 (when the collection was created), while less frequent writers provide a more even distribution of texts across all months. In addition, five features were created for users to simply count the occurrence of some very specific n-grams in all of their documents. This ensures that some of the strongest indicators of depression can still be easily identified even when using averaged document vectors or only a large number of documents. These features were used in boolean form by all of the models described and, without a regard to case, count the following terms:

- The chemical and brand names of common antidepressants available in the United States (e.g.: *Sertraline* or *Zoloft*) obtained from WebMD[4]
- Explicit mentions of a diagnosis including the word *depression* (e.g.: "*I was diagnosed with depression*" or "*I've been diagnosed with anxiety and depression*")
- The term "*my depression*"
- The term "*my anxiety*"
- The term "*my therapist*"

The terms listed were carefully selected based on the training documents and were designed to capture only statements that relate to the author's personal situation, with the exception of antidepressants. Selected terms could be expanded for future work, for example, to include a more comprehensive list of medications or more general expressions of diagnosis (e.g., also including the terms "major depressive disorder" or "MDD"). Although the selected terms are not primarily helpful for early predictions, they are strong indicators to find already diagnosed individuals, which is also essential for the present task.

Figure 4 illustrates the correlation matrix of the complete metadata feature set for the 2017 task and includes the class label information to indicate the relevance of each feature. See Sect. 4.3 for more details on word and grammar usage.

The 2018 task includes the same set of features described above and an additional set of ten features obtained from the LIWC software. These LIWC features have been chosen based on their correlation with the class label in the depression task training data. Another addition to the original feature set is the average length of the *title* field that was also not used in 2017.

The correlation matrix of the used metadata feature set for the 2018 task can be found in Fig. 5. The correlation is colored from red (negative correlation) to blue (positive correlation). The color follows a gradient according to the strength of the correlation. If the ellipse slopes to the right, it is a positive correlation, and if it slopes to the left, it is a negative correlation.. Although some features—especially the pronoun counts—seem redundant at first sight, all of the original features are preserved as they are based on a Part of Speech (POS) tagging using the Python

[4] http://www.webmd.com/depression/guide/depression-medications-antidepressants, accessed on 2021-02-01.

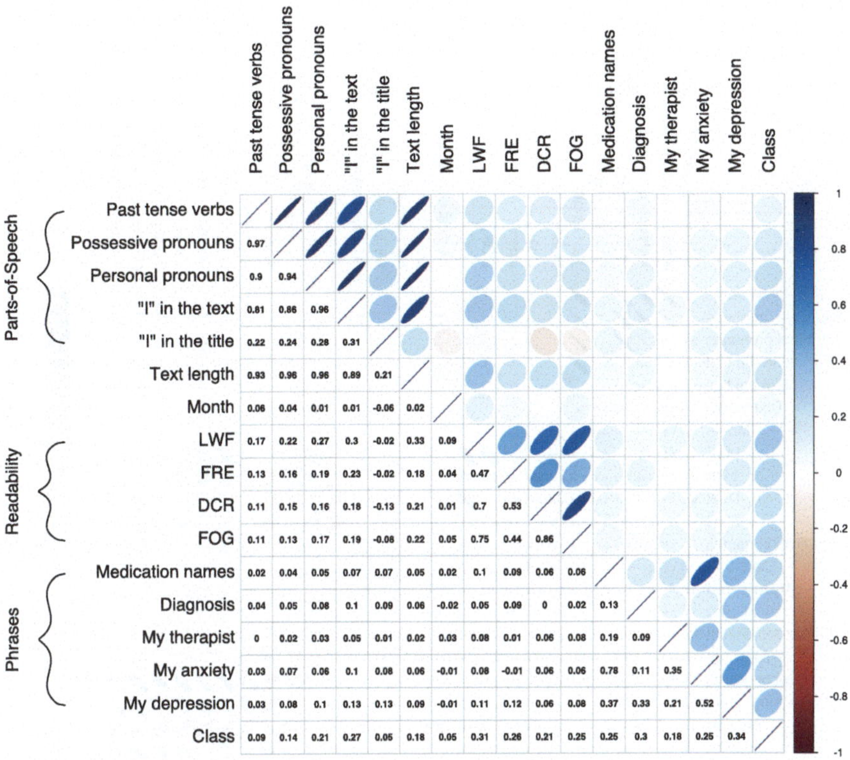

Fig. 4 Correlation matrix of all user features including the class information (nondepressed/depressed) based on the 2017 depression task training data. This plot is best viewed in electronic form. License: Reproduced with authors approval from [72]

NLTK framework[5] while LIWC features are based on a lexicon that also includes abbreviations or common misspellings. Most of the described features are averaged over all documents per user to obtain the final metadata feature vector, except for the counts of specific phrases like medication names or mentioned diagnoses which are summed. Finally, all averaged features are standardized to have unit variance and a mean of 0 and the summed features are converted to flags with a value of 1 for users that have used such a phrase in any document, and −1 otherwise.

Detecting mental health status based on language use dates back to speech studies [10, 79] that found an elevated use of first person singular pronouns in the spoken words of depression patients. Similar research based on written texts [64] reported, for example, more frequent use of the word "I" in particular and more negative emotion words. A recent study [2] also found more "absolutist" words (e.g., "absolutely", "completely", "every", or "nothing") in English forum posts related to depression,

[5] http://www.nltk.org/book/ch05.html, accessed on 2021-02-01.

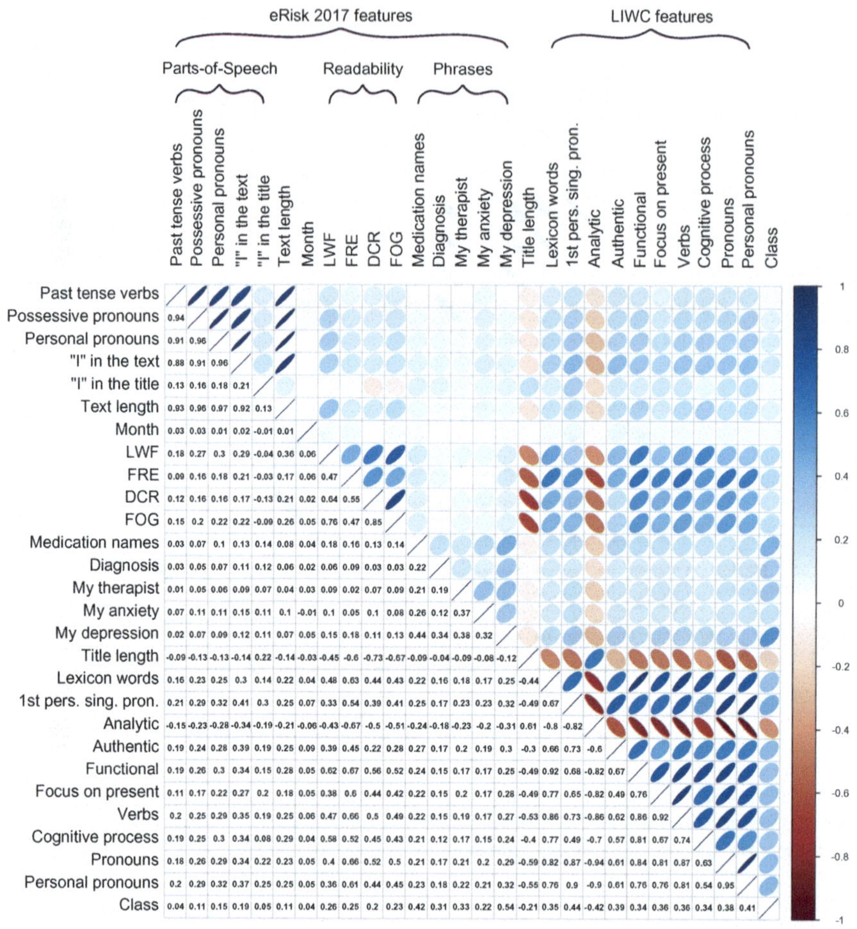

Fig. 5 Correlation matrix of all user features including the class information (nondepressed/depressed) based on the 2018 depression task training data. This plot is best viewed in electronic form. License: Reproduced with authors approval from [73]

anxiety, and suicidal ideation than in posts from completely unrelated areas as well as in posts concerning asthma, diabetes, or cancer.

The findings for these specific datasets confirm that texts by individuals suffering from depression indeed contain more pronouns and especially the word "I". Their texts are also slightly longer and more complex according to three of the four text complexity measures. This likely represents the difference between average users, who often post a large number of short statements, and those who discuss problems and may even be looking for help.

4.2 Readability

Measuring the readability or complexity of a written text is a well-established idea, and different measures exist. Most of them return a result that corresponds to the school years in the US needed to understand a text. The given datasets cannot be used to indicate whether depressed persons write more or less complex texts because of the general difference of text quality between the classes. Since the control subjects were chosen randomly, they often differ drastically from the depressed subjects, who might use Reddit to discuss their problems or generally talk to other people. Messages of the control group often simply consist of news headlines, a single short sentence, or even a single word. Readability metrics can help to distinguish messages containing discussions and explanations from such simple content that is unlikely to help with the identification of depression.

4.3 Word and Grammar Usage

As described in Sect. 4.1, effects of depression on word and grammar usage are well-known and can include, for example, increased usage of pronouns, especially personal pronouns and in particular the word "I", and verbs in past tense. Based on these previous findings, occurrences of the word "I" were counted separately in the text and title of each message in the 2017 eRisk dataset. On top of that, past tense verbs, personal pronouns, and possessive pronouns were counted in the concatenation of text and title by utilizing the default POS tagger. As an alternative to this approach, a total of 93 lexicon-based features can be obtained from the LIWC tool [58]. Besides features referring to a specific POS, this also includes categories like emotions, informal language, or time orientations. LIWC also calculates four summary variables that represent the authenticity, emotional tone, confidence or leadership, and analytical thinking of a text. Section 4.4 describes which of these features have been utilized for the experiments of this work. The five final word usage features were used for the participation in eRisk 2017, see Sect. 5, and aim to count very specific, hand-picked phrases that could be a strong indicator of positive cases. They count the occurrences of the exact phrases "my depression", "my anxiety", and "my therapist" as well as names of some common antidepressants[6] and variations of the phrase "I was diagnosed with depression"[7] (see Sect. 4.1). These very explicit features are less aimed at finding early indications of depression but at predicting the obvious cases correctly, which is important for the given task. In contrast to the other metadata features, this count is summed up over all user documents to make this a strong feature, even if the phrases/word only occur in a few or a single document.

[6] https://www.webmd.com/depression/guide/depression-medications-antidepressants, accessed on 2021-02-08.

[7] Only including the word "I" and an explicit diagnosis as in "I've been diagnosed with anxiety and depression" or "I was diagnosed with major depressive disorder".

Table 4 User based metadata features used in combination with the selected LIWC features

Feature	Type	Description
"I" in the text	Avg.	Only the word "I"
"I" in the title	Avg.	Only the word "I"
Possessive pronouns	Avg.	Based on POS tagging
Personal pronouns	Avg.	Based on POS tagging
Past tense verbs	Avg.	Based on POS tagging
4 readability scores	Avg.	FOG, FRE, LWF, and DCR
Month of the writings	Avg.	
Text length	Avg.	
Title length	Avg.	
Depression	Sum	"My depression"
Anxiety	Sum	"My anxiety"
Therapist	Sum	"My therapist"
Diagnosis	Sum	E.g., "I was diagnosed with depression"
Antidepressants	Sum	E.g., "zoloft" and "paxil"

4.4 *Metadata Feature Summary*

Table 4 summarizes the 17 metadata features that have been described above excluding the features obtained from LIWC. In addition to these, the ten LIWC features with the highest correlation to the class label in the training data have been selected. Because the LIWC lexicon includes several variations, misspellings, and abbreviations, it is accepted that some of these features already occur in the previously described feature set and therefore introduce a slight redundancy. The selected LIWC features are the number of function words, variations of the word "I" (e.g., including abbreviations containing "I" as well as "me" and "myself"), all pronouns, personal pronouns, verbs, words indicating a cognitive process, words with a focus on the present, the total number of lexicon words found, and the two calculated summary variables indicating analytical thinking and authenticity. To build the user-level metadata vector for the experiments described in Sect. 5.10, these features were again averaged over all documents of the same user. The described metadata features result in a 27-dimensional vector per user. The concatenated feature vectors of all users are standardized as described in Sect. 5.10 before being used as input to a classifier. The five counts of specific terms are transformed into boolean flags by representing a value above 0 as 1 and a value of 0 as -1, similar to the previous work [72] using *Long Short Term Memory* (LSTM) [30] networks. As the experiments will show, this set of metadata features alone can lead to very good results on the eRisk 2017 dataset.

4.5 Linguistic Metadata

The knowledge that mental state has various effects on a person's language has driven the development of language analysis tools like LIWC [70], which allows researchers to calculate a total of 93 lexicon-based features for any given text. Similar to the eRisk task at CLEF, social media texts have already been used in a shared task concerning the detection of depression and post-traumatic stress disorder (PTSD) [15]. Apart from shared tasks, several different approaches have been used to detect depression on platforms like Facebook, Twitter, and Reddit [27].

Using linguistic metadata features on a user basis as an additional input to all classification models was one of the main concepts behind this team's participation in the eRisk 2017 task. The detailed description of these features was mentioned in Sect. 4.1. This section will only focus on examining possible additional metadata features. In particular, metadata features based on the emotions, opinions, and sentiments contained in a user's writings. This is based on the assumption that writings containing indications of depression might contain more negative emotions and an overall rather negative sentiment than writings of the control group. Since sentiment analysis is a very broad and active research area [56], a variety of methods could be used to extract a sentiment feature from the Reddit messages. This section focuses on using lexica to calculate the sentiment and emotional content based on the words used in a message.

Various researchers have collected several lexica specific to the task of sentiment or emotion detection. The ones selected for this task are the NRC Emotion Lexicon [50], the Opinion Lexicon,[8] the VADER Sentiment Lexicon [32], and SentiWordNet [4]. The NRC Emotion Lexicon contains 14,182 words that are assigned to one or more of the categories "positive", "negative", "anger", "anticipation", "disgust", "fear", "joy", "sadness", "surprise", and "trust". The respective features for each document are calculated by counting the words of each category and dividing these counts by the total number of lexicon words present in the document. The Opinion Lexicon consists of a list of 2,006 positive and 4,783 negative words that can be used to similarly calculate two features. In contrast, the VADER Sentiment Lexicon contains 7,517 terms (including emoticons) with their average sentiment score based on ten human annotators on a scale between -4 (extremely negative) to $+4$ (extremely positive). A single VADER feature is therefore calculated as the mean sentiment score of a document's words that occur in the lexicon.

While the first three lexica directly consist of word lists with either an associated score or a categorization, SentiWordNet is based on the sets of synonyms (synsets) assigned to any word by WordNet [49] and contains a positivity, negativity, and objectivity score for each synset. Calculating the score for a message therefore requires to first obtain the fitting synset for each word based on the POS it represents in its sentence. POS tagging and the lookups of WordNet and SentiWordNet are all done based on NLTK for this work. The final SentiWordNet score of a message $SWN(d)$ is calculated as:

[8] https://www.cs.uic.edu/~liub/FBS/sentiment-analysis.html#lexicon, accessed on 2021-02-06.

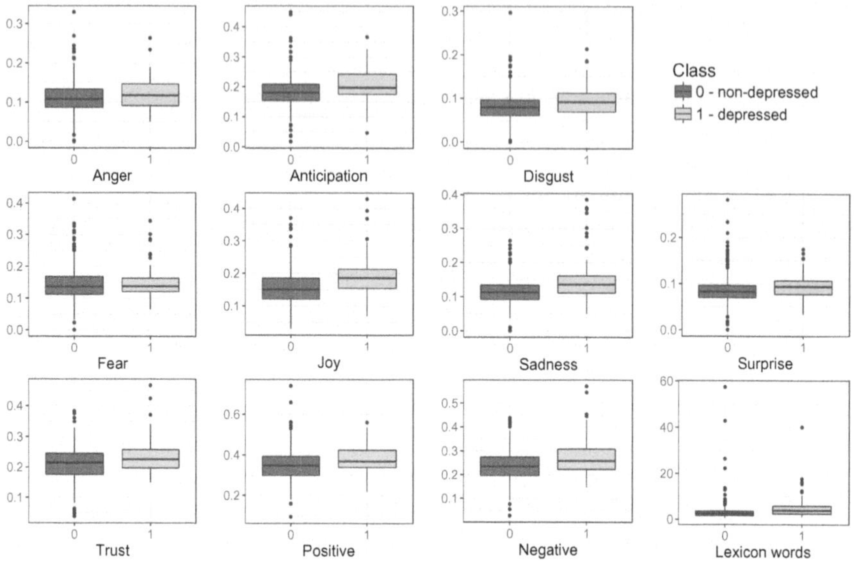

Fig. 6 Boxplot of the user-level emotion features based on the NRC Emotion Lexicon. Reproduced with publishers permission from [71]

$$SWN(d) = \frac{1}{n_w} \cdot \sum_{w \in d} SWN_{pos}(w, POS_w) - SWN_{neg}(w, POS_w) \,, \qquad (6)$$

with n_w denoting the number of words in message d, the part of speech represented by a word POS_w, the positivity score of a word $SWN_{pos}(w, POS_w)$, and the negativity score of a word $SWN_{neg}(w, POS_w)$. Words that do not exist in WordNet are removed from the document before the calculation.

Similar to the other metadata features, the sentiment and emotion features described above are averaged over all documents of a user to obtain a user-level metadata vector. Figure 6 shows boxplots of all features extracted from the NRC Emotion Lexicon and also includes an additional feature based on the number of lexicon words present in the documents. Contrary to the original assumption, all kinds of emotions, as well as positive and negative words, tend to occur more often in documents of depressed users in this dataset. In general, the most indicative feature based on these boxplots seems to be the number of lexicon words present in a document.

Figure 7 displays a correlation matrix of all described sentiment and emotion features and includes the class label information (0 for non-depressed and 1 for depressed). While the correlations among these features show how negative emotions indeed lead to lower VADER and SentiWordNet score and vice versa, all features have a slight positive correlation with the class label. The amount of positive and negative opinion words based on the Opinion Lexicon is also strongly correlated, showing that users with more positive words also use more negative words. This

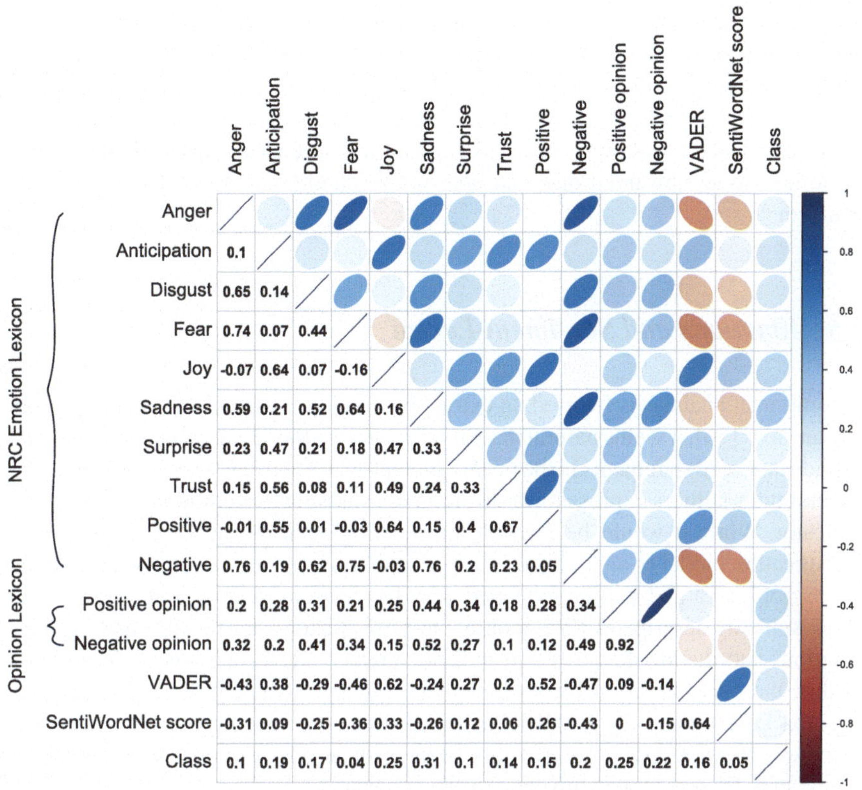

Fig. 7 Correlation matrix of user-based emotion and sentiment features including the class information (non-depressed/depressed) for the 2017 eRisk dataset. Reproduced with publishers permission from [71]

matches the insights given by the above boxplots and shows that all kinds of lexicon words occur more often in the depressed class and that the calculated sentiment scores based on VADER and SentiWordNet have no interesting correlation at all. As this indicates, experiments have shown that these features are not viable to enhance the previous models for early detection of depression based on the eRisk 2017 dataset.

The limited meaning of these features is likely due to the character of this specific dataset. While it could be assumed that depressed individuals indeed use more emotions of any kind in online discussions, the messages of the control group differ too drastically to make any general assumptions based on these observations. Since the control group has been selected randomly and therefore contains messages from all kinds of subReddits, the overall text quality and writing style cannot be compared to the target group. Another dataset used for the detection of anxiety on Reddit [69] was explicitly collected in a way to obtain similar writings in both the control and target group. By only selecting messages from specific subReddits, the researchers considered their observation that "anxiety-related posts are overwhelmingly from a first-person point-of-view" [69]. As the eRisk control group also contains many writings that only contain news headlines, a single short sentence, or even a single word, comparing them to messages of individuals who discuss their personal problems is often difficult. Based on these findings, choosing the control group users more selectively could be an interesting plan for future eRisk tasks. However, this could lead to an unwanted bias that does not resemble real-world data on a social platform.

4.6 Emotions and Sentiment Lexica

As sentiment analysis is focused on extracting opinions, affects, and emotions from written texts [56], it seems natural that knowledge from this area can also be beneficial to find emotional statements in the field of mental health text classification. Especially the emotions authors express towards their personal situation could be an important indicator. While it would be possible to use the output of any kind of sentiment classification model as an additional feature, the work in this section has focused on the use of lexica and will be extended with language models in Sect. 4.9. First of all, the already described LIWC tool includes two features for positive and negative emotions and distinct features that indicate anxiety, anger, or sadness. In addition to this, the NRC Emotion Lexicon and two general sentiment lexica, namely the Opinion Lexicon and the VADER Sentiment Lexicon, have been used. There also exist several other lexica that have not been evaluated, for example from the World Well-Being Project at the University of Pennsylvania.[9]

The corresponding counts or scores obtained from these lexica for the eRisk 2017 dataset were again averaged over all user documents. Unfortunately, for this specific dataset no relevant correlation between these features and the class label could be observed. Indeed, the positive (depressed) class contains slightly more emotions and sentiments of all kinds, which might again indicate the general difference of text quality and content between the depressed subjects and the control group. As the emotion and sentiment features were of no use in this specific case, they were not included in the final set of metadata features used in the experiments of this work. Nevertheless, it can be assumed that they would be more meaningful when used with a text corpus that generally included more sentiment and emotion in both classes by using a control group that more closely resembles the target group.

4.7 Word Embeddings

Neural word embeddings have become a popular and efficient way to model words and interactions between them for text classification tasks. They date back to the con-

[9] http://www.wwbp.org/lexica.html, accessed on 2021-02-09.

cept of distributed word representations [29] that, in contrast to local representations, do not handle each word separately with a single neuron, but use several neurons to represent a word and let each neuron be part of the description of several words. This enables distributed representations to learn general concepts of language instead of just independent word representations. One of the most important and still popular method to train word embeddings was published by Google as Word2Vec [46, 48], which consists of two neural network architectures, namely the Continuous bag-of-words (CBoW) and the (Continuous) Skip-gram (SG) architecture. The concept of Word2Vec was developed further by Facebook and published as fastText in 2017 [8, 33, 47], which also directly offers text classification. While being based on the same two model architectures as Word2Vec, fastText represents words as bags of character n-grams and thus allows to obtain vectorizations even for unknown words. A different approach to learn word embeddings, GloVe, has been published by researchers of the Stanford NLP group [59]. GloVe aims to combine the advantages of local context window approaches like Skip-gram with those of global matrix factorization models like *Latent Semantic Analysis* (LSA) [18].

Pre-trained word vectors obtained from large corpora are available for fastText,[10] GloVe[11] and Google.[12] For this work, a 50-dimensional GloVe model trained on Wikipedia and the Gigaword 5 news corpus as well as a 300-dimensional GloVe model trained on Common Crawl were chosen. In addition, three 300-dimensional pre-trained fastText models based on similar corpora were used.

Finally, to also examine word embeddings that better fit the domain of Reddit messages (or social media platforms in general), an own fastText model was trained on a dataset containing all Reddit comments between October 2007 and May 2015.[13] The total dataset consists of about 1.7 billion messages that have been preprocessed and tokenized in a way that preserves emoticons, punctuation, and words that include special characters (e.g., censored words). One of the preprocessing steps included replacing any references to Reddit users (in the form of /u/<username>) by a generic phrase "ref_user" to prevent any connections to actual users in the resulting word embeddings. Similarly, any reference to a subReddit (in the form of /r/<subReddit>) was replaced by the phrase "ref_subReddit_<subReddit>" to be able to learn a vector representation of them as well that can be regarded as their topic. No stemming or stopword removal of any kind was done. The resulting tokens of each message were lowercased (except for emoticons) and separated with a space to enable fastText to properly treat punctuation.[14] Since the dataset also contains messages written in different languages than English and a sophisticated language detection classifier would have required too much time for so many documents, a

[10] https://fasttext.cc/docs/en/pretrained-vectors.html and https://fasttext.cc/docs/en/english-vectors.html, accessed on 2021-02-08.

[11] http://nlp.stanford.edu/projects/glove, accessed on 2021-02-08.

[12] https://code.google.com/archive/p/word2vec/, accessed on 2021-02-08.

[13] https://www.Reddit.com/r/datasets/comments/3bxlg7/i_have_every_publicly_available_Reddit_comment/, accessed on 2021-02-03.

[14] https://github.com/facebookresearch/fastText/issues/333, accessed on 2021-02-08.

Table 5 Characteristics of the GloVe and fastText Word Embeddings used

Model	Dimension	Corpus tokens (in billion)	Word vectors (in milllion)	Words of eRisk 2017 (%)	Words of eRisk 2018 (%)
GloVe Wiki + News	50	6	0.4	81.9	72.6
GloVe Crawl	300	42	2	93.2	89.9
fastText Wiki	300	?	2.5	81.7	75.9
fastText Wiki + News	300	16	1	79.5	70.0
fastText Crawl	300	600	2	88.5	82.3
fastText Reddit	300	49.9	6	99.7	99.6

simple language detection based on stopword counts was utilized: Only messages with more English stopwords than those from other languages[15] were retained (thus also discarding messages without any stopwords). This resulted in a final training corpus of 1.37 billion messages and a total of 49.9 billion tokens. The C++ implementation of fastText was used to train a 300-dimensional CBoW model without subword information and default values for all other parameters, which contains the 6 million unique tokens that occur at least five times in this corpus. Training took about 26 hours using 12 threads on an Intel Xeon E5-2687W 3.10GHz and needed about 17GB of RAM.

The characteristics of all utilized word embeddings are shown in Table 5. It also contains the number of words each model includes of the words that occur in writings of at least two users of the eRisk 2017 and 2018 datasets after the same preprocessing and tokenization steps as described above. Due to the vocabulary of the 2018 dataset being more extensive than the 2017 dataset, the percentage of the existing words in the embeddings vocabulary got slightly lower. This set of words is used in the experiments described in Sect. 5.10.

As a qualitative analysis of the constructed fastText model, it is possible to examine the nearest neighbors of some hand-picked representative tokens according to cosine similarity. Figure 8 displays six word clouds with the corresponding example token in the middle and its ten (20 in the case of emoticons) nearest neighbors around it. These examples especially illustrate that the model trained on Reddit messages can identify similar emoticons and subReddits, which was not possible using the pre-trained fastText or GloVe models. The closest neighbors of the depression subReddit also include terms like "suicidewatch" and "mmfb" (make me feel better), illustrating relations that were learnt to terms besides other subReddits. It has also learnt similar embeddings for antidepressants like Zoloft. While this as well as similar words to the terms "depression" and "suicidal" can also be observed using the pre-trained

[15] Based on the 2,400 stopwords for 11 languages of the NLTK Python package, http://www.nltk.org/book/ch02.html#annotated-text-corpora, accessed on 2021-02-08.

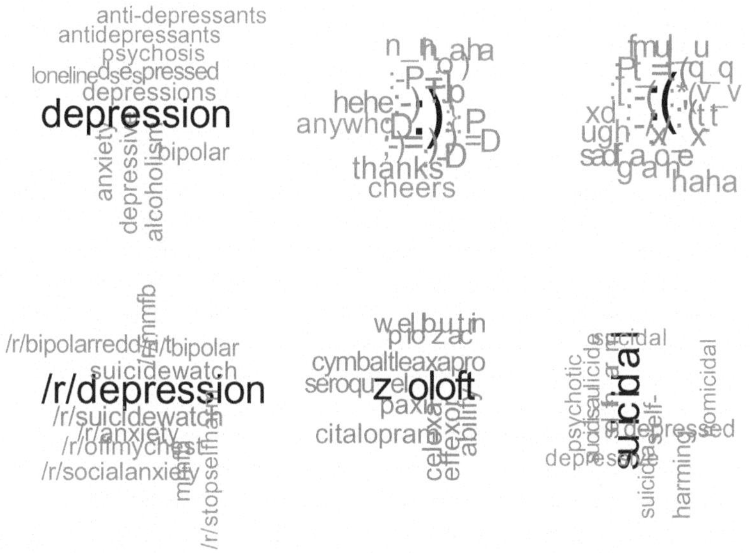

Fig. 8 Nearest neighbors for six hand-picked tokens in the fastText model trained on Reddit comments, for the 2017 dataset, according to cosine similarity. License: Creative Commons CC-BY Trotzek et al. [74]

models, their nearest neighbors seem slightly more medical and from a more neutral perspective (e.g., "ssri" or "sertraline" close to "zoloft", "melancholia" or "insomnia" for "depression", and "deranged" or "delusional" for "suicidal") than those of the model trained on Reddit. The fastText Crawl model also returns neighboring terms like "depression.This" or "depression.What", which might indicate a preprocessing problem concerning punctuation.

To further investigate the extent to which the self-trained fastText Reddit model learnt a general model of the English language, the standard word analogy dataset [46] can be used as one indicator. Table 6 compares results on the word analogy dataset published for state-of-the-art models to the results of the new model trained on Reddit messages. The dataset was originally created to evaluate the word embeddings of Word2Vec and consists of 8,869 semantic as well as 10,675 syntactic analogy questions: Given an analogy (e.g., Athens and Greece) and a third word (e.g., Oslo), word embeddings have to return the fourth word (Norway in this case) as closest vector to the result of $vec(\text{“}Greece\text{”}) - vec(\text{“}Athens\text{”}) + vec(\text{“}Oslo\text{”})$ according to cosine similarity. The Word2Vec results are far from the ones obtained by the state-of-the-art fastText models trained on Wikipedia and news articles. Especially the result in the syntactic category illustrates that even the training on these much less formal documents has lead to a decent model of the English language.

Table 6 Semantic, syntactic, and total accuracies on the word analogy dataset for 300-Dimensional word embeddings

Model	Sem.	Syn.	Total
Word2Vec [48]	63	58	61
GloVe Crawl [59]	82	69	75
fastText Wiki [8]	78	75	76
fastText Wiki + News [47]	**90**	**84**	**87**
fastText Crawl [47]	87	82	85
fastText Reddit	56	74	66

4.8 Neural Network Architecture

Convolutional Neural Networks (CNN) [38] have been utilized to achieve outstanding results, especially in the area of image classification, and are generally viable for data with a grid-like structure [24]. Recently, studies have shown that they can also be used effectively for text classification tasks [81]. The architecture of the simple CNN used for the experiments, which is described later in Sect. 5.5, is based on the one-layer CNN for sentence classification described by Zhang and Wallace [81]. Similar to this sentence classification network, it consisted of only a single convolutional layer but used a total of 100 filters with a height of 2 and a width corresponding to the word vector dimensions. Concatenated Rectified Linear Units (CReLU) [68] are used as activation function for the convolutional layer and the fully-connected layers, resulting in twice as many outputs due to the concatenation with the negated activation. 1-max pooling is used to obtain a single scalar from each filter, which results in a 200-dimensional vector due to the CReLU activation. This output is then propagated through three fully-connected layers with, again, CReLU activation, of which the first one applies dropout to its output. The fourth and final layer applies softmax to the output. As input, the network receives each document of a user individually in the form of the 100 first word vectors per document, while using zero-padding for documents with less than 100 words. This results in a 100×50 or 100×300 dimensional input matrix depending on the used word embedding as described in the previous section. The limitation to 100 words (or even less) is possible as the number of words per document ranges between 1 (when ignoring the empty documents) and 6,487 but has a mean of 34.58 according to the tokenization done for this work. As this results in a separate output for each document per user, the 98th percentile of these outputs is used as the final prediction for the user. This value was chosen instead of the mean to give more weight to documents with a higher probability.

Alternatively to the described model architecture, it was experimented to directly use the metadata features as a second input to the network. An approach similar to the previous one at eRisk 2017 [72], where the metadata features were fed through a fully-connected layer and then concatenated with the output of an LSTM layer, did not lead to better results than just using the text input. The same applies to the idea to use the final 1×50 dimensional vector before the softmax layer as additional input for a metadata classifier like logistic regression (LR). Since the results of networks using the metadata differed only marginally from the text-only network described above, only results of the latter will be reported in the following to reduce the complexity. Future work will be needed to explore better ways to merge the CNN output with the metadata directly. In this work, a simple late fusion ensemble will show that the best results so far can indeed be achieved by combining these features.

4.9 Transformers

Google introduced the first Bidirectional Encoder Representations from Transformers (BERT) [19] which achieved outstanding results in many downstream NLP (natural language processing) tasks. Transformer-based models were pre-trained on large unlabelled corpora to learn a universal representation of the language. After the release of BERT, a robustly optimized BERT pre-training approach (RoBERTa) [39] was introduced. It extends the BERT approach by changing the pre-training procedure. The pre-training phase is longer, uses more data and longer sequences. In addition, the hyperparameters have been improved.

Later results on the eRisk tasks have shown that Transformer models are suitable for the early risk detection and provide good results (see chapter "A Survey of the First Five Years of eRisk: Findings and Conclusions" of this book). However, the training dataset provided is not suitable for this, because the individual posts cannot be assigned with certainty as depressive or non-depressive. For such an assignment, the chronological component is missing, until when a user was still in good health, if applicable.

For example, only the last 5 posts could indicate an impending depressive mood. It would then be counterproductive to annotate all previous posts as depressive. It is therefore planned to combine the results of the Transformers with metadata obtained from LIWC features. The fine-tuning will take place on external data that contains more accurate annotation based on single texts.

5 Chosen Models for the eRisk Tasks, Related Work and Ongoing Work

This section describes the models used in the 2017 and 2018 depression task, related work as well as ongoing work. Two conventional document vectorization models and three models utilizing LSTM, a layer architecture for *Recurrent Neural Networks* (RNN) [24] specialized on sequences of data, have been used for the 2017 task. One of these models also employs LSA as a dimensionality reduction step. All models have been optimized by 5-fold cross-validation on the training data using F_1-Score before the submission for the first chunk of test data and were not modified at a later point. The same applies to the described prediction thresholds chosen by cross-validation to submit predictions each week. The only exception is the final model BCSGE, which was used to get more time for optimization: For the first nine weeks, no predictions were submitted for this model, so only the predictions using all documents at once in the last week were scored. All models used a concatenation of the text and title field of each document as input and did not treat text and title separately. Identified quotes within text contents have been modified by adding a prefix to each quoted word, while the tokenization step includes words, numbers, and emoticons as described in Sect. 2.2.

For the 2018 task, there were also five models submitted. In comparison to the participation in the eRisk 2017 pilot task, the prediction thresholds were simplified. For each model, only a single prediction threshold value was chosen based on cross-validation on the training data to indicate whether a subject is classified as *depressed*. The number of documents already processed for a user is not used anymore as the new models are less prone to predict many false positives after processing only a few documents. In addition, *non-depressed* predictions are now only submitted in the final week because early prediction of these cases has no effect on the score and later writings might still identify them as *depressed*. Selecting viable prediction thresholds is difficult as a balanced result according to both ERDE_o and F_1-Score is often hard to achieve. The goal for this participation was to use rather low thresholds to find *depressed* cases as early as possible without generating too many false positives.

In contrast to the eRisk 2017 participation of this team, only the first model and the final ensemble utilize the updated set of user metadata features described in Sect. 4.1. The bag-of-words (BoW) model, which achieved the best overall F_1-Score as well as second best ERDE_5 and ERDE_{50} score in the previous task [41], is reused with and without metadata features. The Recurrent Neural Network (RNN) using a LSTM layer was not re-evaluated and replaced with a CNN. This decision was based on further research using the eRisk 2017 dataset [74], which showed that the CNN model was able to outperform results of the LSTM models and easier to configure and less prone to overfitting. Since the BoW Ensemble is the same for the 2017 and 2018 tasks, both models are described in the same Sect. 5.1. Next up are alternately the remaining four models for each year's task. Section 5.10 describes the extended research done with CNN's. And finally, Sect. 5.11, expounds the transformer model used.

5.1 Bag-of-Words Ensemble - BCSGA - 2017/2018

The first model in the 2017 and 2018 task utilizes an ensemble of BoW classifiers with different term weightings and n-grams. The term weighting for BoW can generally be split into three components: a *term frequency component* or local weight, a *document frequency component* or global weight, and a *normalization component* [67]. A general term weighting scheme can therefore be given as [80]:

$$t_{t,d} = l_{t,d} \cdot g_t \cdot n_d \ , \tag{7}$$

where $t_{t,d}$ is the calculated weight for term t in document d, $l_{t,d}$ is the local weight of term t in document d, g_t is the global weight of term t for all documents, and n_d is the normalization factor for document d. A common example would be using the *term frequency* (tf) as a local weight and the *inverse document frequency* (idf) as a global weight, resulting in tf-idf weighting [67].

All ensemble models use cosine normalization (l^2-norm) for n_d but varying local and global weights. The first one uses a combination of uni-, bi-, tri-, and 4-grams obtained from the training data: the 200,000 [1-4]-grams with the highest IG (information gain) as given by Eq. 8 are selected and their raw term frequency is used as local weight, while their IG score is used as a global weight.

$$I(U,C) = \sum_{e_t \in \{0,1\}} \sum_{e_c \in \{0,1\}} P(U = e_t, C = e_c) \cdot log_2 \left(\frac{P(U = e_t, C = e_c)}{P(U = e_t) \cdot P(C = e_c)} \right) \ , \tag{8}$$

with the random variable U taking values $e_t = 1$ (the document contains term t) and $e_t = 0$ (the document does not contain term t) and the random variable C taking values $e_c = 1$ (the document is in class c) and $e_c = 0$ (the document is not in class c).

The second BoW utilizes a modified version of tf, namely *augmented term frequency* (atf) [80], multiplied by idf:

$$atf\text{-}idf(t,d) = \left(a + (1-a) \frac{tf_t}{\max(tf)} \right) \cdot \log \frac{n_d}{df(d,t)} \ , \tag{9}$$

with $\max(tf)$ being the maximum frequency of any term in the document, the total number of documents n_d, and the smoothing parameter a, which is set to 0.3 for this model. This BoW, as well as the third one, contains all unigrams of the training corpus. The local weight of the third model consists of the *logarithmic term frequency* ($logtf$) [55] and the global weight is given by *relevance frequency* (rf) [36], which can be combined as:

$$logtf\text{-}rf(t,d) = (1 + \log(tf)) \cdot \log_2 \left(2 + \frac{df_{t,+}}{\max\left(1, df_{t,-}\right)} \right) \ , \tag{10}$$

where $df_{t,+}$ and $df_{t,-}$ is the number of documents in the *depressed/non-depressed* class that contain the term t. The final model of this ensemble uses the hand-crafted user features described in Sect. 4.1.

The BoW model for 2018 is equivalent to the model described above, except for the extended set of metadata features.

All three BoW and the hand-crafted features were each used as input for a separate LR classifier. Due to the imbalanced class distribution, a modified class weight was used for these classifiers similar to the original task paper [40] to increase the cost of false negatives. For the 2017 task it was calculated for the *non-depressed* class as $1/(1+w)$ and for the *depressed* class as $w/(1+w)$, with $w_1 = 2$, $w_2 = 6$, $w_3 = 2$, and $w_4 = 4$ in the order as the different models have been described above. This differs slightly from the 2018 task where it was calculated for the *non-depressed* class as $1/(1+w)$ and for the *depressed* class as $w/(1+w)$, with $w = 2$ for all four models. The final output probabilities were calculated as the unweighted mean of all four LR probabilities. For the 2017 task and each week, this ensemble predicted any user with a probability above 0.5 as *depressed* and users below 0.15 as *non-depressed* and in the final week all users with a probability equal to or less than 0.5 were predicted as *non-depressed*. For the 2018 task and each week any user with a probability above or equal to 0.4 as *depressed* was predicted as depressed, while in the final week all users with a probability less than 0.4 were predicted as *non-depressed*. Those thresholds were determined by testing every threshold value in 0.01 steps.

5.2 Paragraph Vector - BCSGB - 2017

The second model for the 2017 task is based on document vectorization by using *Paragraph Vector* [37], sometimes referred to as *doc2vec*, similar to the previously published *Word2Vec* [46, 48] on which it is based. While *Word2Vec* is used to train embedded word vectors from a large text corpus, *Paragraph Vector* learns vector representations for sentences, paragraphs, or whole documents. It was also found that *Paragraph Vector* can work better for smaller corpora than *Word2Vec*, which potentially makes it a viable option for this task. The two neural network architectures for each of these methods are all based on the probabilistic *Neural Network Language Model* [6].

For the Paragraph Vector classification of eRisk users, two separate models have been trained based on the training documents using the Python implementation in *gensim 1.0.1* [63]:

1. A *Distributed BoW* model with 100 dimensional output, 10 training epochs, a context window of 10 words, negative sampling with 20 noise words, no down-sampling, a learning rate from 0.025 to 1e−4, and all words contained in the documents.
2. A *Distributed Memory* model using the sum of input words with 100 dimensional output, 10 training epochs, a context window of 10, hierarchical softmax, down-sampling of high-frequency words with 1e−4, a learning rate from 0.025 to 1e−4, and all words contained in the documents.

Text content and title of the documents have again been concatenated and each of the resulting texts was used as separate input to Paragraph Vector. The output vectors of these two models were concatenated, as recommended by the developers [37], resulting in a 200 dimensional vector per document. Test documents were vectorized

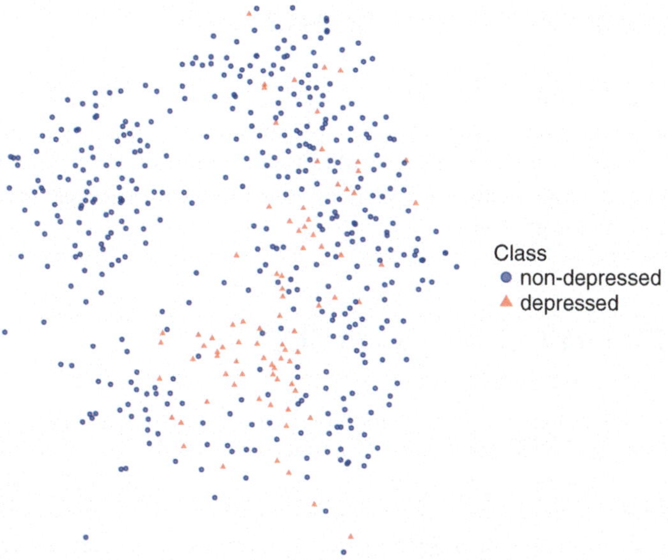

Fig. 9 Plot of the t-SNE reduced averaged document vectors per user for the Paragraph Vector model 2017 (BCSGB). License: Reproduced with authors approval from [72]

using an inference step that only outputs a new document vector and leaves all network weights fixed.

Finally, the average of all documents by each user was calculated to obtain the average topic of everything the user has written. Figure 9 shows a two-dimensional representation of the averaged training document vectors calculated by t-distributed stochastic neighbor (t-SNE) [76]. Even after a reduction to only two dimensions, there is at least one visible cluster of *non-depressed* users and a rather noisy cluster of *depressed* users.

A LR classifier was trained on the 200-dimensional averaged document vectors, using the same class weight equation as in the previous model with $w = 4$. The calculated class probabilities were again averaged with the probabilities obtained from the LR based model on the hand-crafted user features. Since this model depends more on the number of documents it has been trained on, the final predictions were based on the probability as well as the number of documents written by the user to prevent too many false positives. *Depressed* predictions were submitted for probabilities from 0.6 with at least 20 documents, 0.7 with at least 10 documents, and all probabilities above 0.9, while *non-depressed* predictions required a probability below 0.1 with at least 20 documents, 0.05 with at least 10 documents, or a probability below 0.01.

5.3 Bag-of-Words Ensemble - BCSGB - 2018

The second model for the 2018 task is similar to the first one described in Sect. 5.1, but it only includes the three BoW in the ensemble and disregards the metadata features. Again, for the depression task any test subject with a probability of at least 0.4 was predicted as *depressed*, while users with a probability below 0.4 were predicted as *non-depressed* in the final week.

5.4 LSTM with LSA Vectors - BCSGC - 2017

This and the following two models are based on a Tensorflow [1] neural network approach using an LSTM layer and differ from the last three models submitted for the 2018 task. By using sequences of text documents as input, the LSTM network allows to learn a general context of each user's documents while processing them in chronological order. All three LSTM models also use the hand-crafted user features as an additional metadata input and merge them with the LSTM output in a fully connected layer. This again ensures that these features are not lost after document vectorization and averaging. A final softmax layer was used to produce the actual output probabilities, the softsign function [75] was chosen as activation for the LSTM cell, and dropout was added to prevent overfitting. The training steps of this and the following two LSTM models utilized Adam [35] optimizer to minimize the cross-entropy loss.

For this first LSTM approach, LSA was used to reduce the BoW vectorized documents to a viable number of dimensions based on *Singular Value Decomposition* (SVD) [13]. All documents were first transformed into a BoW by selecting only the 10,000 unigrams with the highest IG and using their term frequency multiplied by their IG as term weighting. LSA was then used to reduce these document vectors to 100 dimensions, which retained 90.32% of the original variance in the training dataset. To obtain an equal sequence length for all users that is viable as network input, the document sequences were modified to have a length of 25 documents. For users with fewer documents, zero vectors were appended, while two randomly selected consecutive document vectors were averaged for longer sequences, until the maximum length was reached. Adam was then used with a fixed learning rate of 1e−4, 64 units were added to the LSTM cell, a dropout to keep the probability of 80% was applied, and the network was trained for 300 epochs.

Similar to the previous model, prediction thresholds were based on the network's output probability and the number of documents. *Depressed* predictions required a probability above 0.5 and at least 20 documents, above 0.7 and at least five documents, or above 0.9, while *non-depressed* predictions were submitted for probabilities below 0.05.

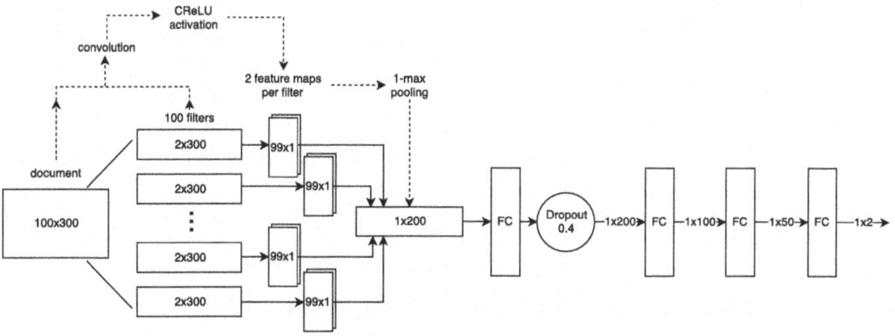

Fig. 10 Architecture of the CNN used for the models 2018 BCSGC and BCSGD (with 300 instead of 50 dimensional word vectors). License: Reproduced with authors approval from [73]

5.5 CNN with GloVe Embeddings - BCSGC - 2018

The implementation has been done based on Tensorflow [1] and the input of this CNN is based on GloVe [59] word embeddings: A 50-dimensional set of word embeddings pre-trained on Wikipedia and News[16] is used to produce a matrix of word vectors for the first 100 words of each document in the dataset. Prior to this vectorization, the documents are preprocessed and tokenized in a way that preserves, for example, emoticons, punctuation, words including special characters, and generally all tokens that occur in the documents of at least two users. Zero-padding is used for documents with less than 100 words. Each document is therefore represented by a 100×50 matrix and is classified independently. Since the number of words per document in the training data ranges between 1 (when ignoring the empty documents) and 6,487 but has a mean of 34.58 according to the tokenization done for this work, the limitation to 100 words (or even fewer to minimize the necessary zero-padding) is viable.

The text classification network architecture used for this work is displayed in Fig. 10, which shows the use of 300 dimensional word vectors (and therefore 100×300 documents) as used for the next model BCSGD. It is similar to the one-layer CNN for sentence classification described by Zhang and Wallace [81] and consists of only a single convolutional layer, 100 filters with an equal height of 2 and a width corresponding to the word embedding dimensions, and uses 1-max pooling to extract a single value from each filter. Due to the usage of the CReLU activation, this finally results in a 200-dimensional vector per document that is propagated through four fully connected layers, of which the first applies dropout to its output and the final one applies softmax. The training steps of this and the following CNN model utilized Adam to minimize the cross-entropy loss. Both models were trained using a learning rate of 1e−4 and a batch size of 10.000 documents. BCSGC was trained for 30 epochs.

[16] http://nlp.stanford.edu/projects/glove, accessed on 2021-02-04.

To obtain a final prediction per user, the 98th percentile of the outputs from all the user's documents is calculated. This ensures that even *depressed* users with very few documents with a high probability can be correctly predicted. Any subject with a final probability of at least 0.4 was predicted as *depressed* in each week, while probabilities below 0.4 again resulted in a *non-depressed* prediction in the final week.

5.6 LSTM with Paragraph Vectors - BCSGD - 2017

This fourth model utilized the same LSTM network as described for the previous one with identical parameters, except for a number of 128 hidden units in the LSTM cell and a training duration of 170 epochs. For the input sequences, documents were vectorized based on the two concatenated Paragraph Vector models of the second approach. Again, the resulting sequences of 200-dimensional document vectors were modified to have a unified length of 25. The model was configured to submit *depressed* predictions for any user with a probability above 0.3 and at least 50 documents, above 0.4 and at least 20 documents, or above 0.7, while probabilities below 0.01 resulted in a *non-depressed* prediction.

5.7 CNN with fastText Embeddings - BCSGD - 2018

The second CNN model is based on the same architecture as the previous one (see Fig. 10) but utilizes 300-dimensional fastText [8, 33, 47] word embeddings. For this model, the fastText word embeddings that were trained on the Reddit corpus (see Sect. 4.7) were utilized.

Similar to the previous CNN model in Sect. 5.5, the resulting 100×300 matrix of word embeddings obtained for each document was classified separately and the 98th percentile of the outputs was used as output for the corresponding user. This model was trained for 25 epochs using the same parameters as BCSGC. The prediction threshold for *depressed* predictions was set to 0.7 for both tasks, leading to a *non-depressed* prediction for probabilities below 0.7 in the final week.

5.8 Late LSTM with Paragraph Vectors - BCSGE - 2017

To have some additional time for model optimization and to compare the impact on the ERDE score, the fifth model was not used to submit any predictions until the last week. It is identical to the fourth model but uses two new 200-dimensional Paragraph Vector models, that were trained on both training and test documents. This is an unsupervised method that uses only text documents without any label

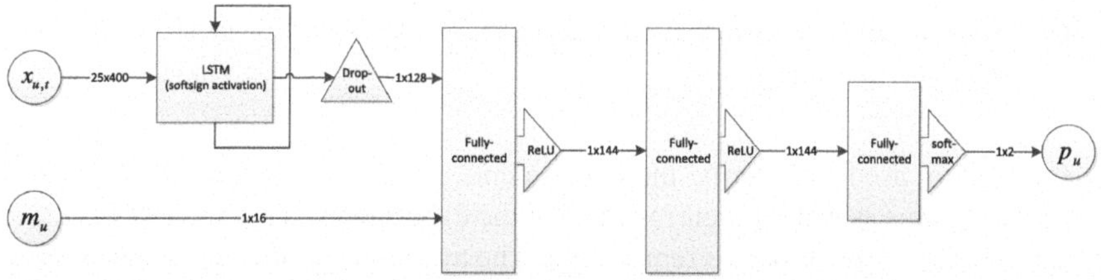

Fig. 11 Network architecture of the final LSTM model 2018 for BCSGE. License: Reproduced with authors approval from [72]

information. Also, this model uses a second fully connected layer before the softmax layer, *Rectified Linear Unit* (ReLU) activation [28] for both fully connected layers, a weight decay factor of 0.001 for all weights in the network, exponential learning rate decay from 1e−4 to 1e−5, a dropout to keep the probability of 70% for LSTM outputs, 128 hidden units in the LSTM, and was trained using batches of 100 users over 130 epochs. The document sequence length was again unified to 25 and a minority oversampling that duplicates each *depressed* user in the training input was used to counter the class imbalance. The final network architecture for this model is displayed in Fig. 11, where m_u represents the metadata for a single user u and $x_{u,t}$ is the sequence of input documents written by this user. In the final week, predictions obtained from this model were submitted based on the same thresholds that were used for the previous one.

5.9 CNN and Bag-of-Words Metadata Ensemble - BCSGE - 2018

The final model consists of a simple late fusion ensemble that has been calculated as the unweighted mean of the outputs obtained from models BCSGA 2018, BCSGC 2018, and BCSGD 2018 - the BoW including metadata and the two CNN models. Although these outputs have not been calibrated (e.g., by using Platt scaling [61]) and can therefore not be seen as directly comparable probabilities. Results from earlier experiments, described in the following Sect. 5.10, have shown that such ensemble was able to improve the results of the separate models. Again, a prediction threshold of at least 0.4 was used for the depression detection task.

5.10 Setup for Extended Experiments Using CNN's and Metadata Features

This section is used to describe the experiments done based on the CNN and the metadata features as well as their results. For the experiments the same process used during the eRisk 2017 task was reproduced. The available test documents were processed in the same ten chunks that contain 10% of the writings obtained from each user. Training is done once on the full training dataset. Afterwards, test chunks are processed in sequential order, while the documents of the previous chunks are always used again. The only exception to this process is the model called "Meta LR Wait" in the following results Sect. 6, which is a LR based model on metadata features that was configured to only submit a prediction after the final chunk. Similar "waiting" models were also utilized by some teams during eRisk 2017 [20, 44] and can be interesting to evaluate the possible F_1-Score, while neglecting the early detection aspect and therefore the ERDE_o scores. Since the models based on metadata use features averaged over all documents of the same user, they were also calculated for each chunk separately, again using documents from earlier chunks as well. An additional parameter for the early detection models is the prediction threshold that determines whether a model is confident enough to predict a subject as positive (depressed) or whether it waits for more data. While these thresholds were based on cross-validation using the training data for this team's participation in the eRisk 2017 task and included the number of documents already read in multiple threshold levels [72], the experiments described are based on a single threshold value that achieved the best test result for the specific model. This is likely to lead to overfitting on the specific test data but also allows comparing the best possible results of the utilized models. Generally, prediction thresholds between 0.5 and 0.7 lead to a balanced result in all scores, while higher thresholds can often maximize ERDE_5 but severely decrease the F_1-Score. This fits the observations described in Sect. 3. Since the correct prediction of so few depressed test subjects affects ERDE_5, it is often best to submit fewer predictions overall and therefore simply minimize false positives. Negative (non-depressed) predictions were only submitted after seeing the final chunk. The models based on user metadata features all utilized the same LR classifier. The 27 features described in Sect. 4.4 were first standardized to have a mean of 0 and unit variance, with the exception of the boolean flag features that already have a value of either -1 or 1. The resulting scaled feature vector was then used to train a LR classifier and later predict probabilities for the test subjects of each chunk.

5.11 Setup for Transformer Experiments

The model was finetuned on a dataset proposed by [45]. Some details of this dataset can be seen in Table 7. The data was collected from the subReddit

Table 7 Some statistics [45] of the dataset used to train the classifiers

Dataset	Class	Users	Posts	Sentences	Years
Users-submissions-200	selfharm	10,319	13,681	131,233	2006–2020
Users-submissions-200	random	15,937	14,913	128,064	2005–2020

Table 8 Details of the transformer model

	Roberta-base
Layers	12
Attention heads	12
Hidden states	768
Parameters	125M

`/r/selfharm`[17] [45]. The non-depressive texts were taken from randomly selected Reddit posts. In this process, care was taken to ensure that they did not belong to any of the depression-related subReddits.

Since the number of available posts increases with each chunk, but the transformer only allows a fixed number of tokens (256 in this case), all posts were concatenated and predicted with a sliding window. Here, each sequence that exceeds the max_seq_length is divided into several windows (subsequences), each with a length of 256 tokens. The final prediction is then the averaged prediction for all its subsequences.

Table 8 shows the details of the used RoBERTa transformer.

Table 9 displays the hyperparameters used to fine-tune the model. Only three epochs were used for the training because the model was transferred to a different kind of dataset.

Some extended tests with the raw probabilities predicted by the model were performed. To further increase the certainty of predictions in the overall decision, when classifying a person as depressed or not depressed, all partially achieved probabilities were multiplied by 1.5 for each chunk. For a second test, a dynamic factor was applied to the probabilities:

$$p_{raw} \cdot \sqrt{\frac{n_{chunk}}{10} + 1} \ , \tag{11}$$

[17] http://www.Reddit.com/r/selfharm, accessed on 2021-02-27.

Table 9 Hyperparameters used for the transformer model during fine-tuning

Hyperparameter	Value
Optimizer	AdamW
Learning rate	2e-5
Polynomial decay	1e-7
Manual seed	42
Max sequence length	256
Warmup steps	100
Adam epsilon	1e-8
Epochs	3
Batch size	16

The idea of this modifier is to give the later chunks, when more data is available, more influence on the final decision. The results for the model and the adjusted probabilities can be seen in Sect. 6.5.

6 Results

This section presents all accomplished results from past, related and ongoing works. This includes all submitted models for the 2017 and 2018 task, as well as non submitted models and an extra section about the use of transformers.

6.1 Results for eRisk 2017

Before discussing the official task results, analyzing the amount of correctly classified depressed individuals using the five BCSG models can give a first insight into the classification performance. The cumulative number of *depressed* predictions and actual true positives per model and week is shown in Fig. 12. A horizontal line marks the total number of 52 *depressed* samples in the test set for reference. It becomes evident that there is still room for improvement. Although each model is able to detect a growing number of depressed users over the ten weeks, the proportion of false positives is large and the number of total true positives ranges between 24 and 38 of the 52 depressed users in the test set. Most true positives were found by the fifth model but at the cost of nearly as much false positives. This could at least partially be influenced by finding better prediction thresholds. Table 10 displays the best $ERDE_5$ and $ERDE_{50}$ scores that are possible for the test data of the task.

The final submissions to the CLEF 2017 early risk detection pilot task were scored using the $ERDE_5$ and $ERDE_{50}$ score for early detection tasks defined by the

Table 10 Best possible $ERDE_o$ scores for the task based on a perfect prediction in the first week for the 2017 test dataset

	Depression
$ERDE_5$	10.60
$ERDE_{50}$	3.74

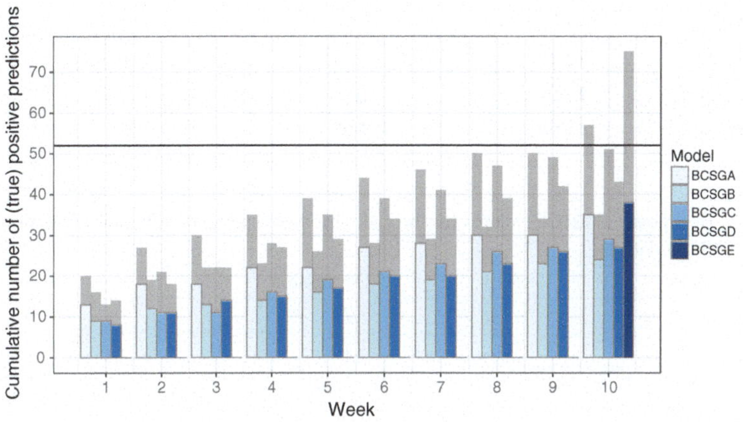

Fig. 12 Cumulative number of *depressed* predictions (blue plus gray bars) and proportion of true positives (blue bars only) per model after each week of the task. A horizontal line marks the 52 *depressed* samples in the test data. All displayed results are based on the 2017 dataset. License: Reproduced with authors approval from [72]

organizers as well as F_1-Score. The scores and the underlying precision and recall values of all the models have been published [41]. In Table 11 the two best results for each individual score are displayed. The highlighted models of BCSG consistently achieved positions in the first ranks and even the fifth model was ranked in the top half according to both ERDE scores by only submitting a prediction in the last week. The achieved ERDE scores for this task cannot be compared to the previously published results by the organizers [40], since the documents had to be processed in weekly chunks for the task and it was not possible to submit predictions before processing a complete chunk. The best results of BCSG could be achieved by using the BoW model BCSGA (first in F_1-Score and second in $ERDE_{50}$) and the Paragraph Vector model BCSGB (first in $ERDE_5$), with the LSTM models close behind.

Since the results for BCSGE are only available for the last week, it was evaluated again for all weeks after the golden truth file was published. For this analysis, separate Paragraph Vector models were trained using the training data and already released test data for each week. If BCSGE had been used from the first week, the results would have been 16.01% in $ERDE_5$, 9.78% in $ERDE_{50}$, and 0.46 in F_1-Score. While this $ERDE_{50}$ score would have been the third best overall, the other scores show that this is still not well optimized and there are too many false positives. Future work will be

Table 11 Best results of the depression task based on the Official evaluation metrics. The models have been chosen to show at least the two best results achieved in each score. All displayed results are based on the 2017 dataset

Model	$ERDE_5$	$ERDE_{50}$	F_1
BCSGA [72]	12.82	**9.69**	**0.64**
BCSGB [72]	**12.70**	10.39	0.55
BCSGC [72]	13.24	10.56	0.56
BCSGD [72]	13.04	10.53	0.57
BCSGE [72]	14.16	12.42	0.60
UArizonaD [65]	**13.07**	10.23	0.45
UNSLA [78]	13.66	**9.68**	**0.59**

Table 12 Best possible $ERDE_o$ scores for the task based on a perfect prediction in the first week for the 2018 test dataset

	Depression
$ERDE_5$	7.78
$ERDE_{50}$	3.79

used to examine the effect of hand-crafted features and preprocessing methods on the prediction results. A quick analysis using the first two models BCSGA and BCSGB has shown that the selected hand-crafted features at least had a slightly positive effect (13.04% in $ERDE_5$, 9.75% in $ERDE_{50}$, and 0.63 in F_1-Score for BCSGA without hand-crafted features), with the exception of the $ERDE_5$ score for BCSGB, which would have been marginally better without hand-crafted features in contrast to a much worse F_1-Score (12.67% in $ERDE_5$, 10.76% in $ERDE_{50}$, and 0.37 in F_1-Score for BCSGB).

6.2 Results for eRisk 2018

Table 12 displays the best $ERDE_5$ and $ERDE_{50}$ scores that are possible for the test data of the task. These results are based on a perfect prediction in the first week of the tasks. As described in Sect. 3, only test users with less than 100 documents (less than 10 per chunk) have any effect on the $ERDE_5$ score. This means that only predicting 26 of the 79 *depressed* test users correctly in the first week and ignoring all others still leads to an $ERDE_5$ score of 7.78 ($F_1 = 0.50$). $ERDE_5$ alone, without the additional F_1-Score, is therefore hard to interpret.

To examine the weekly predictions obtained from the described models, Fig. 13 shows the cumulative number of positive predictions for the task and also visualize the proportion of true positives. This shows that the ensemble indeed lead to the most

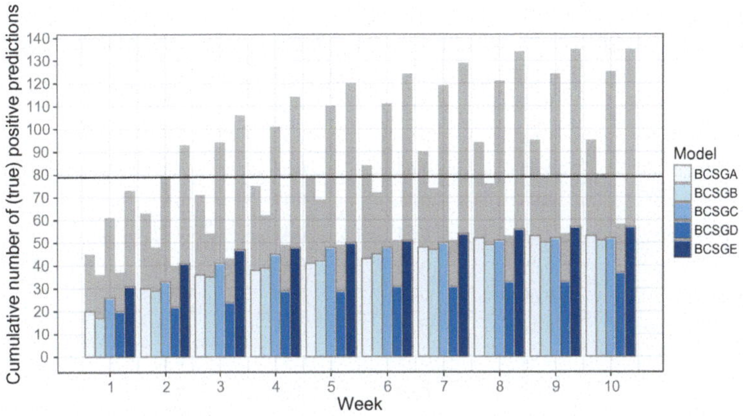

Fig. 13 Cumulative number of *depressed* predictions (blue plus gray bars) and proportion of true positives (blue bars only) per model after each week of the depression task. A horizontal line marks the 79 *depressed* samples in the test data. All displayed results are based on the 2018 dataset. License: Reproduced with authors approval from [72]

true positives but also many false positives. BCSGD seems to perform worse at first sight but indeed achieved a good balance between true and false positives because of its higher prediction threshold. The examination shows a steady progression over the ten weeks for all models.

Table 13 shows the official results [42] of BCSG's models for the depression task and also includes the alternative early detection scores $F_{latency}$ [66] and $\text{ERDE}_o^{\%}$ [74]. $F_{latency}$ was calculated using a value for the parameter p that fits the true positive cost function $P_{latency}$ to return a cost of 0.5 for the median number of documents of the positive test users. This results in a value of $p = 0.0051$ for the depression task (median of 216 documents per *depressed* test user). In contrast to the standard ERDE_o score, $\text{ERDE}_o^{\%}$ is calculated based on the percentage of read documents per user and is therefore easier to interpret in a chunk-based task. Additional results by other teams have been added to these tables to include at least the best two results obtained for each score.

While the direct comparison of BCSGA (BoW with linguistic metadata) and BCSGB (BoW only) shows that the metadata features result in more positive predictions, the actual amount of true positives was only better for the depression task and resulted in a better ERDE_5 score but worse ERDE_{50} and F_1-Score. Similar to the task in 2017, the BoW ensemble again obtained the best results in the depression task. Overall, the models of BCSG achieved the second-best results in ERDE_5 and the best results in all other scores except for another second-best result according to $\text{ERDE}_{50}^{\%}$ in the depression task. As already described in Sect. 3, the ERDE_o score and especially ERDE_5 should be viewed with caution because of the fact that optimizing it can often lead to simply minimizing false positives by only predicting very few users at all. A detailed look at the results and the achieved ERDE_5 scores shows that,

Table 13 Best results of the depression task based on the official evaluation and the alternative metrics $F_{latency}$ and $\text{ERDE}_o^{\%}$. The models have been chosen to show at least the two best results achieved in each score. All displayed results are based on the 2018 dataset

Model	ERDE_5	ERDE_{50}	F_1	$F_{latency}$	$\text{ERDE}_{20}^{\%}$	$\text{ERDE}_{50}^{\%}$
BCSGA [73]	**9.21**	6.68	0.61	0.47	7.08	5.31
BCSGB [73]	9.50	**6.44**	**0.64**	**0.52**	7.17	5.04
BCSGC [73]	9.58	6.96	0.51	0.41	6.89	4.82
BCSGD [73]	9.46	7.08	0.54	0.41	7.32	6.34
BCSGE [73]	9.52	6.49	0.53	0.43	**6.16**	**4.57**
LIIRB [62]	10.03	**7.09**	0.48	0.39	10.66	5.05
UNSLA [22]	**8.78**	7.39	0.38	0.25	7.45	6.96
UNSLD [22]	10.68	7.84	0.45	0.37	**6.23**	**4.52**
UNSLE [22]	9.86	7.60	**0.60**	**0.45**	7.76	5.50

for example, in the first week of the depression task both UNSLA and BCSGA have predicted 45 users as depressed of which 20 were indeed true positives. Still, the resulting ERDE_5 score differs drastically. The predicted users vary in the number of total documents: To be more specific, UNSLA only had five more true positives in the following nine weeks, while BCSGA already had ten more in the second week and a total of 53 in the end. In summary, ERDE_5 produces highly misleading results because of the varying number of documents per user.

6.3 Related Results with CNN and Metadata Features

This section evaluates the results of the models described in Sect. 5.10. Table 14 displays the results achieved in comparison to previously published results for the same 2017 dataset and task. The first three rows in this table represent the best results during the eRisk 2017 task and are therefore solely optimized based on cross-validation over the training data, while the next two results have been achieved after the ground truth was published. All results after these have been achieved after the actual eRisk 2017 task. The models corresponding to the name of a word embedding refer to a CNN using this embedding as input vectorization, the models named "Meta LR" refer to the LR based model on metadata, and the final four results were obtained by calculating the mean of the metadata probabilities and the neural network output. Although these outputs have not been calibrated (e.g., by using Platt scaling [61]), this simple late fusion ensemble lead to the best achieved ERDE_o scores and recall. As expected, the best overall F_1-Score could be obtained by waiting for the last chunk and only then submitting predictions based on the metadata LR. Interestingly, this model would still have achieved the seventh best ERDE_{50} score in the eRisk 2017 task out of 30 submissions, which again illustrates how difficult ERDE_o is to interpret because it is based on the absolute number of documents. The prediction thresholds

Table 14 $ERDE_o$ scores, F_1-Score, precision, and recall of the utilized models and previous publications. The second column displays the prediction threshold (p>). All displayed results are based on the 2017 dataset

Model	$p>$	$ERDE_5$	$ERDE_{50}$	F_1	P	R
UNSLA [78]		13.66	**9.68**	0.59	0.48	**0.79**
FHDO-BCSGA 2017 [72]		12.82	9.69	**0.64**	0.61	0.64
FHDO-BCSGB 2017 [72]		**12.7**	10.39	0.55	**0.69**	0.46
TVT-NB [78]		13.13	**8.17**	0.54	0.42	**0.73**
TVT-RF [78]		**12.30**	8.95	**0.56**	**0.54**	0.58
GloVe W+N	0.5	12.95	**7.57**	0.63	0.56	0.73
GloVe Crawl	0.7	12.98	8.59	0.63	0.58	0.69
fastText Wiki	0.6	13.06	8.17	0.57	0.47	0.71
fastText W+N	0.55	13.11	7.95	0.60	0.49	0.77
fastText Crawl	0.6	13.01	8.60	0.64	0.60	0.67
fastText Reddit	0.7	13.52	8.04	0.62	0.51	**0.79**
fastText Reddit	0.8	12.71	9.23	0.56	0.63	0.50
Meta LR	0.35	12.65	8.57	0.66	0.59	0.73
Meta LR	0.55	**12.35**	9.86	0.65	0.72	0.60
Meta LR Wait	0.35	13.32	11.33	**0.73**	**0.77**	0.69
G W+N + Meta LR	0.45	12.34	8.93	**0.71**	**0.72**	0.69
fT Wiki + Meta LR	0.35	13.52	**7.29**	0.55	0.41	**0.85**
fT Wiki + Meta LR	0.5	**12.13**	8.77	**0.71**	0.71	0.71
fT Reddit + Meta LR	0.55	12.46	8.77	0.67	0.69	0.65

have been chosen to represent the best possible $ERDE_o$ scores that still include a viable F_1-Score. A second threshold has been reported for the self-trained fastText Reddit model and the metadata LR to illustrate to which extent slightly different thresholds can have an effect on $ERDE_o$ scores. As already described, especially optimizing $ERDE_5$ often includes decreasing F_1-Score. The reported results contain the best scores published for this task so far and, importantly, achieve a balanced result among all scores. Although $ERDE_o$ and F_1-Score are difficult to maximize simultaneously, the results show that the described models are able to do so.

In addition to comparing the achieved results to previously published results for this task, Table 15 shows how the same models with the same prediction thresholds would have scored according to the proposed $ERDE_o^{\%}$ score as well as the $F_{latency}$ score from [66]. While the "Meta LR Wait" model is now scored equally bad in both criteria because it had to read all documents, the CNN scores now tend to be better than the ones obtained for the metadata models alone. Still, the best overall $ERDE_o^{\%}$

Table 15 Scores of the above models according to the proposed $\text{ERDE}_o^{\%}$ criterion and the $F_{latency}$ measure from [66]. All displayed results are based on the 2017 dataset

Model	$p>$	$\text{ERDE}_{20}^{\%}$	$\text{ERDE}_{50}^{\%}$	$F_{latency}$
GloVe W+N	0.5	8.70	7.08	**0.52**
GloVe Crawl	0.7	9.44	6.58	0.44
fastText Wiki	0.6	**8.18**	6.69	0.46
fastText W+N	0.55	8.34	6.10	0.49
fastText Crawl	0.6	9.60	7.23	0.48
fastText Reddit	0.7	8.53	**5.53**	0.51
fastText Reddit	0.8	10.21	9.21	0.35
Meta LR	0.35	9.32	7.32	0.43
Meta LR	0.55	10.74	8.74	0.40
Meta LR Wait	0.35	13.32	13.32	0.26
G W+N + Meta LR	0.45	9.68	7.56	0.45
fT Wiki + Meta LR	0.35	**6.40**	**4.78**	**0.49**
fT Wiki + Meta LR	0.5	9.21	7.47	0.48
fT Reddit + Meta LR	0.55	9.46	7.47	0.45

scores could be achieved by the same ensemble. The additional models with higher thresholds that were previously included to obtain a better ERDE_5 score (namely fastText Reddit with $p > 0.8$ and Meta LR with $p > 0.55$) now result in the worst overall $\text{ERDE}_o^{\%}$ scores next to the waiting model. This again indicates that especially optimizations of ERDE_5 do not necessarily mean a better classification result. The 50-dimensional GloVe model achieves the best $F_{latency}$ score, which is also better than the best score reported in the original paper (0.389) for the same dataset [66].

6.4 *Results of Ongoing Work*

For this chapter the previous work done with CNN's and word embeddings, which is described in Sect. 5.10 (based on the eRisk 2017 dataset), was extended for the eRisk 2018 dataset to see if the models can perform equally to the results presented in the previous Sect. 6.3. The achieved results for ERDE_5, ERDE_{50}, F_1-Score, Precision and Recall, are shown in Table 16. For these results the described models in Sect. 6.3 were used as well as the same word embeddings mentioned in Table 5. Only the fastText Reddit embedding differs and was trained with 100 instead of 300 dimensions. The first four rows in Table 16 represent the best results that were reached in the eRisk 2018 task. Only the Meta LR Wait model reached an improved precision score

Table 16 ERDE$_o$ scores, F_1-Score, precision, and recall of the utilized models and previous publications. The second column displays the prediction threshold (p>). All displayed results are based on the 2018 dataset

Model	*p*>	ERDE$_5$	ERDE$_{50}$	F_1	P	R
FHDO-BCSGB [73]		9.50	**6.44**	**0.64**	0.64	0.65
UNSLA [22]		**8.78**	7.39	0.38	0.48	0.32
UDCB [11]		15.79	11.95	0.18	0.10	**0.95**
RKMVERIC [57]		9.81	9.09	0.48	**0.67**	0.38
GloVe W+N	0.45	9.41	7.18	**0.57**	0.66	0.51
GloVe Crawl	0.40	10.12	7.81	0.41	0.30	0.67
fastText Wiki	0.40	10.97	7.26	0.39	0.25	**0.90**
fastText W+N	0.45	9.64	**6.88**	0.52	0.46	0.61
fastText Crawl	0.45	10.31	7.44	0.48	0.35	0.77
fastText Reddit	0.45	10.32	7.11	0.47	0.34	0.76
Meta LR	0.5	**9.33**	7.81	0.48	0.44	0.53
Meta LR Wait	0.60	9.74	8.89	**0.57**	**0.80**	0.44
G W+N + Meta LR	0.55	**9.24**	7.83	**0.52**	**0.61**	0.46
fT Wiki + Meta LR	0.40	9.60	7.61	**0.52**	0.43	**0.65**
fT Reddit + Meta LR	0.55	9.31	7.87	0.50	0.56	0.46
GloVe Crawl + Meta LR	0.35	9.62	**7.21**	0.50	0.40	**0.65**

compared to all other results. The CNN and Meta LR models performed good overall and achieved balanced results among all scores. Again the best F_1-Score was achieved by the Meta LR Wait model with the GloVe W + N embedding performing equally good. Overall the F_1-Scores got worse compared to the results reached using the 2017 dataset.

In addition to comparing the achieved results to previously published results for this task, Table 17 shows how the same models with the same prediction thresholds would have scored according to the proposed ERDE$_o^{\%}$ score as well as the $F_{latency}$ score from [66]. Similar to the comparison between the results shown in Table 14 and Table 16, the results shown in Table 17 did improve a lot on the ERDE$_o^{\%}$ metric, while achieving overall worse results on $F_{latency}$ score compared to the results in Table 15. The GloVe Crawl model reached an improved ERDE$_{20}^{\%}$ score and the fastText Wiki model did reach an improved ERDE$_{50}^{\%}$ score compared to all other results for the given metric. Overall the thresholds used for the results in Table 17 have been slightly lowered, in comparison to Table 15. On both datasets, 2017 and 2018, the GloVo W + N model accomplished the best $F_{latency}$ score.

Table 17 Scores of the above models according to the proposed $ERDE^{\%}_{o}$ criterion and the $F_{latency}$ measure from [66]. All displayed results are based on the 2018 dataset

Model	$p>$	$ERDE^{\%}_{20}$	$ERDE^{\%}_{50}$	$F_{latency}$
GloVe W+N	0.45	7.50	6.28	**0.43**
GloVe Crawl	0.40	**4.64**	4.64	0.34
fastText Wiki	0.40	5.80	**4.27**	0.35
fastText W+N	0.45	6.51	5.48	0.41
fastText Crawl	0.45	6.58	4.94	0.39
fastText Reddit	0.45	6.44	4.67	0.39
Meta LR	0.50	8.13	6.73	0.34
Meta LR Wait	0.60	9.74	9.74	0.29
G W+N + Meta LR	0.55	8.26	7.34	0.34
fT Wiki + Meta LR	0.40	7.81	6.61	**0.38**
fT Reddit + Meta LR	0.55	8.38	7.28	0.33
GloVe Crawl + Meta LR	0.35	**7.36**	**5.71**	**0.38**

Table 18 $ERDE_{o}$ scores, F_1-Score, precision, and recall of the transformer model and previous publications. The second column displays the prediction threshold (p>). All displayed results are based on the 2018 dataset

Model	$p>$	$ERDE_5$	$ERDE_{50}$	F_1	P	R
FHDO-BCSGB [73]		9.50	**6.44**	**0.64**	0.64	0.65
UNSLA [22]		**8.78**	7.39	0.38	0.48	0.32
UDCB [11]		15.79	11.95	0.18	0.10	**0.95**
RKMVERIC [57]		9.81	9.09	0.48	**0.67**	0.38
roberta-base	0.51	**10.55**	9.13	0.37	0.31	0.47
roberta-base Wait	0.50	11.13	9.91	**0.41**	0.29	**0.67**
roberta-base Mod.	0.76	10.75	**8.97**	0.37	0.28	0.53
roberta-base Dyn.	0.71	10.64	10.40	0.40	**0.32**	0.52
roberta-base + Meta LR	0.43	9.99	8.77	**0.58**	0.60	**0.57**
roberta-base + Meta LR	0.65	9.34	7.91	0.52	0.56	0.48
roberta-base Mod. + Meta LR	0.69	9.73	8.87	0.56	**0.81**	0.43
roberta-base Dyn. + Meta LR	0.67	**9.33**	**7.88**	0.53	0.58	0.48

6.5 Results with Transformers

The results achieved with Transformers, based on the models described in Sect. 5.11, are shown in Table 18. The best F_1-Score was achieved with an ensemble model combining the roberta-base and Meta LR probabilities. The F_1-Score of 0.58 was slightly better then the results based on CNN's, shown in Table 16. However the roberta-base model by its own only achieved a F_1-Score of 0.41. Neither of the roberta-base model with modified or dynamic probabilities did perform any better than the normal roberta-base model.

7 Discussion

This section discusses all previous, related and ongoing work, based on the eRisk tasks on early risk detection of depression in 2017 and 2018.

The pilot task for early detection of depression in 2017 has highlighted a variety of challenges posed by this area of research. These challenges include the task of distinguishing actual clinical depression from normal dejected mood as well as other, more or less related mental disorders like anxiety disorders, PTSD, or bipolar disorder.

A particular difficulty with the challenge is that relatives of depressed individuals and therapists offering advice can easily be mistaken for *depressed* cases when giving too much weight to single words or phrases. Drug users (which might indeed be an accompanying factor of depression [9, 34]) and authors posting fictional stories could regularly be spotted as false positives. On the other hand, there are cases of individuals who post hundreds of very ordinary comments but suddenly start expressing their feelings and talk about their depression. It is therefore important to determine a suitable metric.

Both $F_{latency}$ and $\text{ERDE}_o^{\%}$ include ideas to improve the evaluation of early prediction models. $F_{latency}$ contains a cost function that grows less rapidly and incorporates the F_1-Score, which makes it more meaningful when viewed alone. $\text{ERDE}_o^{\%}$ is more viable for chunk-based shared tasks because it is calculated based on the proportion of read documents per user instead of the absolute number, which leads to results that are more interpretable than the standard ERDE_o. A combination of these two ideas could be a promising basis for discussions about future early detection tasks.

The results of the 2017 task show that all chosen approaches, see Sect. 5, are generally suitable for early detection of depression and all of them are of interest for consecutive research. Due to the promising results using Paragraph Vector, optimizing these models and applying similar word and document embedding methods like fastText [8, 33] and GloVe [59] could be a priority for further research and were therefore used on consecutive work. The introduced neural network approaches with LSTM cells have been shown to be viable as well and allow for a variety of possible extensions and optimizations. Better prediction thresholds optimized based on ERDE scores or more specific signals for *depressed* predictions could help in making earlier predictions without too many false positives.

After the first challenge took place, experiments for the eRisk 2017 task for early detection of depression were continued by examining additional user-level metadata features and evaluating a CNN as text-based depression classifier. The results have been reported for the eRisk 2017 and 2018 datasets using these two approaches. A new fastText word embedding has been trained on a large corpus of Reddit comments.

The analysis of the resulting word vectors has shown that the model has learnt features specific to this domain and is viable for general syntactic questions in the English language as shown based on the standard word analogy task.

Those approaches were optimized to obtain the best performance on the eRisk 2017 task for comparison to previously published results and among these models.

For the 2018 depression task, the results had similar F_1-Scores but much better ERDE_o scores based on a test set that was nearly as large as 2017 training and test set combined. Extended tests, based on linguistic metadata [74], on the bigger 2018 dataset, have confirmed that the F_1-Scores overall got worse with the use of more data. The ERDE_o and $\text{ERDE}_o^{\%}$ however did improve notably. Additional experiments will be necessary to find better ways to integrate the metadata features directly into the neural network. On the other hand, utilizing ensembles of more than just two models and calibrating the resulting probabilities seems promising. Combining word embeddings of two models in a single neural network has also not been evaluated yet.

In addition, it could be interesting to provide a dataset with a control group that more closely resembles the depressed group regarding writing style and text quality. This could enable systems to find smaller differences in language use instead of separating users based on the pure text quality. Overall, the eRisk workshop has fostered research in this challenging and has shown that there is room for future improvements.

An examination of lexicon-based sentiment and emotion features as additional linguistic metadata has shown that these features are not helpful for depression detection using this specific dataset. A possible explanation for this fact has been found in the different text quality and style between the depressed users and the control group. The further evaluations of new combinations and prediction thresholds for the same models utilized during the task have provided new insights into the effect of the metadata features and varying thresholds.

The results in Sect. 6.5 have shown that transformers can be suitable for this kind of classification task. Using adjusted probabilities did not noticeably improve the results. However, it is necessary to do much more research with transformers. Using different models or pre-training a language model from scratch on Reddit data can improve the results. Large datasets with single text-based annotations on depression risk are the basic requirement to predict a trend in posts from a user.

8 Conclusion

Depression is the most common mental disorder. Still, it is estimated that only half of the individuals who have any mental disorder are in professional treatment [3]. As a consequence, depression is a major contributor to the nearly 800,000 [54] people who are dying by suicide every year, which makes further research in this area inevitable. Therefore, this work aimed to improve early risk detection of mental health disorders, especially depression. To accomplish this goal, various models were tested, to see if they might fit this specific problem. The use of linguistic metadata, convolutional neural networks, word embeddings, and language models have shown promising results. This means that the general use of NLP can have an impact on improving the early risk detection of mental health disorders and can therefore have a positive influence on treatment accessibility for patients. However, there are limitations to the NLP approach. It is an urgent need to collect more data and find suitable data for control groups to accomplish even more meaningful results. For future research, a promising approach could be a deeper evaluation of the possibility of using emotion and sentiment features, which can be important indicators for signs of depression. Additionally, finding a way to integrate the metadata features into neural network models successfully could be an interesting task for future research. Finally, our results with transformers indicated that this approach could work well. For future works, more transformer models should be considered.

References

1. Abadi, M., Barham, P., Chen, J., Chen, Z., Davis, A., Dean, J., Devin, M., Ghemawat, S., Irving, G., Isard, M., Kudlur, M., Levenberg, J., Monga, R., Moore, S., Murray, D. G., Steiner, B., Tucker, P., Vasudevan, V., Warden, P., Wicke, M., Yu, Y., & Zheng, X. (2016). Tensorflow: A system for large-scale machine learning. In *Proceedings of the 12th USENIX Conference on Operating Systems Design and Implementation* (pp. 265–283). OSDI'16, USENIX Association.
2. Al-Mosaiwi, M., & Johnstone, T. (2018). In an absolute state: Elevated use of absolutist words is a marker specific to anxiety, depression, and suicidal ideation. *Clinical Psychological Science, 6*(4), 529–542. PMID: 30886766.
3. Alonso, J., Codony, M., Kovess, V., Angermeyer, M. C., Katz, S. J., Haro, J. M., De Girolamo, G., De Graaf, R., Demyttenaere, K., Vilagut, G., et al. (2007). Population level of unmet need for mental healthcare in Europe. *British Journal of Psychiatry, 190*(4), 299–306.
4. Baccianella, S., Esuli, A., & Sebastiani, F. (2010). SentiWordNet 3.0: An enhanced lexical resource for sentiment analysis and opinion mining. In *Proceedings of the Seventh International Conference on Language Resources and Evaluation (LREC'10)* (Valletta, Malta). European Language Resources Association (ELRA).
5. Beck, A. T., & Alford, B. A. (2009). *Depression - causes and treatment* (2nd ed.). Philadelphia: University of Pennsylvania Press.
6. Bengio, Y., Ducharme, R., Vincent, P., & Janvin, C. (2003). A neural probabilistic language model. *Journal of Machine Learning Research, 3*, 1137–1155.
7. Berger, M., Wagner, T. H., & Baker, L. C. (2005). Internet use and stigmatized illness. *Social Science & Medicine, 61*(8), 1821–1827.
8. Bojanowski, P., Grave, E., Joulin, A., & Mikolov, T. (2017). Enriching Word Vectors with Subword Information. *Transactions of the Association for Computational Linguistics, 5*, 135–146.
9. Brook, D. W., Brook, J. S., Zhang, C., Cohen, P., & Whiteman, M. (2002). Drug use and the risk of major depressive disorder, alcohol dependence, and substance use disorders. *Archives of General Psychiatry, 59*(11), 1039.
10. Bucci, W., & Freedman, N. (1981). The language of depression. *Bulletin of the Menninger Clinic, 45*(4), 334–58.
11. Cacheda, F., Iglesias, D. F., Nóvoa, F. J., & Carneiro, V. (2018). Analysis and experiments on early detection of depression. In *Working Notes Conference and Labs of the Evaluation Forum CLEF 2018* (vol. 2125). *CEUR Workshop Proceedings*.

12. Chall, J. S., & Dale, E. (1995). *Readability revisited: The new Dale-Chall readability formula*. Brookline Books.
13. Chen, Z. (2018). Singular value decomposition and its applications in image processing. In *Proceedings of the 2018 International Conference on Mathematics and Statistics* (New York, NY, USA), ICoMS 2018 (pp. 16–22). Association for Computing Machinery.
14. Christensen, J. Readability Helps the Level.
15. Coppersmith, G., Dredze, M., Harman, C., Hollingshead, K., & Mitchell, M. (2015) CLPsych 2015 shared task: Depression and PTSD on Twitter. In *Proceedings of the 2nd Workshop on Computational Linguistics and Clinical Psychology: From Linguistic Signal to Clinical Reality* (Denver, Colorado, 05 2015) (pp. 31–39). Association for Computational Linguistics.
16. Dale, E., & Chall, J. S. (1948). A formula for predicting readability. *Educational Research Bulletin, 27*(1), 11–28.
17. De Choudhury, M., Counts, S., & Horvitz, E. (2013). Social Media as a Measurement Tool of Depression in Populations. WebSci '13 (pp. 47–56). Association for Computing Machinery.
18. Deerwester, S., Dumais, S. T., Furnas, G. W., Landauer, T. K., & Harshman, R. (1990). Indexing by latent semantic analysis. *Journal of the American society for information science, 41*(6), 391–407.
19. Devlin, J., Chang, M., Lee, K., & Toutanova, K. (2018). BERT: Pre-training of Deep Bidirectional Transformers for Language Understanding. *CoRR abs/1810.04805*.
20. Farıas-Anzaldúa, A. A., Montes-y Gómez, M., López-Monroy, A. P., & González-Gurrola, L. C. (2017). Uach-inaoe participation at erisk2017. In *Working Notes Conference and Labs of the Evaluation Forum CLEF 2017* (vol. 1866) CEUR Workshop Proceedings.
21. Flesch, R. (1948). A new readability yardstick. *A New Readability Yardstick, 32*(3), 221–233.
22. Funez, D. G., Ucelay, M. J. G., Villegas, M. P., Burdisso, S., Cagnina, L. C., Montes-y Gómez, M., & Errecalde, M. (2018). Unsl's participation at erisk 2018 lab. In *Working Notes Conference and Labs of the Evaluation Forum CLEF 2018* (vol. 2125). CEUR Workshop Proceedings.
23. Gloster, A. T., Lamnisos, D., Lubenko, J., Presti, G., Squatrito, V., Constantinou, M., Nicolaou, C., Papacostas, S., Aydin, G., Chong, Y. Y., Chien, W. T., Cheng, H. Y., Ruiz, F. J., Garcia-Martin, M. B., Obando-Posada, D. P., Segura-Vargas, M. A., Vasiliou, V. S., McHugh, L., Höfer, S., Baban, A., Dias Neto, D., Nunes da Silva, A., Monestès, J.-L., Alvarez-Galvez, J., Paez-Blarrina, M., Montesinos, F., Valdivia-Salas, S., Ori, D., Kleszcz, B., Lappalainen, R., Ivanović, I., Gosar, D., Dionne, F., Merwin, R. M., Kassianos, A. P., & Karekla, M. (2021). Impact of covid-19 pandemic on mental health: An international study. *PLOS ONE, 15*(12) , 1–20.
24. Goodfellow, I., Bengio, Y., & Courville, A. (2016). *Deep learning*. MIT Press.
25. Gowen, K., Deschaine, M., Gruttadara, D., & Markey, D. (2012). Young adults with mental health conditions and social networking websites: Seeking tools to build community. *Psychiatric Rehabilitation Journal, 35*(3), 245–250.
26. Gunning, R. (1952). *The technique of clear writing*. McGraw-Hill.
27. Guntuku, S. C., Yaden, D. B., Kern, M. L., Ungar, L. H., & Eichstaedt, J. C. (2017). Detecting depression and mental illness on social media: An integrative review. *Current Opinion in Behavioral Sciences, 18*, 43–49. Big data in the behavioural sciences.
28. Hahnloser, R., & Seung, H. S. (2001). Permitted and forbidden sets in symmetric threshold-linear networks. In *Advances in neural information processing systems* (vol. 13). MIT Press.
29. Hinton, G. E., McClelland, J. L., & Rumelhart, D. E. (1986). *Distributed representations* (pp. 77–109). Cambridge, MA, USA: MIT Press.
30. Hochreiter, S., & Schmidhuber, J. (1997). Long short-term memory. *Neural Computation, 9*, 1735–1780.
31. Huang, Y., Wei, L., & Chen, Y. (2017). Detection of the Prodromal Phase of Bipolar Disorder from Psychological and Phonological Aspects in Social Media. *CoRR abs/1712.09183*.
32. Hutto, C., & Gilbert, E. (2014). Vader: A parsimonious rule-based model for sentiment analysis of social media text. In *Proceedings of the International AAAI Conference on Web and Social Media* (vol. 8(1)).

33. Joulin, A., Grave, E., Bojanowski, P., & Mikolov, T. (2017). Bag of tricks for efficient text classification. In *Proceedings of the 15th Conference of the European Chapter of the Association for Computational Linguistics (EACL): Volume 2, Short Papers* (Valencia, Spain, April 3–7) (pp. 427–431).
34. Khantzian, E. (1985). The self-medication hypothesis of addictive disorders: Focus on heroin and cocaine dependence. *American Journal of Psychiatry, 142*(11), 1259–1264.
35. Kingma, D. P., & Ba, J. (2015). Adam: A method for stochastic optimization. In *3rd International Conference on Learning Representations, ICLR 2015, San Diego, CA, USA, May 7–9, Conference Track Proceedings*.
36. Lan, M., Tan, C.-L., & Low, H.-B. (2006). Proposing a new term weighting scheme for text categorization. In *Proceedings of the 21st National Conference on Artificial Intelligence - Volume 1* AAAI'06 (pp. 763–768). AAAI Press.
37. Le, Q., & Mikolov, T. (2014). Distributed representations of sentences and documents. In *Proceedings of the 31st International Conference on Machine Learning* (Bejing, China, 22–24 Jun 2014), (vol. 32, pp. 1188–1196). Proceedings of Machine Learning Research, PMLR.
38. Lecun, Y. (1989). *Generalization and network design strategies*. Elsevier.
39. Liu, Y., Ott, M., Goyal, N., Du, J., Joshi, M., Chen, D., Levy, O., Lewis, M., Zettlemoyer, L., & Stoyanov, V. (2019). Roberta: A robustly optimized bert pretraining approach. arXiv:abs/1907.11692.
40. Losada, D. E., & Crestani, F. (2016). A test collection for research on depression and language use. In *Experimental IR Meets Multilinguality, Multimodality, and Interaction - 7th International Conference of the CLEF Association, CLEF 2016, Évora, Portugal, September 5–8, 2016, Proceedings* (vol. 9822, pp. 28–39) Lecture Notes in Computer Science. Springer.
41. Losada, D. E., Crestani, F., & Parapar, J. (2017) eRISK 2017: CLEF lab on early risk prediction on the internet: experimental foundations. In *Experimental IR Meets Multilinguality, Multimodality, and Interaction - 8th International Conference of the CLEF Association, CLEF 2017, Dublin, Ireland, September 11–14, 2017, Proceedings* (vol. 10456, pp. 346–360). Lecture Notes in Computer Science. Springer.
42. Losada, D. E., Crestani, F., & Parapar, J. (2018). Overview of erisk: Early risk prediction on the internet. In *Experimental IR Meets Multilinguality, Multimodality, and Interaction - 9th International Conference of the CLEF Association, CLEF 2018, Avignon, France, September 10-14, 2018, Proceedings* (vol. 11018, pp. 343–361) *Lecture Notes in Computer Science*. Springer.
43. Loyola, J. M., Errecalde, M. L., Escalante, H. J., & Montes-y-Gómez, M. (2017). Learning when to classify for early text classification. In *Computer Science - CACIC 2017 - 23rd Argentine Congress, La Plata, Argentina, October 9–13, 2017, Revised Selected Papers* (vol. 790, pp. 24–34). *Communications in Computer and Information Science*. Springer.
44. Malam, I. A., Arziki, M., Bellazrak, M. N., Benamara, F., El Kaidi, A., Es-Saghir, B., He, Z., Housni, M., Moriceau, V., Mothe, J., et al. (2017). Irit at e-risk. In *Working Notes Conference and Labs of the Evaluation Forum CLEF 2017* (vol. 1866) *CEUR Workshop Proceedings*.
45. Martínez-Castaño, R., Htait, A., Azzopardi, L., & Moshfeghi, Y. (2020). Early risk detection of self-harm and depression severity using bert-based transformers. In *Working Notes of CLEF 2020 - Conference and Labs of the Evaluation Forum, Thessaloniki, Greece, September 22–25, 2020*, (vol. 2696). *CEUR Workshop Proceedings*, CEUR-WS.org.
46. Mikolov, T., Chen, K., Corrado, G. S., & Dean, J. (2013). Efficient estimation of word representations in vector space. In *1st International Conference on Learning Representations (ICLR)* (Scottsdale, Arizona, USA, 2013), vol. abs/1301.3781.
47. Mikolov, T., Grave, E., Bojanowski, P., Puhrsch, C., & Joulin, A. (2018). Advances in pre-training distributed word representations. In *Proceedings of the Eleventh International Conference on Language Resources and Evaluation (LREC 2018)* (Miyazaki, Japan, May 2018).
48. Mikolov, T., Sutskever, I., Chen, K., Corrado, G. S., & Dean, J. (2013). Distributed representations of words and phrases and their compositionality. In *Advances in Neural Information Processing Systems (NIPS)* (Lake Tahoe, Nevada, USA, 2013) (pp. 3111–3119).

49. Miller, G. A. (1995). Wordnet: A lexical database for english. *Communications of the ACM (CACM), 38*(11), 39–41.
50. Mohammad, S. M., & Turney, P. D. (2013). Crowdsourcing a word-emotion association lexicon. *Computational Intelligence, 29*, 3.
51. Nadeem, M. (2016). Identifying Depression on Twitter. *CoRR abs/1607.07384*.
52. Naslund, J. A., Aschbrenner, K. A., Marsch, L. A., & Bartels, S. J. (2016). The future of mental health care: Peer-to-peer support and social media. *Epidemiology and Psychiatric Sciences, 25*(2), 113–122.
53. Naslund, J. A., Grande, S. W., Aschbrenner, K. A., & Elwyn, G. (2014). Naturally occurring peer support through social media: The experiences of individuals with severe mental illness using YouTube. *PLoS One, 9*(10), e110171.
54. Organization, W. H. (2017). Depression and other common mental disorders: Global health estimates. Technical documents.
55. Paltoglou, G., & Thelwall, M. (2010) A study of information retrieval weighting schemes for sentiment analysis. In *Proceedings of the 48th Annual Meeting of the Association for Computational Linguistics* (Uppsala, Sweden, July 2010) (pp. 1386–1395). Association for Computational Linguistics.
56. Pang, B., & Lee, L. (2008). Opinion mining and sentiment analysis. *Foundations and Trends in Information Retrieval, 2*(1–2), 1–135.
57. Paul, S., Jandhyala, S. K., & Basu, T. (2018). Early detection of signs of anorexia and depression over social media using effective machine learning frameworks. In *Working Notes Conference and Labs of the Evaluation Forum CLEF 2018* (vol. 2125) *CEUR Workshop Proceedings*.
58. Pennebaker, J., Mehl, M., & Niederhoffer, K. (2003). Psychological aspects of natural language. Use: Our words, our selves. *Annual Review of Psychology, 54*, 547–77.
59. Pennington, J., Socher, R., & Manning, C. (2014). Glove: Global Vectors for Word Representation. In *Proceedings of the 2014 Conference on Empirical Methods in Natural Language Processing (EMNLP)* (Doha, Qatar, October 25–29 2014) (pp. 1532–1543).
60. Pfefferbaum, B., & North, C. S. (2020). Mental health and the covid-19 pandemic. *New England Journal of Medicine, 383*(6), 510–512.
61. Platt, J. C. (1999). Probabilistic outputs for support vector machines and comparisons to regularized likelihood methods. In *Advances in Large Margin Classifiers* (pp. 61–74). MIT Press.
62. Ramiandrisoa, F., Mothe, J., Benamara, F., & Moriceau, V. (2018). Irit at e-risk 2018. In *Working Notes Conference and Labs of the Evaluation Forum CLEF 2018* (vol. 2125). *CEUR Workshop Proceedings*.
63. Řehůřek, R., & Sojka, P. (2010). Software framework for topic modelling with large corpora. In *Proceedings of LREC 2010 workshop New Challenges for NLP Frameworks* (Valletta, Malta, 2010) (pp. 46–50). University of Malta.
64. Rude, S., Gortner, E.-M., & Pennebaker, J. (2004). Language use of depressed and depression-vulnerable college students. *Cognition and Emotion, 18*(8), 1121–1133.
65. Sadeque, F., Xu, D., & Bethard, S. (2017). Uarizona at the clef erisk 2017 pilot task: Linear and recurrent models for early depression detection. In *Working Notes Conference and Labs of the Evaluation Forum CLEF 2017* (vol. 1866). *CEUR Workshop Proceedings*.
66. Sadeque, F., Xu, D., & Bethard, S. (2018). Measuring the latency of depression detection in social media. In *Proceedings of the Eleventh ACM International Conference on Web Search and Data Mining* (New York, NY, USA, 2018), WSDM '18 (pp. 495–503). Association for Computing Machinery.
67. Salton, G., & Buckley, C. (1988). Term-weighting approaches in automatic text retrieval. *Information Processing & Management, 24*(5), 513–523.
68. Shang, W., Sohn, K., Almeida, D., & Lee, H. (2016). Understanding and improving convolutional neural networks via concatenated rectified linear units. In *Proceedings of the 33nd International Conference on Machine Learning, ICML* (New York City, New York, USA, 2016) (vol. 48, pp. 2217–2225). *JMLR Workshop and Conference Proceedings*, JMLR.org.
69. Shen, J. H., & Rudzicz, F. (2017). Detecting anxiety through Reddit. In *Proceedings of the Fourth Workshop on Computational Linguistics and Clinical Psychology* (Vancouver, BC, Aug. 2017) (pp. 58–65). Association for Computational Linguistics.

70. Tausczik, Y. R., & Pennebaker, J. W. (2010). The psychological meaning of words: LIWC and computerized text analysis methods. *Journal of Language and Social Psychology, 29*(1), 24–54.
71. Trotzek, M., Koitka, S., & Friedrich, C. M. (2017). Early detection of depression based on linguistic metadata augmented classifiers revisited - best of the erisk lab submission. In *Experimental IR Meets Multilinguality, Multimodality, and Interaction - 9th International Conference of the CLEF Association, CLEF 2018, Avignon, France, September 10–14, 2018, Proceedings* (vol. 11018, pp. 191–202). *Lecture Notes in Computer Science*. Springer.
72. Trotzek, M., Koitka, S., & Friedrich, C. M. (2017). Linguistic metadata augmented classifiers at the CLEF 2017 task for early detection of depression. In *Working Notes of CLEF 2017 - Conference and Labs of the Evaluation Forum, Dublin, Ireland, September 11–14, 2017* (vol. 1866). *CEUR Workshop Proceedings*, CEUR-WS.org.
73. Trotzek, M., Koitka, S., & Friedrich, C. M. (2018). Word embeddings and linguistic metadata at the CLEF 2018 tasks for early detection of depression and anorexia. In *Working Notes of CLEF 2018 - Conference and Labs of the Evaluation Forum, Avignon, France, September 10–14, 2018* (vol. 2125). *CEUR Workshop Proceedings*, CEUR-WS.org.
74. Trotzek, M., Koitka, S., & Friedrich, C. M. (2020). Utilizing neural networks and linguistic metadata for early detection of depression indications in text sequences. *IEEE Transactions on Knowledge and Data Engineering, 32*(3), 588–601.
75. Turian, J. P., Bergstra, J., & Bengio, Y. (2009). Quadratic features and deep architectures for chunking. In *Proceedings of North American Chapter of the Association for Computational Linguistics (NAACL HLT 2009)* (pp. 245–248). The Association for Computational Linguistics.
76. van der Maaten, L., & Hinton, G. (2008). Visualizing data using t-sne. *Journal of Machine Learning Research, 9*(86), 2579–2605.
77. Vaswani, A., Shazeer, N., Parmar, N., Uszkoreit, J., Jones, L., Gomez, A. N., Kaiser, L. u., & Polosukhin, I. (2017). Attention is all you need. In *Advances in Neural Information Processing Systems* (vol. 30). Curran Associates, Inc.
78. Villegas, M. P., Funez, D. G., Ucelay, M. J. G., Cagnina, L., & Errecalde, M. (2017). Unsl's participation at erisk 2017: Pilot task on early detection of depression. In *Working Notes Conference and Labs of the Evaluation Forum CLEF 2017* (vol. 1866). *CEUR Workshop Proceedings*.
79. Weintraub, W. (1981). *Verbal Behavior: Adaptation and Psychopathology*. Springer Publishing Company.
80. Wu, H., & Gu, X. (2014). Reducing over-weighting in supervised term weighting for sentiment analysis. In *Proceedings of COLING 2014, the 25th International Conference on Computational Linguistics: Technical Papers* (Dublin, Ireland, Aug. 2014) (pp. 1322–1330). Dublin City University and Association for Computational Linguistics.
81. Zhang, Y., & Wallace, B. (2017). A sensitivity analysis of (and practitioners' guide to) convolutional neural networks for sentence classification. In *Proceedings of the Eighth International Joint Conference on Natural Language Processing (Volume 1: Long Papers)* (Taipei, Taiwan, Nov. 2017) (pp. 253–263). Asian Federation of Natural Language Processing.

Comparison of Machine Learning Models for Early Depression Detection from Users' Posts

Josiane Mothe, Faneva Ramiandrisoa, and Md Zia Ullah

Abstract With around 300 millions people worldwide suffering from depression, the detection of this disorder is crucial and a challenge for individual and public health. As with many diseases, early detection means better medical management; the use of social media messages as potential clues to depression is an opportunity to assist in this early detection by automatic means. This chapter is based on the participation of the CNRS IRIT laboratory in the early detection of depressive people (eRisk) task at the CLEF evaluation forum. Early depression detection differs from depression detection in that it considers temporality; the system must make its decision about a user's possible depression with as little data as possible. In this chapter we re-evaluate the models we have developed for our participation at eRisk over the years on the different collections, to obtain a more robust comparison. We also add new models. We use well-established classification methods, such as Logistic regression, Random forest, and Support Vector Machine (SVM). The users' data from which the system should detect if they are depressed, are represented as vectors composed of (a) various task-oriented features including depression related lexicons and (b) word and document embeddings, extracted from the users' posts. We perform an ablation study to analyze the most important features for our models. We also use BERT deep learning architecture for comparison purposes, both for depression detection and early depression detection. According to our results, well-established machine learning models are still better than more modern models for -early- detection of depression.

J. Mothe (✉)
ESPE, Univ. Toulouse Jean-Jaurès, Univ. de Toulouse, IRIT, UMR5505 CNRS, 118 Rte de Narbonne, Toulouse, France
e-mail: josiane.mothe@irit.fr

F. Ramiandrisoa · M. Z. Ullah
Univ. de Toulouse, IRIT, UMR5505 CNRS, 118 Rte de Narbonne, Toulouse, France
e-mail: r.faneva.mahery@gmail.com

M. Z. Ullah
e-mail: mdzia.ullah@irit.fr

F. Crestani et al. (eds.), *Early Detection of Mental Health Disorders by Social Media Monitoring*, Studies in Computational Intelligence 1018,
https://doi.org/10.1007/978-3-031-04431-1_5

1 Introduction

According to the World Health Organization (WHO), the number of people with mental disorders worldwide is increasing day by day; the most common mental disorders are depression and anxiety. Globally, the number of people suffering from depression is more than 300 million over the world (See Fig. 1); this corresponds to an increase of more than 18% between 2005 and 2015.[1] The WHO has also found that depression affects more women than men. Using the same data, the BMC Medicine journal found that France is the most affected country with a rate of 21% followed by the United States (19.2%).[2] In France, it is estimated that nearly one person in five suffered or will suffer from depression during their lifetime. Thus, the detection of this disorder is crucial and constitutes a challenge for individual and public health.

Clinical factors are key to detect patients at risk. Some studies have also shown that depressed people use particular linguistic expressions [12, 23, 31]. Depressed people would use some specific linguistic patterns such as excessive use of personal pronouns, past tense or negative emotions. People's writings can therefore be used as cues to try to detect their psychological state and if they are possibly depressed.

In recent years, the emergence of social networks such as Facebook, Twitter or Reddit has allowed people to share their personal experiences, ideas or thoughts in a simple way. According to Bhavani and Kulkarni [19], people prefer to express themselves online rather than offline. This phenomenon has generated a lot of data which is an opportunity for many research topics, and therefore also for the med-

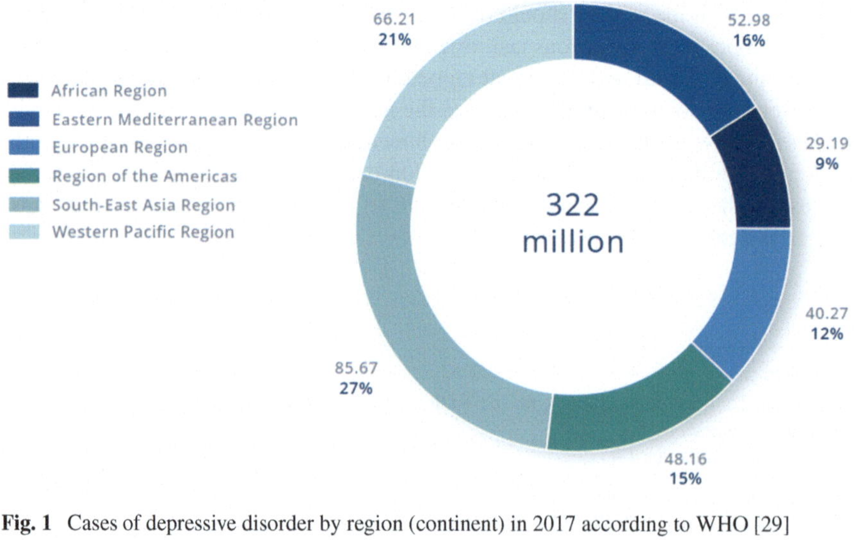

Fig. 1 Cases of depressive disorder by region (continent) in 2017 according to WHO [29]

[1] https://www.la-depression.org/, accessed January 28, 2021.

[2] http://www.doctissimo.fr/psychologie/news/la-france-pays-le-plus-touche-par-la-depression, accessed January 28, 2021.

ical field [8]. Besides, a study by Marriott and Buchanan [25] reports there is no significant difference between an individual's online and offline personality in terms of authenticity. Social media is thus a good source for studying the ability of an automatic system to help on the detection of depressed people. It becomes possible to study the writings of these users in order to try to detect depressed users based on linguistic indicators.

Most approaches in the literature to detect depression on social networks use supervised learning methods trained on manually annotated datasets. Different groups of features have been used such as the use of emoticons [45], the time of publication on the social network [5] and the themes mentioned [38]. Different machine learning techniques have been applied to this type of problem, from well-established categorization techniques to more recent deep learning models [16]. Nonetheless, these studies consider different datasets and there is no detailed analysis to compare different models and different types of features for early detection of depression.

Early depression detection implies that time is considered; the idea is to detect the early signals in the texts. Social media posts are generally time-stamped and thus early detection is technically possible. The challenge then is to re-consider the models and features used for depression detection for the task of early detection. Early detection means less information from each user to train the models; this may impact more on some models than others. In the experiments, this is introduced through chunks of texts where the first chunk contains the first part of the users' posts. This notion is further detailed in Chap. 2 of the book.

In this chapter, we present a supervised learning approach for -early- detection of depression. This work has started on the eRisk task datasets of the 2017 and 2018 editions (see Chap. 2). On the one hand, we used well-established classifiers including Random forest and Support vector machines. On the other hand, we used the more recently developed BERT modeling [10]. With the first type of models, we need to define the features that will be used in the vectors representing the information. We re-used some features from the literature and also considered new features in our models. We also investigate the use of word and document embeddings in this chapter. BERT learns the semantic relationships between the words in a sentence to create language representations which are later used as features (instead of manually defining a set of features, which implies a certain level of domain knowledge). Considering the impressive results of BERT-based models, we hypothesize that BERT will be better on the condition that it has enough information to be fine-tuned, while well-established models will better answer the early detection of depression. This chapter presents the multiple models we developed and evaluated on the task of depression detection and early depression detection. We also deeply analyze these results in order to provide useful insights into the advantages of the different versions of the models.

This chapter is organized as follows: Sect. 2 presents features and models used to identify signs of depression from social media in related work. Section 3 details the data modeling, that is to say, the features we use to build the models to be trained for early detection of depression. Section 4 describes the different machine learning models that we use to detect depression. The experimental framework, collection statistics, and the evaluation metrics are stated in Sect. 5. Section 6 presents the results on 2017 and 2018 eRisk challenge datasets and includes a deep analysis of the results obtained by the different machine learning models as well as the most important features for feature-based models. Section 7 presents a visualization of the predictions of a model using Random Forest on early detection of depression. Section 8 concludes this chapter.

2 Related Work

Most of the work on the identification of depression on social media attempts to make the diagnosis process automatic. Many of these studies are based on supervised learning methods and use techniques such as statistical methods and natural language processing.

Approaches based on statistical methods collect statistical elements by quantifying activity on social networking platforms, social isolation, number of friends, user network based on users' interests or mutual connections, etc. As for approaches that use natural language processing techniques, they are mainly based on linguistic/semantic analysis of posts such as analysis of emotions expressed, sentence structure, etc. Some studies combine both types of features [4, 5].

In the case of postpartum depression (a mood disorder that can affect mothers after childbirth), De Choudhury et al. [4] defined several measures to characterize the differences between mothers with postpartum depression and those without, that they evaluated on Facebook posts of 165 users from which 28 with postpartum depression. The authors defined 49 characteristics that they grouped into 4 categories: *user characteristics* which include characteristics that measure social network activity such as the number of posts per day, *social capital* which includes measures on the interaction with others such as the number of mentions of the word *love* for friends' posts, *content characteristics* that are computed from the content of publications such as emotion analysis and *linguistic style* that measures behavioral changes based on the use of linguistic styles in publications. Considering t-test, the authors found that 35 of the 49 characteristics significantly distinguish between the two groups. They developed several regression models to predict whether a mother is at risk of postpartum depression. On the prenatal data, the model using all characteristics achieved the best result, however, their best model overall was the one based on prenatal data combined with postnatal data. In our work, we were inspired or adapted some characteristics from De Choudhury et al. *content characteristics* and *linguistic style* categories.

In another study, De Choudhury et al. [5] defined several features and feature categories to characterize Twitter users concerning depression. The authors crowdsourced 476 volunteer Twitter user' accounts of which 171 had a high CES-D[3] score used as a cue to automatically detect depression. The authors defined 43 charac-

[3] CES-D stands for Center for Epidemiologic Studies Depression who provides a questionnaire that can be used to detect depression [35].

teristics that they grouped into the following categories: *engagement*, *self-centered social graph (self-centered network)*, *emotion*, *language style* and *depression language*. Four more demographic characteristics were considered: *age*, *gender*, *level of education* and *income*. The authors then analyzed the data to try to distinguish between depressed and non-depressed behaviors. The authors found that those with depression engage in less social activity, display more negative emotions, pay more attention to themselves, show an increase in relational and medical concerns, and express more religious thoughts. They also found that even though their egocentric networks are small, depressed users appear to belong to closely grouped networks and are generally very connected to their network. De Choudhury et al. [5] also created several models, using different combinations of characteristics and different classification methods to predict whether a user is depressed or not based on their tweets. They found that the SVM classifier trained with features, reduced in size with the principal component analysis method, provided the best result with an accuracy of 0.70 and a precision of 0.74. In our work, we adapted some of the characteristics from the *emotion*, *commitment* and *depression language* groups .

The work carried in the eRisk task (see Chap. 2 of this book) are closer to ours than the ones from De Choudhury et al. [5]. eRisk differs from the above-mentioned work in that it aims to detect as early as possible signs of depression from users' texts, in this case, Reddit[4] forum posts. For early detection, the temporality is considered by dividing the set of chronologically ordered posts of a given user into 10 partitions (also called chunks) containing 10% of the user's texts each. Hence, early depression detection is to predict whether a user is depressed by using as few partitions as possible. Early detection is measured by $ERDE_x$ which has been defined for the eRisk task (see Sect. 2 in Chap. 2 for more details) in addition to recall, precision, and F_1 measures.

Trotzek et al. [41] developed five models for early depression detection for eRisk 2017. All these models use linguistic meta-information extracted from each user's texts and combine them with classifiers based on a bag-of-words, paragraph vector, latent semantic analysis, and recurrent neural networks. Their bag of word model performed the best considering the F_1 measure while their model based on paragraph vectors performed best considering the precision and the $ERDE_5$. In eRisk 2018, the same authors used four machine learning models, two are based on convolutional neural network; the other two are based on features computed from the user's texts either considering bags of words or a combination of linguistic metadata and bags of words. They also considered an ensemble model that combines the results obtained from three (two models based on convolutional neural network and one features based model) of these four models [43]. The model that considers bags of words only performed the best according to the $ERDE_{50}$ and F_1 measure in 2018. They also obtained the best result on the $ERDE_5$ and $ERDE_{50}$ for eRisk 2017 dataset after the competition, with another ensemble model which combines a convolutional neural

[4] Reddit is a social news aggregation, web content rating, and discussion website (https://www.reddit.com).

network-based model using fastText as word embedding [17] trained on Wikipedia articles and a model based on linguistic features [41].

Funez et al. [13] proposed a model based on concise semantic analysis [22] which extracts a few concepts from category labels, here depressed versus non-depressed. Each term is then represented as a vector in this concept space and a text or a set of texts is represented as the centroid of the vectors terms it is composed of. This is used to represent each user considering their posts. For early depression detection, the authors considered the temporal difference of the representation of the users by using previous posts (first chunk) and current posts. They named their model Temporal Variation of Terms (TVT). TVT model obtained better performance for $ERDE_5$ and $ERDE_{50}$ measures than the standard bag-of-words model on eRisk 2017.

Later, Funez et al. [14] proposed a variant of TVT called FTVT (Flexible Temporal Variation of Terms) where the number of posts used is flexible. Their other model, SIC, incrementally reads documents and estimates the evidence that document words provide depressive and/or non-depressive labels. SIC classifies a user as depressive as soon as the accumulated evidence of the depressive class surpasses the evidence of the other one.

For their participation to eRisk 2018, Funez et al. submitted five models, three of which are variants of their FTVT approach (hyper-parameter values are changed), from which one obtained the best $ERDE_5$, and two are variants from their SIC approach.

Burdisso et al. [2] proposed the SS3 model which builds for each category (depressed vs. non-depressed) a dictionary of words with their frequency on the training set. The dictionary is incrementally updated as new posts are considered. During the classification phase, SS3 calculates a score that measures the relationship between a word w and a category c based on these word frequencies. For classification, SS3 first divides the text into blocks (e.g., paragraphs), then each block is further divided into smaller blocks until the word level is reached. Then, SS3 calculates the $\overrightarrow{gv}$ vector for each word. These vectors are aggregated (e.g., sum, maximum, etc.) to generate the vectors for the upper block in a recursive process up to the input text. Finally, the texts are classified using these vectors according to the category with the highest value. The authors obtained the best result by considering the $ERDE_5$ measure on eRisk 2017. They also proposed $SS3^{\Delta}$, which differs from SS3 on the classification policy. With $SS3^{\Delta}$, they got the best result considering the $ERDE_{50}$ measure. Burdisso et al. improved SS3 with $\tau-$SS3 [1] which dynamically recognizes useful patterns on text streams, i.e., it can learn and recognize n-grams of variable lengths. $\tau-$SS3 performed the best considering $ERDE_{50}$ on the 2018 edition.

Table 1 presents the results participants obtained for the early depression detection task at eRisk (marked-up with a "*") as well as other results that have been obtained using the eRisk datasets, but after the competition ends.

Table 1 Results on the eRisk task from participants -marked with *- as well as post challenge results. Bold font highlights the best run for the considered collection and measure for an official participation. Best models are different according to the collection and measure

Models		$ERDE_5$ (%)	$ERDE_{50}$ (%)	F_1	P	R
2017						
Trotzek [41]	FHDOA*	12.82	9.69	**0.64**	0.61	0.67
	FHDOB*	**12.70**	10.39	0.55	**0.69**	0.46
UArizona* [40]		17.93	12.74	0.34	0.21	**0.92**
UNSL* [44]		13.66	**9.68**	0.59	0.48	0.79
TVT [13]		13.13	8.17	0.54	0.42	0.73
SS3 [2]		12.60	8.12	0.52	0.44	0.63
τ−SS3 [1]		12.60	7.70	0.55	0.43	0.77
Trotzek [41]	(a)	12.13	8.77	0.71	0.71	0.71
	(b)	13.52	7.29	0.55	0.41	0.85
	(c)	13.32	11.33	0.73	0.77	0.69
2018						
FTVT* [14]		**8.78**	7.39	0.38	0.48	0.32
BCSGB* [43]		9.50	**6.44**	**0.64**	0.64	0.65
RKMVERIC* [32]		9.81	9.08	0.48	**0.67**	0.38
UDCB* [3]		15.79	11.95	0.18	0.10	**0.95**
τ−SS3 [1]		9.48	6.17	–	–	–

3 Information Modeling

For depression detection, the objective is to detect whether users are predicted to be depressed giving their posts. For early depression detection, the objective is close to the previous one, but the detection should be based on a minimum number of posts considering their chronological order. To tackle this problem, we rely on supervised machine learning techniques whose principle is to learn a decision function from a set of labeled examples. In the case of depression detection, an example is a user described by a list of features and the binary label, indicating whether the user is depressed or not.

Considering eRisk data, we have no information on the users for anonymity reasons, which is often the case when considering personal data, but we know their posts. User features have thus to be extracted from a series of user's posts, either all the posts for depression detection, or a subset of them for early depression detection. To extract the user features, we considered two approaches: feature-based and word/document embedding based. We then successively use the two representations on well-establish machine learning algorithms (see Sect. 4.1) to learn the model for predicting depression.

3.1 Feature-Based Representation

The features we considered are many (256 in total). They come either from the literature [4, 5, 41] or from our own developments [16, 24, 36, 37].

We categorized these features into six meta-categories (META1 to META6), each of which are divided in turn into categories (numbered with roman numerals from I to XVI). This hierarchical representation of features will be used for deep analysis of the impact of features on the results. The six meta-categories are as follows: representation of full texts, lexicons on depression, temporal aspects, writing style, emotion, and lexical categories. These meta-categories, the associated categories, and features are detailed in Table 2.

Whatever the feature is, its value is calculated by averaging the number of occurrences found at the post level over all the user' posts to consider; values are normalized.

3.1.1 META_1: Representation of Full Texts

Group I: These features are extracted from posts known to be written by people annotated as depressed in eRisk 2017 training set. We extracted the 50 most frequent uni-grams from the depressed users' texts and learnt a first model (Random forest based) whose task was to detect depressed users. We then selected the 18 uni-grams that the chi-squared ranking filter considers as the most important. Although these terms may be collection-dependent, we kept them across the models.
Group II: They correspond to the frequency of Part-Of-Speech categories (adjectives, verbs, adverbs, and nouns). According to De Choudhury et al., people who want to commit suicide were characterized with a higher use of verbs, adjectives, and adverbs, but lower use of nouns [5]. We used these cues as detection characteristics for depression even though a depressed person is not necessarily suicidal. The World Health Organization has shown that depression is one of the major causes of suicide in the world.[5]

3.1.2 META_2: Lexicons Related to Depression

Group III: Depressed users often mention depression symptoms and antidepressants names in their texts. We used the list of depressive symptoms and antidepressant names obtained from [5] and Wikipedia.[6] The value of this characteristic is the normalized frequency of the uni-grams from the lists. Depressed users use group of words such as "want to die" (tri-grams) or "to take my own life" (5-g), etc. We used the 25 3-g and 25 5-g which were the most frequent expressions of a potentially suicidal thought, from a collection of tweets by Colombo et al. [6].

[5] https://www.who.int/news-room/fact-sheets/detail/depression.

[6] http://en.wikipedia.org/wiki/List_of_antidepressants accessed on 23/02/2017.

Table 2 Description of the features used to represent the users' posts. Similar types of features are grouped into categories; and similar categories are further grouped into meta-categories

Cat.	Number	Name	Hypothesis or tool/resource used
$META_1$: Representation of full texts			
I	1–18	Bag-of-words	18 most frequent uni-grams in the eRisk 2017 training set [16]
II	19–22	Part-Of-Speech frequency	Higher usage of adjectives, verbs, adverbs, and lower usage of nouns [5]
$META_2$: Lexicons on depression			
III	23	Depression symptoms and related drugs	From Wikipedia list[1] and [5]
	24	Relevant 3-g	25 3-g [6]
	25	Relevant 5-g	25 5-g [6]
IV	26	Frequency of "depress"	Depressed people talk often about the depression
	27	Related words to depression	Words: "sleep," "depress," and "sad"
V	28	Drugs name	The chemical and brand names of antidepressants from WebMD available in United States[2] [41]
$META_3$:Temporality			
VI	29	Temporal expressions	High use of words that refer to past: last, before, ago, ...[28]
VII	30	Ratio of Posting Time	High frequency of publications in deep night (00 pm - 07 am) [5]
	31–34	Season of a year (4 seasons in total)	Frequency of publications in season (one season corresponds to 3 months)
VIII	35	Past frequency	Combination of temporal expressions and past tense verbs
	36	Past tense verbs	Depressive people talk more about the past
	37	Past tense auxiliaries	Same motivation as above

(continued)

Table 2 (continued)

Cat.	Number	Name	Hypothesis or tool/resource used
META4: Writing style			
IX	38	Average number of posts	Depressed users have a much lower number of posts
	39	Average number of words per post	Posts of depressed user are more longer
	40	Minimum number of posts	Generally depressive users have a lower value
	41	Average number of comments	Depressed users have a much lower number of comments
	42	Average number of words per comment	Comments of depressed and non depressed users have different means
X	43	Gunning Fog Index	Estimate of the years of education that a person needs to understand the text at first reading [41]
	44	Flesch Reading Ease	Measure how difficult to understand a text is [41]
	45	Linsear Write Formula	Developed for the U.S. Air Force to calculate the readability of their technical manuals [41]
	46	New Dale-Chall Readability	Measure the difficulty of comprehension that persons encounter when reading a text. It is inspired from Flesch Reading Ease measure [41]
XI	47–51	First person pronouns	High use of : *I, me, myself, mine, my*
	52	*I* subject of *be*	High use of *I'm* [39]
	53	All first person pronouns	Sum of frequency of each first pronoun [45]
	54	*I* in subjective context	Depressive users refers to themselves frequently (all *I* targeted by an adjective)
XII	55	Over-generalization	Depressed users tend to use intense quantifiers and superlatives [28]
XIII	56	Negation	Depressive users use more negative words like: *no, not, didn't, can't*, ..., etc.
XIV	57	Capitalized	Depressive users tend to put emphasis on the target they mention
	58	Punctuation marks	! or ? or any combination of both tend to express doubt and surprise [45]
	59	Emoticons	Another way to express sentiment or feeling [45]
META5: Emotion			
XV	60	Emotions	Frequency of emotions from specific categories: anger, fear, surprise, sadness and disgust
	61–62	Sentiment	Use of NRC-Sentiment-Emotion-Lexicons[3] [27] to trace the polarity in users writings
META6: Lexical categories			
XVI	63–256	Empath	All 194 Empath categories [4] [11]

[1] http://en.wikipedia.org/wiki/List_of_antidepressants, accessed on 23/02/2017
[2] http://www.webmd.com/depression/guide/depression-medications-antidepressants, accessed on 10/01/2018
[3] http://saifmohammad.com/WebPages/NRC-Emotion-Lexicon.htm, accessed on 23/02/2017
[4] http://empath.stanford.edu

Group IV: The first feature of this group corresponds to the "depression" term and its syntactic variants. The next feature is the frequency of the words: "sleep," "depress," and "sad."
Group V: A list of antidepressants from WebMD available in United States,[7] [41].

3.1.3 META$_3$: Temporality

Group VI: Depressed users often talk about the past [28]. We used a list of English words referring to the past: yesterday, last, before, ago, past, back, earlier, later, nostalgia.
Group VII: Depressed users tend to post publications late at night [5]. We capture the ratio of publications between 12am (midnight) and 7am. We also calculate the characteristic seasons of a year by dividing the 12 months of the year into 4 seasons (season 1: December, January, and February; season 2: March, April, and May; etc.). Each season corresponds to a characteristic, thus considering the seasonality of depression [30].
Group VIII: The features in this group (past frequency, past tense verbs, and past tense auxiliaries) make allusion to the past.

3.1.4 META$_4$: Writing Style

Group IX: This group gathers different features related to the number of posts and the number of words per post.
Group X: These features measure the readability of the posts, thus the complexity of the sentences and texts.
Group XI: These features are related to the first person use in the posts.
Group XII: Depressed persons are prone to over-generalize [28]. For example, instead of criticizing someone who has hurt them, a depressed person may write "all men/women are xx."
Group XIII: When suffering from depression, people usually express with much more negative feeling in their writings than healthy individuals. We therefore decided to consider this characteristic.
Group XIV: Depressed people are more likely to focus on the target they mention. The use of capitalized words is one way of expressing this emphasis. Their writings are a true reflection of their moods. In this case, special punctuation marks, such as question marks or exclamation marks, tend to encourage users to express their doubts or surprises towards a target [46]. Emoticons are another way of expressing how people feel. Xinyu Wang et al. [45] have shown that taking emoticons into account is important in detecting depression.

---

[7] http://www.webmd.com/depression/guide/depression-medications-antidepressants accessed on 10/01/2018.

3.1.5 META$_5$: Emotion

Group XV: Depression is closely related to emotions and sentiments. Depressed people tend to be more subjective about what they mention or write, which is why we have assumed that it is useful to trace the polarity and emotions of their texts.

3.1.6 META$_6$: Lexical Categories

Group XVI: The idea here is to analyze the publication through lexical categories. For this, we used the empath python library[8] that analyzes texts through lexical categories.

3.1.7 Embedding Representation

A user is represented by a vector built from the history of posts available. Here, we use embeddings based representation both at the word level from Word2Vec [26] and at the sentence level with a combination of two Doc2Vec [20] variants.

Word embedding refers to the representation of a word in a semantic space as a vector of numerical values. Words that are semantically and syntactically similar tend to be close in this embedding space. Document embedding refers to the representation of a document's content using a vector of numerical values. The goal of Doc2Vec is to create a vector representation of a document/paragraph/sentence, disregarding of its length. The Doc2Vec model can work very well when trained on a small corpus compared to Word2Vec [42].

To represent users from their posts/comments at the word level, we use the pre-trained Word-vector which was trained on GoogleNews corpus using Word2Vec model [26] following the Skip-gram architecture with negative sampling and a window size of 10 words. The pre-trained model contains 300-dimensional vectors for 3 million words and phrases. We first extract the word vector from Word2Vec model for each word in a post. When we could not find a word in the model, we represent it with a zero vector of 300 dimension. We average the word vectors of every word from a post in row-wise. Then, for a given user, we aggregate all the vectors from that user's posts by averaging the corresponding vectors. This average aggregated vector is considered as the vector representation for that user.

To represent users from their posts/comments at the sentence level, we use the Sentence-vector which is a combination of two Doc2Vec variants trained using Doc2Vec [20] model based on Word2Vec. First, we extract a sentence embedding vector for each post from two Doc2Vec model variants, (a) distributed memory model and (b) distributed bag-of-words model (see Fig. 2). Then for a given user, we aggregate all the vectors from that user's posts/comments by averaging the vectors; we thus calculate the centroid vector for each user.

[8] http://empath.stanford.edu.

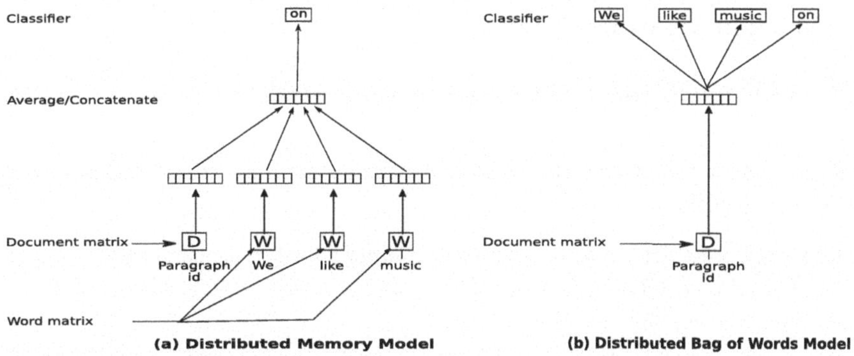

Fig. 2 Doc2Vec models inspired from [20]

More specifically, we trained the two following Doc2Vec model variants (see Fig. 2) with the dataset of 2017 and 2018 separately, thus creating 4 models (see Sect. 5):

- A distributed memory model which is an extension of Word2Vec CBOW model: instead of using only words to predict the next word, this Doc2Vec model adds another input feature vector which is unique to the paragraph (ID of the paragraph in the Fig. 2a). During training, the word matrix *W* and the paragraph matrix *D* are trained (i.e., change their weight), and at the end, a column in the paragraph matrix *D* represents a unique vector of a paragraph.
- A distributed bag-of-words model which is similar to the Word2Vec skip-gram model but uses the paragraph matrix to classify all the words from the document (see Fig. 2b). Instead of predicting the next word, it uses the paragraph matrix to classify all the words in a paragraph. Specifically, during the training phase, a classifier is trained to decide whether the words belong to the paragraph or not. This model consumes less memory, as there is no need to save word vectors as in the distributed memory model.

Mikolov et al. [20] recommend using a combination of the two models (i.e. distributed memory model and distributed bag-of-words model) to represent a text/document; although distributed memory model generally achieves state-of-the-art performances for most tasks [7]. To represent a sentence/post, we concatenate the two vectors of 100 dimension representing the sentence/post, obtained by the two Doc2Vec model variants, thus forming a single vector of 200 dimensions.

4 Machine Learning Models

4.1 Well-Established Machine Learning Models

We consider the following well-established machine learning (ML) algorithms from different categories:

- Random Forest (RF): a Random forest classifier with 100 decision trees,
- SGD_Logloss (SGD-log) logistic regression: a stochastic gradient descent classifier trained using the "log" loss function,
- SVM_Linear (SVM-$linear$): a support vector machine classifier with the linear kernel,
- SVM_RBF (SVM-rbf): a support vector machine classifier with the RBF kernel,
- Neural network (NN): a multi-layer perceptron classifier where the configuration is one hidden layer with 100 units, the Relu activation function, and the "log" loss function using LBFGS optimizer,
- K-nearest-neighbor (KNN): a 3-nearest neighbors classifier.

Unless otherwise stated, we kept the default values of the respective hyper-parameters of all machine learning algorithms from Scikit-learn (version 0.22.1) [33]. To produce the results of all machine learning algorithms, we used the random_state= 42 (the scikit-learn parameter that handles the random seed for the models and which is required for RF for sampling of the features and the randomness of the bootstrapping of the samples, SGD for shuffling the data, SVM for probability estimate, NN controls).

These classical classifiers are not designed to solve detection problems at the earliest possible time while we deal with such problems in this work. Early detection problems integrate a time dimension in the classification, in other words, they use data streams as input. That is, at a given instant t, only a partition of the data is available for classification; the further forward in time, the more data is available. The objective is to be able to decide accurately using the minimum amount of data, i.e. as quickly as possible over time.

To allow classifiers to deal with the early detection problem, we adopt a classification process where we integrate the time dimension outside the classifiers. This process consists of training classifiers without taking into account the time dimension, in other words, using all the data available in the training corpus, and consider the time dimension during the test stage. More precisely during the test stage, when only the first posts are considered (i.e., chunk 1), and for a given user, a trained classifier makes its decision on the user using only the data available at this stage. If the user is predicted as depressed then the classification process stops, otherwise the classifier predicts the user again using the data available at the first stage plus the one available at the second stage (i.e. chunk 1 and chunk 2). This process is repeated and in the end, if the user is still not predicted as depressed when using all the data, then the user is considered as non-depressed. In eRisk, one stage (or chunk) contains partial data of a user, only 10% of users' writings, chronologically ordered.

4.2 BERT-Based Model

BERT (Bidirectional Encoder Representations from Transformers) is a pre-trained language representation model [10]. BERT model architecture is a multi-layer bidirectional transformer encoder, which considers both left and right contexts in all of its layers. BERT is pre-trained on large corpus using a masking technique: given a sentence, 15% of the input words are masked and during training, the goal is to predict these words. This technique overcomes the limitation of unidirectional processing and is also superior to language models that combine right-to-left and left-to-right processing, see [10, 34].

Pre-trained Google BERTs are freely available on github.[9] The BERT_{Base} model contains 12 layers of size 768, 12 self-attention heads and 110M parameters, while the BERT_{Large} model contains 24 layers of size 1,024, 16 self-attention heads and 340M parameters. BERT can be fine-tuned to answer specific downstream tasks. BERT_{Base} model has two variants: $\text{BERT}_{Base-cased}$ which is case sensitive and makes a difference between for example "english" and "English" words, and $\text{BERT}_{Base-uncased}$ which is not case sensitive.

In this work, we fine-tune Google's $\text{BERT}_{Base-uncased}$ pre-trained model on the training data using an 80/20 subdivision where 20% percent of the training set is used as the validation set. This 80/20 subdivision of training set is performed following the stratified fashion using Scikit-learn's "train_test_split" function where the random_state is 42. We add two additional dense layers (512 and 2 units, respectively) at the end of the 12-layer pre-trained network. During the fine-tuning, we freeze all parameters of the first 12-layers of the network (pre-trained part) but allow learning the new added two layers. We use cross-entropy loss function, AdamW optimizer, 1e−5 learning rate, 32 batch size, 10 epochs, and a maximum of 128 tokens per sentence. Training is repeated on the entire training dataset across epochs. We store the model checkpoint if the validation loss is lower than training loss after each epoch. We name this BERT's fine-tuned model as "BERT-fine-tuned-natural."

The depression dataset is unbalanced since the majority of the posts/comments are not depressive individually and collectively over all users. To tackle the unbalance issue, we balance the classes when fine-tuning the Google's $\text{BERT}_{Base-uncased}$ pre-trained model. The balancing is done via weighting the classes in the loss function. Therefore, we first compute the class weights for the labels in the training set and pass these weights to the loss function [18]. We keep all the hyper-parameters exactly the same as "BERT-fine-tuned-natural." We name this fine-tuned model as "BERT-fine-tuned-balanced."

During testing stage, we evaluate both "BERT-fine-tuned-natural" and "BERT-fine-tuned-balanced" models. We use our BERT-fine-tuned model (either "BERT-fine-tuned-natural" or "BERT-fine-tuned-balanced") to obtain the predicted probability for the testing samples. We assume that all the posts/comments written by a user labeled as depressed are also depressed. In the end, we need to classify the user as depressed or not. To tackle the early detection problem for a user, we follow a

[9] https://github.com/google-research/bert, accessed on 02/02/2021.

cumulative approach and also consider two aggregation functions (i.e., maximum or mean) to calculate the probabilities. We apply the first aggregation function (maximum or mean) on the predicted probabilities for the posts/comments of each chunk by a user. Then, when combining two or more chunks, we again apply the second aggregation function (maximum or mean) on the first aggregated values of two or more chunks by a user. Moreover, to tackle the detection problem for a user, we apply the same aggregation strategy that we use for early detection.

5 Experimental Framework

We developed a series of experiments whose objective is to compare different models on the eRisk depression task. More precisely we aim at comparing well-established machine learning methods with the more recent BERT model. With regard to well-established machine learning, we also investigate the variety of features we described in Sect. 3. For this, we used some eRisk collections as well as different evaluation measures. More details about the collections and metrics can be found in Chap. 2.

5.1 Collections

In the evaluation stage, we use the two collections available for early depression detection: CLEF eRisk 2017 and 2018 collections. eRisk 2018 has more users and more posts for both depressed and non-depressed users than eRisk 2017. The data is naturally non-balanced considering depressed vs. non-depressed users. The proportion of users belonging to the two classes on the training and testing datasets are similar (Table 3).

Table 3 Distribution of training and test data from the eRisk 2017 and 2018 collection on early depression detection task

Number		Training		Test	
		Depressed	Non-depressed	Depressed	Non-depressed
2017	Users	83	403	52	349
	Posts	4,911	91,381	1,928	65,735
	Comments	25,940	172,791	16,778	151,930
2018	Users	135	752	79	741
	Posts	6,839	157,116	7,672	169,930
	Comments	42,718	324,721	32,993	333,852

6 Results and Discussion

We first evaluate the models considering a standard depression detection task. In that case, we are not considering early detection, but rather, the system has to predict depression considering the entire set of texts written by the user (Sect. 6.1). Then, we consider early depression detection where the moment in which decisions are taken is crucial (Sects. from 6.2 to 6.4 and 7).

6.1 Depression Detection

In this section, we present the results for depression detection, that is to say without considering its early detection. From the set of user's posts, the system has to predict whether the user is depressed or not. We thus trained each model on the training set and run them on the entire test set, without considering post chunks or partitions.

Table 4 presents the results where machine learning models use:

- 256 features and well-established machine learning algorithms (RF, SGD-log, SVM-$linear$, SVM-rbf, Neural network (NN), KNN) (first block),
- Doc2Vec based embeddings with the same well-established machine learning algorithms (second block),
- Word2Vec based embeddings with the same well-established machine learning algorithms (third block), and
- BERT model (fourth block).

We can observe that some of the well-established algorithms perform strangely bad when considering the representation with 256 features. We suspect this is due to the sparsity of some of the features that lead to model overfitting. We can also observe that when considering the threshold as 0.5 on the output probability of the classification algorithm, precision is favored compared to recall for those machine learning models. Both the 256 feature models and Word2Vec reach a precision of around 0.7 on the 2017 collection. For the 2018 collection, the 256 features model and Doc2Vec yielded the best precision (0.71 and 0.84, respectively). When considering F_1 measure, that combines recall and precision, RF with 256 features is consistently the best. Overall, RF with the 256 feature representation is more robust across the collections and thus we would recommend it when considering well-established machine learning models. Moreover, on the eRisk 2017 dataset, KNN classifier achieves the second best F_1.

Now, when considering BERT variants, the best F_1 measure is obtained for Balanced-mean-mean and the second best by Natural-max-max. Whatever the version, recall is generally favored (except for one configuration) compared to precision when considering the threshold on the output probability of the classification algorithm as 0.5. Recall is up to 1 for balanced versions on both collections, however, in those cases precision is low. As a result when considering F_1 measure, still the RF

Table 4 Well-Established machine learning (ML) methods for detecting depression using the 256 features listed in Table 2, Word2Vec, Doc2Vec, and BERT-based representations for eRisk 2017 and 2018 collections. We considered the threshold on the output probability of the classification algorithm as 0.5 to decide whether the user is depressed or not

		2017			2018		
	ML model	P	R	F_1	P	R	F_1
256	RF	**0.73**	**0.46**	**0.56**	**0.71**	**0.46**	**0.55**
	SGD-log	0.17	0.10	0.12	0.32	0.27	0.29
	SVM-*linear*	**0.73**	0.15	0.25	0.67	0.23	0.34
	SVM-*rbf*	0.00	0.00	0.00	0.62	0.10	0.17
	NN	0.00	0.00	0.00	0.00	0.00	0.00
	KNN	0.23	0.17	0.20	0.15	0.10	0.12
Word2Vec	RF	0.63	0.37	0.46	0.54	0.34	0.42
	SGD-log	**0.73**	0.15	0.25	**0.61**	0.32	0.42
	SVM-*linear*	0.48	0.31	0.38	0.56	0.35	0.43
	SVM-*rbf*	0.47	0.31	0.37	**0.61**	0.35	**0.45**
	NN	0.46	**0.50**	**0.48**	0.36	0.41	0.38
	KNN	0.43	0.38	0.40	0.48	**0.43**	**0.45**
Doc2Vec	RF	**.60**	0.35	0.44	0.71	0.38	0.50
	SGD-log	0.41	**0.75**	**0.53**	0.76	0.41	**0.53**
	SVM-*linear*	0.57	0.23	0.33	**0.84**	0.33	0.47
	SVM-*rbf*	0.57	0.23	0.33	**0.84**	0.33	0.47
	NN	0.49	0.58	**0.53**	0.42	**0.65**	0.51
	KNN	0.53	0.46	0.49	0.52	0.46	0.49
BERT (Fine-tuned)	Natural-max-max	0.25	0.79	0.38	0.25	0.82	0.38
	Natural-max-mean	**0.42**	0.19	0.26	0.62	0.19	0.29
	Natural-mean-max	0.33	0.02	0.04	**0.80**	0.10	0.18
	Natural-mean-mean	0.00	0.00	0.00	0.00	0.00	0.00
	Balanced-max-max	0.13	**1.0**	0.23	0.10	**1.0**	0.18
	Balanced-max-mean	0.14	0.98	0.24	0.10	**1.0**	0.19
	Balanced-mean-max	0.20	0.94	0.33	0.18	0.94	0.31
	Balanced-mean-mean	0.33	0.79	**0.47**	0.32	0.70	**0.44**

using 256 features remains the best. BERT results are rather disappointing. It might be because not enough data is available. Considering these results, we do not expect BERT to perform well when considering early detection, where not enough data is available for proper fine-tuning.

On the variants of BERT that we analyzed, we can see that the trade-off between recall and precision is slightly changed for the different versions. The consistently best across collections is the "Balanced-mean-mean" version for balanced distribution (eighth row of fourth block). Since the model is trained on a balanced distribution by weighting the classes, the predicted score is balanced towards both the positive and control classes. That's why, if we apply the mean aggregation function on the predicted probabilities of posts/comments for each chunk by a user, we obtained a robust estimate on the positive class. When combining multiple chunks by applying the mean function again, we obtained the best overall estimate across chunks. If we rely on the mean of predicted probabilities for the positive class for the balanced model, it produces the best performance across collections for the BERT variants.

Regarding the balanced distribution models, we can see that the greedy max function on the predicted probabilities of posts/comments of each chunk by a user (first max in the names of Table 4, fourth block) makes the aggregated score higher than the threshold (0.5). That means, even if the output probability of a single post/comment of a chunk by a user is higher than 0.5, the user is predicted as depressive. Then, whatever the aggregation function applied when combining multiple chunks for a user (fifth and sixth rows of block 4; Balanced-max-max and Balanced-max-mean), it makes the recall closer to 1, but the precision closer to 0.1.

In the case of the model trained on natural distribution ("imbalanced model"), the predicted class is biased to the control class and only a few posts/comments are classified as positive class. If we apply the greedy maximum function on the predicted probabilities of posts/comments for each chunk by a user, we obtained the maximum probability for the rarely predicted positive class. When combining multiple chunks if we apply the maximum function again, we obtained the best predicted probability across chunks. Since the network is biased towards the control class if we rely on the maximum function both across the posts/comments in a chunk and across chunks for the rare positive class, it produces a comparatively better performance (first row of block 4; Natural-max-max). We can also see that the mean function on the predicted probabilities of posts/comments for each chunk makes the mean aggregated score lower, perhaps lower than the threshold (0.5). This indeed makes the recall closer to 0 whatever the aggregation function (mean/max) is applied later to combine multiple chunks (3rd and 4th rows of block 4 in Table 4; Natural-mean-max and Natural-mean-mean).

The weak performance of BERT compared to other models on both collections could be linked to the missing annotations at the posts/comments level, e.g., if a user only became ill during the course of their history. In this case, all posts are still annotated as depressive while only the later posts/comments should be annotated as depressive. This annotation problem may have an impact on the BERT fine-tuning. We keep this problem for future study.

6.2 Early Depression Detection

In this section, we present the results for early depression detection. We trained the models on the entire training set and run the obtained models by steps on the chunks of the test set: first using the first chunk only, then the first two chunks, then the first three chunks, and until the system uses the entire test set. The system decides at each step. At each step, if the system is confident enough on the predicted score, then it can decide to predict the user as depressed (1), otherwise, it waits for more information. When the system gets all the data (last step) of test set, it has to decide for all the remaining users depressed (1) or non-depressed (2).

Table 5 presents the results with the same blocks as in Table 4. We can observe that when compared to Table 4 and keeping the same prediction probability 0.5, precision slightly decreases while recall slightly increases, resulting in a slightly improved F_1 measure; this holds for both collections and for most of the models using well-established machine learning, whatever the representation is (256 features, Word2Vec or Doc2Vec). The fact that precision decreases is due to the fact that some decisions are taken with the limited number of posts processed on the user. As expected from previous results in Table 4, Random forest with 256 features is the most stable across collections and thus would be the preferred model. It also has among the smallest ERDE values, showing that it is effective for early detection. With regard to BERT, the results are consistent with the one we obtained for -not early- depression detection. That means, for balanced distribution, "Balanced-mean-mean" or "Balanced-mean-max" version (seventh or eighth row of the fourth block) achieves good performance whereas "Natural-max-max" or "Natural-max-mean" version produces better for natural distribution (first or second row of the fourth block).

6.3 Simplified Models

In this section, we focused on simplified models trained using a smaller number of significant features. In Table 2, we can see a list of 256 individual features, 16 groups, and 6 meta-groups of features. We hypothesize that some of those features could be important features to detect early depression while other features could on the contrary be noisy. To extract the important features, we applied the Chi-square (Chi2) feature selection [21] on the training set of each collection individually. We found that 126 features are selected for 2017 collection while 156 features are selected for 2018 collection. With these features only, we then trained the models on the training set and tested the obtained models on the chunks of the test set in a cumulative approach for early depression detection. We present the results in Table 6.

For 2017 collection, we can see that the model with feature selection (Chi2) does not improve the performance compared to the model with 256 features. However, on 2018 collection the feature selection model improves the F_1 and $ERDE_{50}$ measures slightly.

Table 5 Performance of the early depression detection using the well-established machine learning (ML) methods using the 256 features listed in Table 2, Word2Vec, Doc2Vec, and BERT based representation for eRisk 2017 and 2018 collections. We considered the threshold on the output probability of the classification algorithm as 0.5 to decide whether the user is depressed or not

		2017					2018				
	ML model	P	R	F_1	$ERDE_5$ (%)	$ERDE_{50}$ (%)	P	R	F_1	$ERDE_5$ (%)	$ERDE_{50}$ (%)
256	RF	**0.63**	**0.62**	**0.62**	**12.71**	**9.48**	**0.65**	**0.53**	**0.58**	**9.41**	**7.19**
	SGD-log	0.16	0.29	0.21	15.46	13.25	0.28	0.38	0.32	9.53	8.33
	SVM-*linear*	0.21	0.31	0.25	14.61	13.45	0.57	0.27	0.36	9.82	9.21
	SVM-*rbf*	0.00	0.00	0.00	13.10	13.10	0.62	0.10	0.17	9.69	9.69
	NN	0.03	0.04	0.04	14.78	14.53	0.04	0.08	0.05	11.21	11.21
	KNN	0.21	0.50	0.30	14.91	11.09	0.20	0.46	0.28	10.45	8.40
Word2Vec	RF	**.44**	0.58	**0.50**	13.24	**9.20**	0.33	0.46	0.38	9.36	7.17
	SGD-log	0.41	0.35	0.38	**12.61**	9.82	0.35	0.41	0.38	**8.77**	7.12
	SVM-*linear*	0.36	0.46	0.40	12.98	9.62	0.32	0.49	0.39	8.98	6.94
	SVM-*rbf*	0.37	0.44	0.40	12.88	9.53	**0.39**	0.52	**0.45**	8.87	**6.35**
	NN	0.27	0.67	0.39	14.19	9.78	0.22	**0.68**	0.33	10.59	7.55
	KNN	0.34	**0.81**	0.48	14.29	8.85	0.23	0.57	0.33	10.04	7.91
Doc2Vec	RF	**0.53**	0.50	**0.51**	12.73	9.73	0.56	0.51	**0.53**	8.92	6.58
	SGD-log	0.27	**0.87**	0.41	15.05	9.40	.40	0.56	0.46	8.92	6.64
	SVM-*linear*	0.42	0.37	0.39	**12.29**	10.07	0.49	0.43	0.46	8.74	6.89
	SVM-*rbf*	0.45	0.38	0.42	12.37	9.76	**0.58**	0.48	0.52	**8.51**	**6.55**
	NN	0.30	0.71	0.42	14.32	10.76	0.23	**0.81**	0.36	10.52	7.41
	KNN	0.34	0.62	0.44	13.69	9.83	0.36	0.67	0.46	9.50	6.83
BERT (Fine-tuned)	Natural-max-max	0.25	0.79	0.38	16.59	11.86	0.25	0.82	0.38	11.45	8.65
	Natural-max-mean	0.32	0.42	0.36	14.16	12.24	0.39	0.46	**0.42**	10.11	8.83
	Natural-mean-max	0.33	0.02	0.04	12.79	12.78	0.80	0.10	0.18	**9.32**	8.68
	Natural-mean-mean	**1.0**	0.02	0.04	**12.72**	12.72	**1.0**	0.01	0.02	9.60	9.51
	Balanced-max-max	0.13	**1.0**	0.23	21.64	14.99	0.10	**1.0**	0.18	16.30	12.41
	Balanced-max-mean	0.13	**1.0**	0.24	21.30	14.64	0.10	**1.0**	0.18	16.08	12.13
	Balanced-mean-max	0.20	0.94	0.33	16.60	10.45	0.18	0.94	0.31	11.64	8.18
	Balanced-mean-mean	0.27	0.90	**0.41**	14.55	**8.87**	0.22	0.76	0.34	10.35	**7.24**

Table 6 Performance of the early depression detection using the well-established machine learning (ML) methods based on the features selected from Table 2 using Chi2 technique for eRisk 2017 and 2018 collections. We considered the threshold on the output probability of the classification algorithm as 0.5 to decide whether the user is depressed or not

		2017					2018				
	ML model	P	R	F_1	$ERDE_5$ (%)	$ERDE_{50}$ (%)	P	R	F_1	$ERDE_5$ (%)	$ERDE_{50}$ (%)
256	RF	**0.63**	**0.62**	**0.62**	**12.71**	**9.48**	**0.65**	0.53	0.58	**9.41**	7.19
Chi2	RF	0.60	**0.62**	0.61	12.76	9.54	0.63	0.56	**0.59**	**9.41**	**6.65**

6.4 *Ablation Analysis*

In the ablation analysis, we considered Random forest with feature-based models. On the one hand, we consider the reference model, the one that uses all the 256 features, to which we removed some features (exclusion). On the other hand, we considered models where a limited set of features are considered (inclusion). We conducted the analysis at the meta-level as well as at the category-level.

6.4.1 Meta Level Analysis

In the *exclusion analysis*, from the reference model (first row, Table 7), we removed one meta category of features, considering successively each of the six meta categories. This approach helps in understanding which are the less and most influencing meta categories. If the results decrease when removing a meta category of features, that means that the corresponding features are important. If the results are stable when removing a category of features, that means either that other features cover well the modeled phenomenon or that the features are not important. To be able to distinguish between these two options, we add the inclusion analysis. In the *inclusion analysis*, we built a model that contains the features of a single meta category each time.

From Table 7, we can see that the model that includes all the features is among the best for both collections. Each measure aims at providing different insights on the model capability. Recall and precision are inversely related while F_1 measure combines them. When focusing on F_1 measure, we can observe that excluding META_6 (lexical categories) is not consistently problematic: it is for 2017 dataset, where both recall and precision decrease, but not for the 2018 dataset where precision only decreases but recall increases. Overall, when considering F_1 measure, recall and precision, removing one of the meta categories does not affect the results. This shows that the features from different categories have some kind of redundancy although there are not of the same nature. The same type of conclusion can be drawn when analyzing the early detection measures. META_5 (emoticons) does not help much on early detection, when removed (Exclusion), results improved for both collections. We

Table 7 Ablation study of the meta group of features both in exclusion and inclusion strategy using the Random forest classifier. We considered the threshold on the output probability of the classification algorithm as 0.5 to decide whether the user is depressed or not

	Features	Exclusion					Inclusion				
		P	R	F_1	ERDE$_5$ (%)	ERDE$_{50}$ (%)	P	R	F_1	ERDE$_5$ (%)	ERDE$_{50}$ (%)
2017	All	0.63	**0.62**	**0.62**	**12.71**	**9.48**	0.63	**0.62**	0.62	**12.71**	9.48
	- META$_1$	0.60	**0.62**	0.61	12.91	9.78	0.50	0.52	0.51	13.45	10.35
	- META$_2$	0.61	0.60	0.60	12.73	9.75	0.39	0.50	0.44	13.51	11.30
	- META$_3$	**0.68**	0.58	**0.62**	12.79	9.56	0.12	**0.62**	0.20	18.47	14.95
	- META$_4$	0.61	0.58	0.59	13.08	10.09	0.26	0.58	0.36	14.80	11.79
	- META$_5$	0.67	0.58	**0.62**	12.99	10.46	0.20	0.23	0.21	14.52	13.77
	- META$_6$	0.60	0.58	0.59	12.81	10.12	**0.70**	**0.62**	**0.65**	12.80	**9.19**
2018	All	**0.65**	0.53	0.58	9.41	7.19	**0.65**	0.53	**0.58**	9.41	7.19
	- META$_1$	0.65	0.49	0.56	9.62	7.08	0.49	0.47	0.48	**9.38**	**7.04**
	- META$_2$	0.57	0.54	0.56	9.40	**6.60**	0.32	0.66	0.43	10.64	8.38
	- META$_3$	0.63	0.53	0.58	9.44	6.88	0.10	**0.68**	0.18	13.32	11.06
	- META$_4$	0.62	0.54	0.58	9.43	6.89	0.21	0.53	0.30	10.13	7.62
	- META$_5$	**0.66**	0.57	**0.61**	9.29	6.73	0.08	0.09	0.09	10.55	10.06
	- META$_6$	0.60	**0.63**	**0.61**	**9.12**	6.74	0.59	0.49	0.54	9.76	7.15

can also see that in general not considering the full-text representation (Exclusion META$_1$) hurts the results the most, for almost all the measures. That means that focused features such as lexicons, writing style and emoticons, are not enough, still the entire text is useful.

Now when considering a limited number of features (Inclusion), we can see that some meta categories are more helpful than others and they can be complementary. For example, META$_3$ (temporality) features help for recall for both collections but are not enough to obtain acceptable precision. On the other hand, META$_1$ features are key for early detection (lowest ERDE for the model that uses these features) while META$_3$ features are not (high ERDE). We can also see that model with only META$_6$ (lexical categories) produces the best overall result for Precision and F_1 measures for the 2017 collection. With the META$_6$ features, the inclusion result is also quite convincing for the 2018 collection (Table 7, last row).

6.4.2 Category Level Analysis

The results of the ablation study of the category of features are detailed in Table 8. When considering the exclusion of a category of features, we can see that Part-Of-Speech features (category II) could be omitted, either results improved like on 2017 or they are stable like on 2018 data. The results are consistently better when omitting the readability features (category X) as well. When considering only category II or only category X, we can also see that the resulting models are poorly performing.

Table 8 Ablation study of the category of features defined in Table 2 considering both exclusion and inclusion strategy using the Random forest classifier. We considered the threshold on the output probability of the classification algorithm as 0.5 to decide whether the user is depressed or not

	Features	Exclusion					Inclusion				
		P	R	F_1	$ERDE_5$ (%)	$ERDE_{50}$ (%)	P	R	F_1	$ERDE_5$ (%)	$ERDE_{50}$ (%)
2017	All	0.63	**0.62**	0.62	12.71	9.48	0.63	0.62	0.62	**12.71**	9.48
	- I	0.62	0.54	0.58	12.97	10.03	0.47	0.54	0.50	13.17	9.98
	- II	**0.70**	**0.62**	**0.65**	12.72	9.37	0.38	0.58	0.46	13.86	10.12
	- III	0.66	0.60	0.63	12.80	9.87	0.18	0.52	0.27	15.85	13.14
	- IV	0.67	**0.62**	0.64	12.68	**9.13**	0.50	0.62	0.55	13.53	11.50
	- V	0.62	0.56	0.59	12.70	10.13	0.55	0.12	0.19	13.13	12.63
	- VI	0.67	**0.62**	0.64	12.82	9.19	0.44	0.13	0.21	12.84	11.79
	- VII	0.65	**0.62**	0.63	12.72	9.41	0.13	0.73	0.23	18.88	14.62
	- VIII	0.62	0.58	0.60	12.69	9.93	0.25	0.65	0.36	15.29	10.99
	- IX	0.64	0.58	0.61	12.82	9.66	0.19	0.44	0.26	15.27	12.24
	- X	**0.70**	**0.62**	**0.65**	**12.55**	9.25	0.25	0.56	0.34	14.59	11.94
	- XI	0.66	0.56	0.60	12.58	9.41	0.41	0.52	0.46	14.17	11.73
	- XII	0.65	**0.62**	0.63	12.84	9.22	0.14	**0.90**	0.24	21.66	17.54
	- XIII	0.66	0.60	0.63	12.61	10.12	0.15	0.83	0.25	20.73	17.67
	- XIV	0.63	**0.62**	0.62	12.94	9.47	0.27	0.50	0.35	14.77	11.27
	- XV	0.67	0.58	0.62	12.99	10.46	0.20	0.23	0.21	14.52	13.77
	- XVI	0.60	0.58	0.59	12.81	10.12	**0.70**	0.62	**0.65**	12.80	**9.19**
2018	All	0.65	0.53	0.58	9.41	7.19	**0.65**	0.53	**0.58**	**9.41**	7.19
	- I	0.59	0.49	0.54	9.15	7.02	0.50	0.46	0.48	9.70	7.25
	- II	0.65	0.52	0.58	9.34	6.84	0.29	0.44	0.35	9.82	7.41
	- III	0.60	0.56	0.58	9.39	6.82	0.17	0.63	0.27	11.88	9.83
	- IV	0.62	0.56	0.59	9.44	**6.66**	0.40	0.63	0.49	10.21	8.14
	- V	0.60	0.51	0.55	9.49	**6.66**	0.47	0.28	0.35	9.89	9.32
	- VI	0.58	0.51	0.54	9.50	6.80	0.06	0.01	0.02	9.73	9.70
	- VII	**0.71**	0.49	0.58	9.53	7.02	0.09	0.68	0.16	14.40	11.79
	- VIII	0.58	0.51	0.54	9.40	7.17	0.23	0.57	0.33	10.73	8.71
	- IX	0.65	0.51	0.57	9.58	7.33	0.16	0.41	0.23	10.39	8.73
	- X	0.66	0.53	0.59	9.38	6.97	0.22	0.52	0.31	10.23	8.07
	- XI	0.62	0.53	0.57	9.34	7.13	0.37	0.49	0.42	9.81	7.61
	- XII	0.60	0.52	0.56	9.56	6.78	0.10	0.76	0.18	15.61	13.29
	- XIII	0.60	0.53	0.56	9.44	6.79	0.10	**0.80**	0.18	15.59	13.36
	- XIV	0.59	0.52	0.55	9.58	6.79	0.22	0.39	0.28	10.38	8.60
	- XV	0.66	0.57	**0.61**	9.29	6.73	0.08	0.09	0.09	10.55	10.06
	- XVI	0.60	**0.63**	**0.61**	**9.12**	6.74	0.59	0.49	0.54	9.76	**7.15**

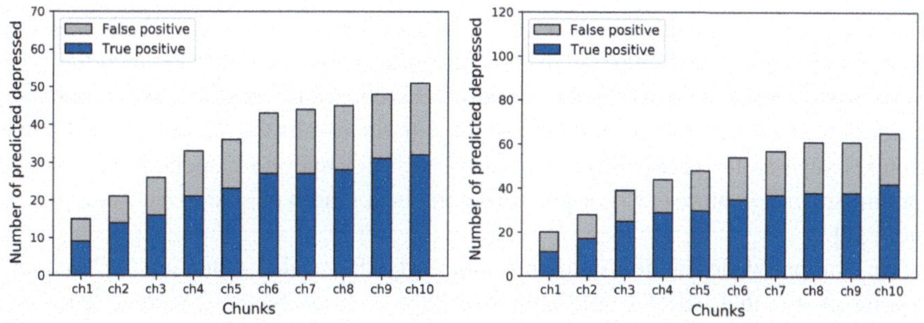

(a) 2017 (b) 2018

Fig. 3 The number of correctly predicted depressed users increases—256 features model with Random forest on eRisk data: **a** 2017 and **b** 2018

Reversely, we can observe that the lexical features (category XVI) are very useful: without this category, the results decrease both for precision and recall on eRisk 2017 and for precision on eRisk 2018. While the results are already quite high when these features are the only considered (inclusion study), the best overall result on 2017 collection and strong performance for 2018 collection. When considering the inclusion analysis, we can also observe that the textual representation (bag-of-words and POS (category I)) is also quite useful just by itself. With regard to the other categories, things are less definite (Table 8).

7 Visualization of Early Detection

The number of depressed predictions (true positives and false positives) per chunk is shown in Fig. 3 for the 256 feature model using Random forest. These are the users for which the system has made a decision on a given chunk. We mention both true positives (detected depressed users) and false positives (users detected as depressed while they are not).

8 Conclusion

In this chapter, we compared different models for learning from annotated examples to detect possible depression of users. Both the examples to train the models and the examples to test the prediction are composed of users' textual posts.

We first compared different ways of representing users: either considering some intuitive and domain-related features or considering straightforward word or document embeddings which does not need any domain expertise. We found that the results are better using domain-specific features although document embeddings are close. Document embeddings are most of the cases better than word embedding.

We also compared six well-established machine learning methods. We found that Random forest is the best. This is consistent with the results we obtained in different contexts such as for predicting the diffusion of information on social media using domain-specific features [15] or predicting the best search engine to use for a given query [9].

We compared depression detection and early depression detection. While our hypothesis was that BERT would outperform the well-established machine learning methods for depression detection, this is not the case. The data available is not enough for proper fine-tuning, even when not considering early detection to fine-tune properly the models.

The feature ablation analysis that we conducted informed us of the counter-intuitive result that emotion features are not efficient and can be omitted; this is probably due to the fact they are too sparse and not much used by the users-at least in the dataset we used for evaluation. De Choudhury et al. [4] also noticed that emotion is not significant for depression detection on Facebook data, but in their other study [5], where they used Twitter the emotion feature is significant for depression detection, especially negative emotion.

Acknowledgements This work is partially supported by the PREVISION project, which has received funding from the European Union's Horizon 2020 research and innovation programme under GA No 833115 (https://cordis.europa.eu/project/id/833115). The paper reflects the authors' view and the Commission is not responsible for any use that may be made of the information it contains.

References

1. Burdisso, S. G., Errecalde, M., & Montes-y-Gómez, M. (2019). *t-ss3: a text classifier with dynamic n-grams for early risk detection over text streams*. arxiv:1911.06147.
2. Burdisso, S. G., Errecalde, M., & Montes-y-Gómez, M. (2019). A text classification framework for simple and effective early depression detection over social media streams. *Expert System Application, 133*, 182–197.
3. Cacheda, F., Iglesias, D. F., Nóvoa, F. J., & Carneiro, V. (2018). Analysis and experiments on early detection of depression. In *Working Notes of CLEF 2018—Conference and Labs of the Evaluation Forum, Avignon, France, September 10–14, 2018*.
4. Choudhury, M. D., Counts, S., Horvitz, E., & Hoff, A. (2014). Characterizing and predicting postpartum depression from shared facebook data. In *Computer Supported Cooperative Work, CSCW '14, Baltimore, MD, USA, February 15–19, 2014* (pp. 626–638).
5. Choudhury, M. D., Gamon, M., Counts, S., & Horvitz, E. (2013). Predicting depression via social media. In *Proceedings of the Seventh International Conference on Weblogs and Social Media*.
6. Colombo, G. B., Burnap, P., Hodorog, A., & Scourfield, J. (2016). Analysing the connectivity and communication of suicidal users on twitter. *Computer Communications, 73*, 291–300.
7. Dai, A. M., Olah, C., & Le, Q. V. (2015). *Document embedding with paragraph vectors*. arXiv:1507.07998.

8. Dalloux, C., Claveau, V., Cuggia, M., Bouzillé, G., & Grabar, N. (2020). Supervised learning for the ICD-10 coding of french clinical narratives. In *Digital Personalized Health and Medicine—Proceedings of MIE 2020, Medical Informatics Europe, Geneva, Switzerland, April 28–May 1, 2020* (2020) (pp. 427–431).
9. Deveaud, R., Mothe, J., Ullah, M. Z., & Nie, J.-Y. (2018). Learning to adaptively rank document retrieval system configurations. *ACM Transactions on Information Systems (TOIS), 37*(1), 1–41.
10. Devlin, J., Chang, M.-W., Lee, K., & Toutanova, K. (2018). *Bert: Pre-training of deep bidirectional transformers for language understanding*. arXiv:1810.04805.
11. Fast, E., Chen, B., & Bernstein, M. S. (2016). Empath: Understanding topic signals in large-scale text. In *Proceedings of the 2016 CHI Conference on Human Factors in Computing Systems, San Jose, CA, USA, May 7–12, 2016* (2016) (pp. 4647–4657).
12. France, D. J., Shiavi, R. G., Silverman, S. E., Silverman, M. K., & Wilkes, D. M. (2000). Acoustical properties of speech as indicators of depression and suicidal risk. *IEEE Transactions on Biomedical Engineering, 47*(7), 829–837.
13. Funez, D. G., Errecalde, M. L., Villegas, M. P., Ucelay, M. J. G., & Cagnina, L. C. (2017). Temporal variation of terms as concept space for early risk prediction. In *Working Notes of CLEF 2017—Conference and Labs of the Evaluation Forum, Dublin, Ireland, September 11–14, 2017.*
14. Funez, D. G., Ucelay, M. J. G., Villegas, M. P., Burdisso, S., Cagnina, L. C., Montes-y-Gómez, M., & Errecalde, M. (2018). Unsl's participation at erisk 2018 lab. In *Working Notes of CLEF 2018—Conference and Labs of the Evaluation Forum, Avignon, France, September 10–14, 2018.*
15. Hoang, T. B. N., & Mothe, J. (2018). Predicting information diffusion on twitter-analysis of predictive features. *Journal of Computational Science, 28*, 257–264.
16. Iarivony Faneva, R. (2020). *Extraction et fouille de données textuelles: application à la détection de la dépression, de l'anorexie et de l'agressivité dans les réseaux sociaux*. Ph.D. thesis, Université de Toulouse.
17. Joulin, A., Grave, E., Bojanowski, P., & Mikolov, T. (2017). Bag of tricks for efficient text classification. In *Proceedings of the 15th Conference of the European Chapter of the Association for Computational Linguistics, EACL 2017, Valencia, Spain, April 3–7, 2017, Volume 2: Short Papers* (pp. 427–431).
18. King, G., & Zeng, L. (2001). Logistic regression in rare events data. *Political Analysis, 9*(2), 137–163.
19. Kulkarni, A. B. K. (2018). Early detection of depression. Master's thesis, University of Houston.
20. Le, Q., & Mikolov, T. (2014). Distributed representations of sentences and documents. In *International Conference on Machine Learning*, PMLR (pp. 1188–1196).
21. Li, J., Cheng, K., Wang, S., Morstatter, F., Trevino, R. P., Tang, J., & Liu, H. (2017). Feature selection: A data perspective. *ACM Computing Surveys, 50*, 6.
22. Li, Z., Xiong, Z., Zhang, Y., Liu, C., & Li, K. (2011). Fast text categorization using concise semantic analysis. *Pattern Recognition Letters, 32*(3), 441–448.
23. Low, L. A., Maddage, N. C., Lech, M., Sheeber, L., & Allen, N. B. (2011). Detection of clinical depression in adolescents' speech during family interactions. *IEEE Transactions on Biomedical Engineering, 58*(3), 574–586.
24. Malam, I. A., Arziki, M., Bellazrak, M. N., Benamara, F., Kaidi, A. E., Es-Saghir, B., He, Z., Housni, M., Moriceau, V., Mothe, J., & Ramiandrisoa, F. (2017). IRIT at e-risk. In *Working Notes of CLEF 2017—Conference and Labs of the Evaluation Forum, Dublin, Ireland, September 11–14, 2017.*
25. Marriott, T. C., & Buchanan, T. (2014). The true self online: Personality correlates of preference for self-expression online, and observer ratings of personality online and offline. *Computers in Human Behavior, 32*, 171–177.
26. Mikolov, T., Sutskever, I., Chen, K., Corrado, G. S., & Dean, J. (2013). Distributed representations of words and phrases and their compositionality. In C. J. C. Burges, L. Bottou, M. Welling, Z. Ghahramani, & K. Q. Weinberger, Eds. *Advances in Neural Information Processing Systems* (vol. 26). Curran Associates, Inc.

27. Mohammad, S., & Turney, P. D. (2013). Crowdsourcing a word-emotion association lexicon. *Computational Intelligence, 29*, 3.
28. Mowery, D., Park, A., Conway, M., & Bryan, C. (2016). Towards automatically classifying depressive symptoms from twitter data for population health. In *Proceedings of the Workshop on Computational Modeling of People's Opinions, Personality, and Emotions in Social Media* (pp. 182–191).
29. Organization, W. H., et al. (2017). Depression and other common mental disorders: Global health estimates. 2017. *Geneva: WHO*.
30. Øverland, S., Woicik, W., Sikora, L., Whittaker, K., Heli, H., Skjelkvåle, F. S., Sivertsen, B., & Colman, I. (2020). Seasonality and symptoms of depression: A systematic review of the literature. *Epidemiology and Psychiatric Sciences, 29*.
31. Ozdas, A., Shiavi, R. G., Silverman, S. E., Silverman, M. K., & Wilkes, D. M. (2004). Investigation of vocal jitter and glottal flow spectrum as possible cues for depression and near-term suicidal risk. *IEEE Transactions on Biomedical Engineering, 51*(9), 1530–1540.
32. Paul, S., Jandhyala, S. K., & Basu, T. (2018). Early detection of signs of anorexia and depression over social media using effective machine learning frameworks. In *Working Notes of CLEF 2018—Conference and Labs of the Evaluation Forum, Avignon, France, September 10–14, 2018*.
33. Pedregosa, F., Varoquaux, G., Gramfort, A., Michel, V., Thirion, B., Grisel, O., Blondel, M., Prettenhofer, P., Weiss, R., Dubourg, V., et al. (2011). Scikit-learn: Machine learning in python. *The Journal of Machine Learning Research, 12*, 2825–2830.
34. Peters, M., Neumann, M., Iyyer, M., Gardner, M., Clark, C., Lee, K., & Zettlemoyer, L. (2018). Deep contextualized word representations. In *Proceedings of the 2018 Conference of the North American Chapter of the Association for Computational Linguistics: Human Language Technologies, Volume 1 (Long Papers)* (pp. 2227–2237).
35. Radloff, L. (2015). A self-report depression scale for research in the general population. *Applied Psychological Measurement, 1*, 413–449.
36. Ramiandrisoa, F., & Mothe, J. (2020). Early detection of depression and anorexia from social media: A machine learning approach. In *Proceedings of the Joint Conference of the Information Retrieval Communities in Europe (CIRCLE 2020), Samatan, Gers, France, July 6–9, 2020*.
37. Ramiandrisoa, F., Mothe, J., Benamara, F., & Moriceau, V. (2018). IRIT at e-risk 2018. In *Working Notes of CLEF 2018—Conference and Labs of the Evaluation Forum, Avignon, France, September 10–14, 2018*.
38. Resnik, P., Armstrong, W., Claudino, L. M. B., Nguyen, T., Nguyen, V., & Boyd-Graber, J. L. (2015). Beyond LDA: exploring supervised topic modeling for depression-related language in Twitter. In *Proceedings of CLPsych@NAACL-HLT*.
39. Rude, S., Gortner, E., & Pennebaker, J. (2004). Language use of depressed and depression-vulnerable college students. *Cognition & Emotion, 18*(8), 1121–1133.
40. Sadeque, F., Xu, D., & Bethard, S. (2017). Uarizona at the CLEF erisk 2017 pilot task: Linear and recurrent models for early depression detection. In *Working Notes of CLEF 2017—Conference and Labs of the Evaluation Forum, Dublin, Ireland, September 11–14, 2017*.
41. Trotzek, M., Koitka, S., & Friedrich, C. M. (2017). Linguistic metadata augmented classifiers at the CLEF 2017 task for early detection of depression. In *Working Notes of CLEF 2017—Conference and Labs of the Evaluation Forum, Dublin, Ireland, September 11–14, 2017*.
42. Trotzek, M., Koitka, S., & Friedrich, C. M. (2018). Utilizing neural networks and linguistic metadata for early detection of depression indications in text sequences. *IEEE Transactions on Knowledge and Data Engineering, 32*(3), 588–601.
43. Trotzek, M., Koitka, S., and Friedrich, C. M. (2018). Word embeddings and linguistic metadata at the CLEF 2018 tasks for early detection of depression and anorexia. In *Working Notes of CLEF 2018—Conference and Labs of the Evaluation Forum, Avignon, France, September 10–14, 2018*.
44. Villegas, M. P., Funez, D. G., Ucelay, M. J. G., Cagnina, L. C., & Errecalde, M. L. (2017). LIDIC—unsl's participation at erisk 2017: Pilot task on early detection of depression. In *Working Notes of CLEF 2017—Conference and Labs of the Evaluation Forum, Dublin, Ireland, September 11–14, 2017*.

45. Wang, X., Zhang, C., Ji, Y., Sun, L., Wu, L., Bao, Z. A., & depression detection model based on sentiment analysis in micro-blog social network. In Trends and Applications in Knowledge Discovery and Data Mining - PAKDD,. (2013). International Workshops: DMApps, DANTH, QIMIE, BDM, CDA, CloudSD, Gold Coast, QLD, Australia, April 14–17, 2013. *Revised Selected Papers, 2013*, 201–213.
46. Xue, Y., Li, Q., Jin, L., Feng, L., Clifton, D. A., & Clifford, G. D. (2014). Detecting adolescent psychological pressures from micro-blog. In *Proceedings of the Health Information Science—Third International Conference, HIS 2014, Shenzhen, China, April 22–23, 2014* (pp. 83–94).

Quick and (Maybe Not So) Easy Detection of Anorexia in Social Media: *To Explainability and Beyond*

Hessam Amini, Elham Mohammadi, and Leila Kosseim

Abstract This book chapter overviews our participation to the first sub-task of eRisk 2019 shared task, which was focused on the task of early detection of anorexia in Reddit posts. Our approach was to utilize several attention-based neural sub-models to extract features and predict class probabilities, which were later used as input features to a Support Vector Machine (SVM) making the final classification. Our submission, named *CLaC* achieved F1 and latency-weighted F1 scores of 0.7073 and 0.6908 respectively, allowing it to rank first in terms of these metrics, and achieved competitive results based on other evaluation metrics. This book chapter also extends our participation to eRisk 2019, and includes the additional experiments that were performed on the model in order to evaluate it in terms of explainability.

1 Introduction

In the last decade, the use of social media to express personal thoughts, emotions, and ideas has become more and more prevalent. The analysis of online data can be useful for many purposes, such as business and marketing, political planning, prediction of stock market [10], as well as enhancing awareness of emergencies [33]. Another noteworthy line of research has focused on the detection of toxicity, hate speech, aggression and cyber bullying on online platforms; an effort that could facilitate timely interventions in violent situations [8, 30].

In healthcare applications, online posts have been used for detecting disease outbreaks [23], finding smoking patterns [29], and the identification of adverse drug

H. Amini (✉) · E. Mohammadi · L. Kosseim
Computational Linguistics at Concordia (CLaC) Laboratory, Department of Computer Science and Software Engineering, Concordia University, Montreal, QC H3G 1M8, Canada
e-mail: hessam.amini@mail.concordia.ca

E. Mohammadi
e-mail: elham.mohammadi@mail.concordia.ca

L. Kosseim
e-mail: leila.kosseim@concordia.ca

F. Crestani et al. (eds.), *Early Detection of Mental Health Disorders by Social Media Monitoring*, Studies in Computational Intelligence 1018,
https://doi.org/10.1007/978-3-031-04431-1_6

reactions [32]. Another useful application is the automatic detection of mental health issues, a relatively recent field which has attracted the attention of many researchers in Natural Language Processing (NLP). Corpora from Twitter, Facebook, blogs and online forums, and Reddit are used as resources to detect various mental health problems, such as anxiety, depression, suicide ideation, and eating disorders [3].

Although automatically monitoring online forums to detect cases of mental health issues is beneficial, the elapsed time between the first signs of a mental issue and the actual detection of a potential victim can play a crucial role. Earlier detection of a harmful behavior can help moderators better handle the situation. However, to the best of our knowledge, not much research has specifically addressed the task of early detection of mental health issues.

The eRisk shared task [16] was created with the goal of addressing issues related to early risk detection of mental health problems. According to [16], early detection can be useful in many applications from the identification of potential sexual offenders to the detection of victims of suicidal tendencies, making intervention possible before it is too late. Losada et al. [16] argues that while current risk assessment approaches often aim at detecting harmful behavior after the fact, it is very important to consider the timing of risk detection and to minimize the time between the observation of the first evidence of destructive behavior and triggering an alarm. To that end, the organizers of the eRisk shared task have encouraged the development of approaches which model the process rather than the outcome, as well as developing reliable evaluation metrics and test collections tailored to early risk detection.

The aim of this book chapter is to overview our participation to the eRisk 2019 shared task [18] and study the approach designed for the early detection of anorexia, in terms of explainability. In that sense, this work will be considered as an extension to Mohammadi et al. [22].

2 Related Work

Many researchers have used corpora from Twitter, Facebook, Reddit, blogs and online forums as resources to experiment with classification tasks pertaining to mental health issues [3].

Pestian et al. [27] experimented with different machine learning methods for suicide note classification. The features used in the study included words, part of speech tags, readability scores, and emotions. The best accuracy of 74% was achieved by a logistic regression model.

DeVault et al. [9] studied the symptoms of psychological distress in dialogues with a virtual agent. The use of a Naïve Bayes classifier for the detection of post-traumatic stress disorder (PTSD) and distress yielded a 20% improvement over the baseline accuracy of 53.5%, and showed that the automatic assessment of psychological distress is indeed possible.

More recently, Jackson et al. [12] used clinical texts obtained through the Clinical Record Interactive Search[1] to extract symptoms of severe mental illness. The authors made use of TextHunter [1] (a natural language processing information extraction tool) and an SVM classifier, and were able to classify 38 symptoms with an F1-score of 85%.

Shen and Rudzicz [28] used different feature sets including word2vec embedding, latent Dirichlet allocation topic modelling, lexico-syntactic features, and n-grams (unigrams and bigrams) to detect anxiety in Reddit posts. Initially, the authors compared the results achieved by an SVM and a 2-layer neural network. Though both classifiers performed well, the SVM yielded marginally better results. However, they achieved their best result of 98% accuracy using the neural network with n-gram probabilities and word embeddings combined with Linguistic Inquiry and Word Count (LIWC) features.

Coppersmith et al. [6] explored the automatic detection of post-traumatic stress disorder (PTSD), depression, bipolar disorder, and seasonal affective disorder (SAD) in Twitter data, using LIWC features and character and word n-grams, and found the latter resulting in superior performance.

Benton et al. [2] used multi-task learning to predict suicide risk and a variety of mental health conditions from Twitter data, including anxiety, depression, PTSD, and schizophrenia. It was found that a multi-task framework can be effectively used in cases with limited data.

Apart from individual efforts, shared tasks (e.g. [7, 20, 21, 34]) have also been organized to encourage the development of common benchmarks (datasets and metrics) and the comparison of approaches for the detection of distress in online textual data.

All of the previous work described above used a classic classification approach that does not measure how early the detection is performed. On the other hand, the eRisk shared tasks [16–19] focus on the early detection of mental health issues. In the first edition of eRisk [16], the data set used was a collection of social media posts and comments from depressed and non-depressed authors, recorded chronologically. As evaluation metric, Early Risk Detection Error (ERDE) was used, an error measure which assigns a penalty to late decisions and rewards early ones [15]. As it was the first edition of this shared task, many teams focused on making accurate rather than early decisions, with the highest F1-score being 64% and the lowest $ERDE_{50}$ score being 9.68% [16].

The second eRisk shared task [17] included two sub-tasks: Early risk detection of depression and early risk detection of anorexia. Like the year before, the ERDE evaluation metric was used as the main metric alongside F1, precision, and recall [17]. The best performing systems, in both sub-tasks, were designed by Trotzek et al. [31]. Their team experimented with different variations of bag of words features and a Convolutional Neural Network (CNN) [14] as well as ensemble models. In the depression sub-task, their system achieved an F1-score of 64% and an $ERDE_{50}$ of

[1] https://crisnetwork.co.

6.44%. In the anorexia sub-task, they achieved an F1-score of 85% and an $ERDE_{50}$ of 5.96%.

In eRisk 2019, the release of the data in the testing phase was changed from chunk-based (i.e. the method used in the previous eRisk shared tasks) to one-by-one. In this process, a decision by the models could be emitted at any point, but once a user was detected as positive by a model, it was not possible to revert back to negative after having more observations. The new evaluation metric *latency-weighted F1* was introduced by the organizers as the official metric, which was essentially an F1 score in time series, with an incremental penalty factor over time. The main reason for introducing a new evaluation metric was the fact that, ERDE was not capable of properly handling the new testing scheme, as the penalty factor in ERDE increased very quickly in one-by-one release of test data. The first sub-task of eRisk 2019 was focused on the early detection of anorexia, where our submission [22] achieved the highest latency-weighted F1 score of 0.6908 and significantly outperformed the second team with a margin of around 6%.

In this book chapter, we will revisit our participation to eRisk 2019 shared task, and will summarize the designed approach and results. We will also study our model in terms of its capability to provide explainability.

3 System Overview

Figure 1 shows the architecture of the model that we used for the eRisk 2019 shared task. The full model includes 8 different neural sub-models, followed by a fusion component, which concatenates the neural features and predicted class probabilities from different sub-models, and forwards them to a final SVM classifier.

This section will provide a more detailed explanation of the different components of the model.

3.1 Sub-models

As shown in Fig. 1, each sub-model includes an input layer that receives as input the posts by a user, and vectorizes its tokens using an embedding layer. The output of the input layer is then fed to a hidden layer, which is followed by a post-level attention/pooling layer that creates a representation of the post from its constituent tokens. The user-level attention layer is responsible for calculating the vector representation of the user, using her/his online posts. Finally, the output (classification) layer predicts the probability distribution of the positive and negative classes (i.e. anorexic versus non-anorexic).

Our main focus during the development of the sub-models was to include diversity of information sources, so that the final ensemble model can incorporate different points of views when performing the final classification.

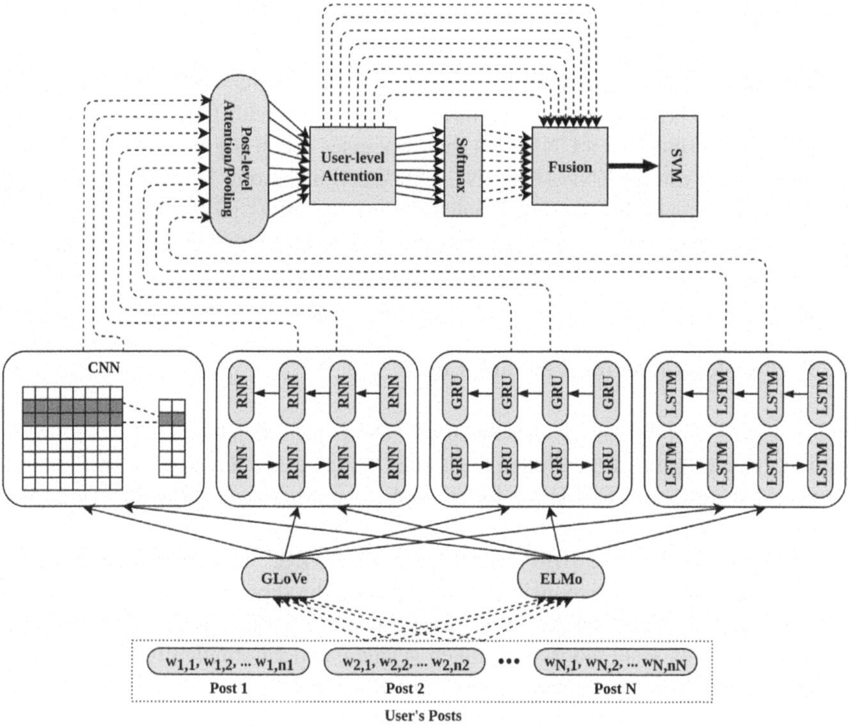

Fig. 1 Architecture of the model. The number of arrows between components corresponds to the number of sub-models that move in that flow. The rounded-corner boxes represent the components that work at the post level, while the sharp-corner boxes are user-level components. The solid lines represent neural connections; while the dotted lines show the flow of data without the existence of a neural connection. The bold arrow between the Fusion and SVM corresponds to the flow of data that exists only in the final model

3.1.1 Input Layer

The inputs to the model are the online posts of each user. Each post is first tokenized and the tokens are sent to the word embedder, in order to be converted into dense vectors. As shown in Fig. 1, these token vectors are then fed to the hidden layer.

Two different pretrained word embeddings were experimented with. The first word embedder was the 300d version of GloVe [26] that was pretrained on 840B tokens of web data from Common Crawl. The second word embedder was the original 1024d version of ELMo, which was pretrained on the 1 Billion Word Language Model Benchmark [4]. These two word embeddings were used in order to provide our ensemble model with sub-models that utilize both contextual (ELMo) and non-contextual (GloVe) word embedders in their input layer.

3.1.2 Hidden Layer

The hidden layer is responsible for processing the token vectors, generated by the input layer. As shown in Fig. 1, we have experimented with four hidden architectures in our sub-models: a CNN [14] that processes token n-grams separately, and a Bidirectional Vanilla RNN (BiRNN), a Bidirectional Long Short-Term Memory (BiLSTM) [11] and a Bidirectional Gated Recurrent Unit (BiGRU) [5], all of which process token vectors sequentially, from first to last and vice-versa, by taking into account the preceding and following tokens, respectively.

3.1.3 Post-level Attention/Pooling Layer

Following [31], for the sub-models that use CNN in the hidden layer, a max pooling is applied to the outputs of the hidden layer after being passed through a Concatenated Rectified Linear Unit (CReLU, i.e. ReLU applied on the concatenation of each vector and its negative).

In the models that use BiRNN, BiLSTM, or BiGRU in their hidden layer, an attention mechanism is responsible for computing the representation of a post (P) by weighted-averaging over the outputs of the hidden layer for each token in the post, where the weights assigned to each token is calculated automatically. The function used by the attention mechanism can be shown in Eq. 1:

$$P = \sum_{t=1}^{n} y_t \omega_t \tag{1}$$

where y_t represents the output of the recurrent hidden layer at time-step t, and ω_t is the weight assigned to the output in that time-step.

In our model, the attention mechanism uses an N-to-1 feed-forward layer (with the weights w, where N is equal to the size of the output vectors of the recurrent hidden layer) to map the output of the hidden layer at each time-step (e.g. y_t) to a scalar (e.g. v_t):

$$v_t = y_t \times w \tag{2}$$

These scalars are then concatenated, and softmax is applied to the resulting vector. The resulting vector from the softmax will include the weights that are used by the attention mechanism:

$$\omega = Softmax([v_1, v_2, v_3, \ldots, v_n]) \tag{3}$$

3.1.4 User-level Attention Mechanism

Knowing that the posts by a user do not contribute equally to evaluate her/his mental state [31], a user-level attention mechanism is used to have the system learn to automatically detect the contribution of each post to the final classification of the user.

The mechanism of the user-level attention is similar to the post-level attention mechanism, but it computes a vector representation of a user from the representation of her/his posts (resulting from the post-level attention/pooling).

3.1.5 Output (Classification) Layer

The final layer in the sub-models is a feed-forward fully-connected layer that maps the output of the user-level attention to a vector with size 2 (corresponding to the *negative* and *positive* classes). At the end of this layer, a softmax activation function gives as the output, the predicted probability distribution over the classes *negative* and *positive*.

3.2 Ensemble Model

As shown in Fig. 1, the ensemble model is composed of several neural sub-models, a fusion component, and a final SVM classifier. The fusion component concatenates the outputs of the user-level attention units (which will subsequently be referred to as neural features), and the predicted probability distributions of the two classes, resulting from the softmax activation functions from all its constituent sub-models. The output of the fusion component is taken as the final representation of a user. This representation is finally fed to an SVM classifier to perform the ensemble classification.

4 Experimental Setup

This section describes our experiments with the above model for our participation to the eRisk 2019 shared task [18].

4.1 Sub-models Implementation

PyTorch [24] was used to implement and train the sub-models. The Adam optimizer [13] was used, and the learning rate was set to 5×10^{-4}. Cross-entropy was

Table 1 Hyperparameter values used in the 8 sub-models

#	Name	Hyperparameters
1	CNN-GloVe	100 bigram convolution filters, trained for 10 epochs
2	CNN-ELMo	200 unigram filters and 50 bigram convolution filters, trained for 6 epochs
3	BiRNN-GloVe	one layer of 64 vanilla RNN units, trained for 14 epochs
4	BiRNN-ELMo	one layer of 50 vanilla RNN units, trained for 13 epochs
5	BiLSTM-GloVe	one layer of 32 bidirectional LSTM units, trained for 31 epochs
6	BiLSTM-ELMo	one layer of 64 bidirectional LSTM units, trained for 14 epochs
7	BiGRU-GloVe	one layer of 64 bidirectional GRUs, trained for 14 epochs
8	BiGRU-ELMo	one layer of 64 bidirectional GRUs, trained for 8 epochs

used as the loss function, and in order to handle the imbalanced distribution of the positive and negative classes in the training set (see Table 2.1), weights proportional to the inverse of the number of samples of each class were assigned to the classes. Due to limitations in terms of computational resources, mini-batches with a maximum size of 128 were used at the post level for each user and only the first 100 tokens of the posts were used.[2] In order to minimize the amount of padding in the batches, posts with similar number of tokens were assigned to the same batch.

In order to fine-tune the other hyperparameters of the sub-models (including the number and size of convolutional filters, number of recurrent units, and number of training epochs), each sub-model was individually trained on the training set and optimized on the validation set (see Table 2.1), based on F1 score. The specifics of the 8 different sub-models are shown in Table 1. Since each sub-model is composed of a unique pair of hidden layer and word embedding type, they will later be referred to as *<hidden-type>-<embedding-type>* (see the second column of Table 1).

[2] This limit only truncated a small number of posts, as the average length was ~37.47 tokens in the eRisk 2018 task 2 data.

4.2 *Ensemble Classifiers*

Scikit-learn [25] was used to develop the SVM classifier used in the ensemble model. Three different versions of ensemble classifiers were developed:

1. **Ens-Feat** is the version of the ensemble model that only utilizes the neural features. The SVM classifier in this version uses a sigmoid kernel. The γ and C parameters in the SVM were set to *auto* (i.e. 1/<number-of-features>) and 4, respectively.
2. **Ens-Prob** uses only the predicted class probabilities from the softmax activation function at the end of the neural sub-models. It utilizes a polynomial kernel with the degree of 1. The γ and C parameters in the SVM were set to *scale* (i.e. 1/[<number-of-features> × <variance-of-features>]) and 1, respectively.
3. **Ens-All** utilizes both neural features and predicted class probabilities in its SVM classifier, that uses a sigmoid kernel, and has its values of γ and C set to *auto* and 2, respectively.

4.3 *Submitted Runs*

Based on the results on the validation set, 5 runs were submitted to the shared task server. For the 1st and 2nd runs, *CNN-GloVe* and *CNN-ELMo* were used, respectively, as stand-alone models,[3] and *Ens-Feat*, *Ens-Prob*, and *Ens-All* comprised the 3rd, 4th and 5th runs.

5 Shared Task Results

Table 2 shows the official results of our submissions, as well as selected runs from other teams (as reported in [18]) that achieved the best result in terms of one of the official evaluation metrics, or achieved competitive results. For the results of our team (*CLaC*), we indicate in Table 2 the specific name of the models used in the five submitted runs.

As shown in Table 2, the model *Ens-All* achieved the highest F1 (0.7073) and latency-weighted F1 (0.6908) scores of all participants' runs. This was in line with our intuition that using an ensemble model that makes use of both neural features and predicted class probabilities from the 8 sub-models has a higher capability of detecting the correct class after observing a small number of writings. The results also show that the *CNN-ELMo* model can achieve F1 and latency-weighted F1 scores that are competitive to *Ens-All*, and outperforms *Ens-Feat* and *Ens-Prob* based on

[3] These two sub-models achieved the most promising results among all the sub-models, during the training phase.

these two metrics. The *CNN-ELMo* model also resulted in the best recall, $ERDE_5$ and $ERDE_{50}$, showing the potential of this model to be used independently for the task of early risk detection of anorexia.

Table 2, also shows that all our models, except *CNN-GloVe* (run 0) achieved significantly superior performances in terms of F1 score and latency-weighted F1 (teams *lirmm* and *INAOE-CIMAT* achieved the next best F1 and latency-weighted F1 scores). Run 1 of team *lirmm* achieved the highest precision. The best recall was achieved by run 2 of the team *Fazl*. Runs 0 and 4 of the team *UNSL* achieved the highest $ERDE_5$ and $ERDE_{50}$, respectively, where we could achieve competitive results using the *CNN-ELMo* model.

Finally, by comparing the results achieved by *CNN-GloVe* and *CNN-ELMo* in Table 2, we can observe the advantages of using ELMo to extract context-sensitive embeddings in achieving a better performance.

Although our systems achieved the best or competitive results according to different evaluation metrics, our implementation of the inference system could have been more efficient. In our system, at every iteration, all the available posts were processed again by the model. As the release of the test data was in a one by one fashion, our approach resulted in a time complexity which was quadratic to the number of posts. Considering that the majority of the processing time in our system was happening in running the ELMo embedder, this approach was not efficient enough to handle 2000 iterations in a timely manner.

Knowing that the post-level-representation computation component of our model (i.e. everything before the user-level attention component) was decoupled across posts, this aspect could have been leveraged in order to have the post representations

Table 2 Official results on the first sub-task of the eRisk 2019 shared task. *#writings*: maximum number of writings (Reddit posts) that were processed for a user, *P*: Precision, *R*: Recall, *l-w F1*: Latency-Weighted F1 score

Team	Model	Run	#writings	P	R	F1	$ERDE_5$ (%)	$ERDE_{50}$ (%)	l-w F1
CLaC	CNN-GloVe	0	109	0.45	0.74	0.56	6.72	3.93	0.54
CLaC	CNN-ELMo	1	109	0.61	0.82	0.70	5.73	3.13	0.69
CLaC	Ens-Feat	2	109	0.60	0.81	0.69	6.02	3.13	0.68
CLaC	Ens-Prob	3	109	0.63	0.76	0.69	6.27	3.55	0.68
CLaC	Ens-All	4	109	0.64	0.79	**0.71**	6.25	3.43	**0.69**
lirmm		0	2024	0.74	0.63	0.68	9.13	5.14	0.63
lirmm		1	2024	**0.77**	0.60	0.68	9.10	5.51	0.62
Fazl		2	2001	0.09	**1**	0.16	17.11	11.22	0.14
UNSL		0	2000	0.42	0.78	0.55	**5.54**	3.92	0.55
UNSL		4	2000	0.31	0.92	0.47	6.14	**2.97**	0.46
INAOE-CIMAT		3	2000	0.67	0.68	0.68	9.17	4.57	0.63

calculated only once and cached. Using this approach, at each iteration, the representations of the newly available posts would have been computed, and would have been passed to the user-level attention along with the retrieved post representations from the previous iterations. This would have reduced the time complexity to linear, making it more efficient to be able to handle all the 2000 iterations.

6 Explainability Analysis

We decided to study our approach a bit further, and investigate the usefulness of the user-level attention component as a means to explain our model's behavior. Due to achieving comparable results to the best performing model, i.e. the *Ens-All*, we focused our experiments on the *CNN-ELMo* model. Furthermore, in order to have an exclusive focus on explainability, early prediction was not included as a factor in these experiments. As a result, testing was done by utilizing the full test set.

6.1 Experiments

For our new set of experiments, first, we passed the posts for each user in the test set to the previously trained *CNN-ELMo* model. Utilizing the weights assigned by the user-level attention component of this model to every user's different posts, we ranked the posts of each user from the highest-weighted to the lowest-weighted. Then we monitored the performance of our model in the following two scenarios:

(1) When feeding only the n top weighted posts to the model: the n was gradually increased from 1 (i.e. only the top-weighted post from a user) to 1000.
(2) When doing scenario 1, but by having the user level attention mechanism being replaced with an average pooling layer.

Using the 2 scenarios mentioned above, we were able to monitor the performance of the model when only top-weighted posts from each user were provided. We could also evaluate the effect of the user-level attention through ablation.

6.2 Results and Discussion

The results from the experiments are shown visually in Fig. 2, and the original numerical data is provided in Table 3.

Looking at the solid lines in Fig. 2, it can be observed that increasing the number of available posts per user will generally lead to improvement in terms of accuracy, precision, and F1 of the model with the user-level attention (scenario 1), while leading to a drop in the recall. The solid lines also show that, as the number of available

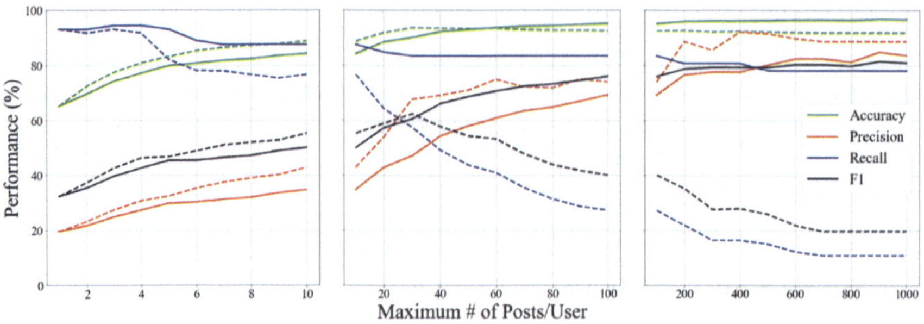

Fig. 2 Performance of the model in terms of the maximum number of highly-weighted posts from each user that have been provided during inference. The solid lines correspond to the model with user-level attention (scenario 1), while the dotted lines correspond to the model with user-level average pooling (scenario 2)

posts increases, the performance measures gradually converge to their final values, which is when all the posts by users are available. We hypothesize that the gradual improvement in precision and drop in recall is due to the behavior of the user-level attention that was used to rank a user's writings by assigning weights to posts based on the amount of signal indicating a user being anorexic. As a result, when a low number of highly-weighted posts is passed to the model, the model has a higher tendency to predict the author as anorexic leading to higher recall. We also believe that the convergence in the performance measures is because the lowest-weighted posts play a very small role in the model's prediction.

As the dotted lines in Fig. 2 show, increasing the maximum number of available posts from 1 to 10 will lead to gradual improvements in accuracy, precision, and F1, while causing a drop in the recall. It is hypothesized that, in general, the 10 highest-weighted posts include the necessary information for the model to make a prediction. It can also be observed that, the model with average pooling even achieves better improvements in terms of F1 and accuracy than the model with the user-level attention. We believe this is because the model with the user-level attention tends to get biased towards specific posts.

Looking at Table 3 and Fig. 2, it can be observed that, starting at 30 posts, the F1 score achieved by the model with the average pooling starts to deteriorate. The same thing happens to the accuracy of this model at 50 posts. Comparing the results with the ones achieved by the model with the user-level attention, it can be observed that the model with the user-level attention is more capable in handling a higher number of posts.

Finally, the rapid drop in the recall of the model with average pooling when increasing the number of available posts can be observed. This shows that, with a higher number of posts available for a user, this model loses its capability to recognize the patterns that are useful in the detection of anorexia. This observation is also aligned with the hypothesis that the weights assigned to posts by the user-level attention generally correlate with the level of signals for anorexia that the posts emit.

Table 3 Performance of the model (in percentage) in terms of the maximum number of highly-weighted posts from each user that have been used during inference. The columns titled *with Average Pooling* belong to the model in which the user-level attention mechanism is ablated. The last row belongs to the case when all the posts from each user are provided for the system

Max # of	With attention (Scenario 1)				With avg pool (Scenario 2)			
Posts/User	A	P	R	F1	A	P	R	F1
1	65.15	19.60	93.15	32.38	65.15	19.60	93.15	32.38
2	69.57	21.86	93.15	35.42	72.39	23.43	91.78	37.33
3	74.23	25.09	94.52	39.65	77.55	27.64	93.15	42.63
4	77.18	27.49	94.52	42.59	80.61	30.59	91.78	45.89
5	79.88	29.96	93.15	45.33	83.19	32.61	82.19	46.69
6	80.74	30.37	89.04	45.30	85.28	35.40	78.08	48.72
7	81.84	31.53	87.67	46.38	86.63	38.00	78.08	51.12
8	82.33	32.16	87.67	47.06	87.24	39.16	76.71	51.85
9	83.56	33.86	87.67	48.85	87.85	40.44	75.34	52.63
10	84.29	34.97	87.67	50.00	88.83	43.08	76.71	55.17
20	88.59	43.06	84.93	57.14	91.90	54.02	64.38	58.75
30	90.18	47.29	83.56	60.40	93.74	67.74	57.53	62.22
40	92.27	54.46	83.56	65.95	93.50	69.23	49.31	57.60
50	93.13	58.09	83.56	68.54	93.37	71.11	43.84	54.24
60	93.74	61.00	83.56	70.52	93.50	75.00	41.10	53.10
70	94.23	63.54	83.56	72.19	93.01	72.22	35.62	47.71
80	94.48	64.89	83.56	73.05	92.76	71.87	31.51	43.81
90	94.85	67.03	83.56	74.39	92.76	75.00	28.77	41.58
100	95.21	69.32	83.56	75.78	92.64	74.07	27.40	40.00
200	96.07	76.62	80.82	78.67	92.76	88.89	21.92	35.16
300	96.19	77.63	80.82	79.19	92.27	85.71	16.44	27.59
400	96.20	77.63	80.82	79.19	92.39	92.31	16.44	27.91
500	96.32	80.28	78.08	79.17	92.27	91.67	15.07	25.88
600	96.56	82.61	78.08	80.28	92.02	90.00	12.33	21.69
700	96.56	82.61	78.08	80.28	91.90	88.89	10.96	19.51
800	96.44	81.43	78.08	79.72	91.90	88.89	10.96	19.51
900	96.81	85.07	78.08	81.43	91.90	88.88	10.96	19.51
1000	96.69	83.82	78.08	80.85	91.90	88.88	10.96	19.51
2000 (all)	96.93	86.36	78.08	82.01	91.90	88.89	10.96	19.51

Table 4 Average weights assigned by the user-level attention mechanism to the *n*th highest weighted posts for users detected by the system as anorexic (W_p) or non-anorexic (W_n)

Rank	W_p	W_n	W_p/W_n
1st	0.388	0.056	6.96
2nd	0.124	0.034	3.66
3rd	0.067	0.026	2.62
4th	0.047	0.021	2.18
5th	0.035	0.019	1.86
6th	0.029	0.017	1.70
7th	0.024	0.015	1.59
8th	0.019	0.014	1.31
9th	0.016	0.013	1.23
10th	0.015	0.012	1.20

In order to further validate the explainability of the of user-level attention, we studied the values of the highest weights assigned by the attention mechanism. We focused on two categories of users: predicted by the model as positive (i.e. true positive and false positive), and predicted by the model as negative (i.e. true negative and false negative). For each category, we averaged the n-th highest weights assigned to the posts by the user-level attention. The results for this analysis is provided in Table 4.

As indicated in Table 4, in case users are predicted by the model as anorexic, the weights assigned to the highest weighted posts are, on average, 6.96 times greater in comparison to the users detected by the model as non-anorexic. This magnitude drops in lower-ranked posts and gradually converges to 1. This could convey that, the model is generally more likely to predict the anorexic label for a user, if the user-level attention mechanism assigns a high weight to a post by this user. It can also indicate that, in cases where the model makes a positive prediction, it has heavily relied on the evidence that it finds from a limited number of posts which it deems as important. This observation is also in support of the hypothesis that the weights assigned to posts by the user-level attention correlate with the amount of anorexia signals that the model finds in posts.

6.3 *Further Analysis*

We dug a bit deeper into the model, in order to evaluate the amount of contribution by the n-grams to the importance weights assigned to each post by the attention mechanism. Considering that the model utilizes unigram and bigram CNN encoders, we know that the model only uses these as initial information sources; hence, we focus our study on these n-grams only. Our approach is described as follows:

We start by considering only one convolution component with k kernels with a specific window size n. If it is applied over a post p containing N n-grams, and the output is fed to a CReLU layer, the output of the CReLU y would have the size $N \times 2k$. We consider y_i as the i-th column in y ($i \in [1 \ldots 2k]$), hence the length of y_i is equal to N. Equation 4 shows the formula to trace where the max element in y_i came from:

$$t_i^p = \text{argmax}(y_i) \tag{4}$$

Then, once the post representation is calculated by applying a max pooling to the output of the CReLU, we compute an *element-level contribution value* ECV_i^p by multiplying the element by its corresponding weight within the attention layer. Having ω_i as the attention layer's weight corresponding to the i-th element in the post representation, ECV_i^p is computed using Eq. 5.

$$ECV_i^p = \max(y_i) \times \omega_i \tag{5}$$

We then compute a *post-level contribution value* for each unique n-gram W within p. For each W, the post-level contribution value PCV_W^p is computed by summing over the ECV_i^ps for the values of i where the t_i^p-th n-gram is equal to W:

$$PCV_W^p = \sum_{i, w_{t_i^p} = W} ECW_i^p \tag{6}$$

The final *contribution value* for n-gram W is computed by averaging over the PCV_W^ps accross posts that actually include this n-gram. The process is shown in Eq. 7:

$$CV_W = \frac{1}{|P_W|} \sum_{p \in P_W} PCV_W^p \tag{7}$$

We ran the aforementioned method for both the unigram and bigram CNN encoders, and then ranked all the unigrams and bigrams based on their contribution value. We found that 99 out of the first 100 ranked n-grams are the names of mental or physical illnesses. The first rank belonged to the word "anorexia", and it was followed by "leukaemia", "dystonia", "leukemia", "preeclampsia", "poliosis", "anemia", "dyslexia", "osteosarcoma", and "insomnia". It is also interesting to find that the misspelled word "annorexia" was ranked 23rd based on the contribution value. This is mainly because of ELMo's good handling of morphological issues, which does not let the misspelled words be considered as out of vocabulary, but rather generates a meaningful embedding for them.

It was also observed that 85 out of the top 100 bigrams had all one thing in common, and it was having the word "weight" as their second token. The top bigram was "gain weight", and it was followed by "appropriate weight", "gained weight", "major weight", "versus weight", "muscle weight", "gaining weight", "good weight", "unwanted weight", "healthy weight", and so on. Overall, the unigrams were given higher ranks than the bigrams, with the highest-ranked bigram, "gain weight" showing up in the 81st rank. We also observed that the 15 top bigrams among the top 100, which did not include the word "weight" seemed generally irrelevant to the task (e.g. "fight fight", "video comparison", or "4-d chess") and may have merely been considered important by the model, due to their frequent occurrence within posts by anorexic users in the training data, and do not seem informative on their own.

Overall, the following observations have been made:

- The model considers the mentioning of the names of mental or physical illnesses as very important clues.
- The model relies more on unigrams than bigrams. This is supported by the overall higher contribution values of unigrams in comparison to the bigrams, the very shallow scope of the top bigrams, and the existence of possibly irrelevant bigrams among the top ones.

Observing the model's narrow scope of focus on specific unigrams and bigrams and keeping in mind the same model was the most-performing deep learning model in the task of early detection of anorexia, it is observed that the task of detection of anorexia is an n-gram triggered task in most cases and not a lot of contextual information is required for the model in order to make the correct prediction. However, this also implies that the model is biased on specific unigrams and bigrams, and may potentially make a wrong prediction merely based on observing those unigrams and bigrams in someone's social media posts. We believe that the use of recurrent models in the ensemble approach has helped to some extent in overcoming this limitation with the *CNN-ELMo* model, and has resulted in a slightly better performance in the *Ens-All* model. But we believe that further work needs to be done in order to develop a model that can better leverage contextual information, while still paying enough attention to the triggering n-grams.

7 Conclusion

This book chapter overviewed our participation to the first sub-task of eRisk 2019, and presented the ensemble approach which was used to detect anorexia in social media. The ensemble model utilized neural features alongside predicted class probabilities which are output by 8 different neural sub-models. Using this model and under the team name *CLaC*, our submission ranked first in terms of F1 and latency-weighted F1 scores in the first sub-task of eRisk 2019.

This book chapter also extended our paper at eRisk 2019 [22], and presented the experiments that were done in order to evaluate the explainability of the model. The experimentation results showed that the the user-level attention mechanism assigned weights to the posts based on the amount of anorexia signals that were present in posts. This capability could be leveraged in a real-life use case to provide a limited set of most signalling posts in order for the experts in clinical psychology to validate the model's predictions.

We also found out that, despite the model's high performance, it has limitations in terms of capturing useful information at the intra-post level, as it mainly focuses on the existence of certain unigrams and bigrams. A future direction for this research would be to develop a model that better captures contextual information in posts, while also not missing out on the important n-grams that are relevant in the detection of anorexia.

Acknowledgements This work was financially supported by the Natural Sciences and Engineering Research Council of Canada (NSERC).

References

1. Ball, M., Patel, R., Hayes, R. D., Dobson, R. J., & Stewart, R. (2014). TextHunter – a user friendly tool for extracting generic concepts from free text in clinical research. In *AMIA Annual Symposium Proceedings*, vol. 2014 (p. 729). American Medical Informatics Association.
2. Benton, A., Mitchell, M., & Hovy, D. (2017). *Multitask Learning for Mental Health Conditions with Limited Social Media Data* (pp. 152–162).
3. Calvo, R. A., Milne, D. N., Hussain, M. S., & Christensen, H. (2017). Natural language processing in mental health applications using non-clinical texts. *Natural Language Engineering, 23*(5), 649–685.
4. Chelba, C., Mikolov, T., Schuster, M., Ge, Q., Brants, T., Koehn, P., & Robinson, T. (2013). *One Billion Word Benchmark for Measuring Progress in Statistical Language Modeling.*
5. Cho, K., van Merrienboer, B., Gulcehre, C., Bahdanau, D., Bougares, F., Schwenk, H., & Bengio, Y. (2014). *Learning Phrase Representations using RNN Encoder–Decoder for Statistical Machine Translation* (pp. 1724–1734).
6. Coppersmith, G., Dredze, M., & Harman, C. (2014). *Quantifying Mental Health Signals in Twitter* (pp. 51–60).
7. Coppersmith, G., Dredze, M., Harman, C., Hollingshead, K., & Mitchell, M. (2015). *CLPsych 2015 Shared Task: Depression and PTSD on Twitter* (pp. 31–39).
8. Davidson, T., Warmsley, D., Macy, M., & Weber, I. (2017). *Automated Hate Speech Detection and the Problem of Offensive Language.*
9. DeVault, D., Georgila, K., Artstein, R., Morbini, F., Traum, D., Scherer, S., Morency, L.-P., et al. (2013). *Verbal Indicators of Psychological Distress in Interactive Dialogue with a Virtual Human.*
10. Giatsoglou, M., Vozalis, M. G., Diamantaras, K., Vakali, A., Sarigiannidis, G., & Chatzisavvas, K. C. (2017). Sentiment analysis leveraging emotions and word embeddings. *Expert Systems with Applications, 69*, 214–224.
11. Hochreiter, S., & Schmidhuber, J. (1997). Long short-term memory. *Neural Computation, 9*(8), 1735–1780.
12. Jackson, R. G., Patel, R., Jayatilleke, N., Kolliakou, A., Ball, M., Gorrell, G., Roberts, A., Dobson, R. J., & Stewart, R. (2017). Natural language processing to extract symptoms of severe mental illness from clinical text: The clinical record interactive search comprehensive data extraction (cris-code) project. *BMJ open, 7*(1), e012012.
13. Kingma, D. P., & Ba, J. (2014). *Adam: A Method for Stochastic Optimization.*
14. LeCun, Y., Haffner, P., Bottou, L., & Bengio, Y. (1999). *Object Recognition with Gradient-Based Learning* (pp. 319–345). In Shape: Contour and Grouping in Computer Vision.
15. Losada, D. E., & Crestani, F. *A Test Collection for Research on Depression and Language Use* (pp. 28–39).

16. Losada, D. E., Crestani, F., & Parapar, J. (2017). *eRisk*. Experimental foundations: CLEF lab on early risk prediction on the internet.
17. Losada, D. E., Crestani, F., & Parapar, J. (2018). *Overview of eRisk 2018: Early Risk Prediction on the Internet (extended lab overview)*.
18. Losada, D. E., Crestani, F., and Parapar, J. (2019). *Overview of eRisk 2019: Early Risk Prediction on the Internet*.
19. Losada, D. E., Crestani, F., and Parapar, J. (2020). *Overview of eRisk at CLEF 2020: Early Risk Prediction on the Internet*.
20. Lynn, V., Goodman, A., Niederhoffer, K., Loveys, K., Resnik, P., and Schwartz, H. A. (2018). *CLPsych 2018 Shared Task: Predicting Current and Future Psychological Health from Childhood Essays* (pp. 37–46).
21. Milne, D. N., Pink, G., Hachey, B., & Calvo, R. A. (2016). *CLPsych 2016 Shared Task: Triaging Content in Online Peer-Support Forums* (pp. 118–127).
22. Mohammadi, E., Amini, H., & Kosseim, L. (2019). *Quick and (maybe not so) Easy Detection of Anorexia in Social Media Posts*.
23. Ofoghi, B., Mann, M., & Verspoor, K. Towards early discovery of salient health threats: A social media emotion classification technique. In *Biocomputing 2016: Proceedings of the Pacific Symposium*, Kohala Coast, Hawaii, January 2016 (pp. 504–515).
24. Paszke, A., Gross, S., Chintala, S., Chanan, G., Yang, E., DeVito, Z., Lin, Z., Desmaison, A., Antiga, L., & Lerer, A. (2017). Automatic differentiation in PyTorch. In *NIPS 2017 Autodiff Workshop*, Long Beach, CA, USA, January 2017.
25. Pedregosa, F., Varoquaux, G., Gramfort, A., Michel, V., Thirion, B., Grisel, O., Blondel, M., Prettenhofer, P., Weiss, R., Dubourg, V., Vanderplas, J., Passos, A., Cournapeau, D., Brucher, M., Perrot, M., & Duchesnay, E. Scikit-learn: Machine learning in Python. *Journal of Machine Learning Research 12*, 2825–2830 (2011).
26. Pennington, J., Socher, R., & Manning, C. (2014). *GloVe: Global Vectors for Word Representation* (pp. 1532–1543).
27. Pestian, J., Nasrallah, H., Matykiewicz, P., Bennett, A., & Leenaars, A. Suicide note classification using natural language processing: A content analysis. *Biomedical Informatics Insights, 3*, BII–S4706 (2010).
28. Shen, J. H., & Rudzicz, F. (2017). *Detecting Anxiety Through Reddit* pp. 58–65.
29. Struik, L. L., & Baskerville, N. B. (2014). The role of facebook in crush the crave, a mobile-and social media-based smoking cessation intervention: Qualitative framework analysis of posts. *Journal of medical Internet Research, 16*, 7.
30. Thompson, J. J., Leung, B. H., Blair, M. R., & Taboada, M. (2017). Sentiment analysis of player chat messaging in the video game StarCraft 2: Extending a lexicon-based model. *Knowledge-Based Systems, 137*, 149–162.
31. Trotzek, M., Koitka, S., & Friedrich, C. M. (2018). *Word Embeddings and Linguistic Metadata at the CLEF 2018 Tasks for Early Detection of Depression and Anorexia*.
32. Yang, C. C., Jiang, L., Yang, H., & Tang, X. Detecting signals of adverse drug reactions from health consumer contributed content in social media. In *Proceedings of ACM SIGKDD Workshop on Health Informatics (HI-KDD 2012)*, Beijing, China, August 2012.
33. Yin, J., Karimi, S., Lampert, A., Cameron, M., Robinson, B., & Power, R. (2015). *Using Social Media to Enhance Emergency Situation Awareness*.
34. Zirikly, A., Resnik, P., Uzuner, Ö., & Hollingshead, K. (2019). *CLPsych 2019 Shared Task: Predicting the Degree of Suicide Risk in Reddit Posts* (pp. 24–33).

Two Simple and Domain-independent Approaches for Early Detection of Anorexia

Sergio Burdisso, Leticia Cagnina, Marcelo Errecalde, and Manuel Montes-y-Gómez

Abstract In this chapter, we describe the participation of our research team in the eRisk addressing the two editions of the early anorexia detection task. We used two domain-independent approaches to address this task. The first approach is based on a temporal-aware document representation, whereas the second one consists of a simple, interpretable, and novel text classification model specially designed for addressing early risk detection scenarios. Regarding the obtained results, in the first edition, we achieved the best $ERDE_5$ value among all participant models using the first approach, whereas with the second one, the best precision (0.91). Besides, using the latter approach, in the second edition, we were able to achieve the best values for both $ERDE_5$ and $ERDE_{50}$, and also promising results in terms of the ranking-based metrics, obtaining the best values, consistently, across all four rankings.

S. Burdisso (✉) · L. Cagnina · M. Errecalde
Universidad Nacional de San Luis (UNSL), San Luis, Argentina
e-mail: sburdisso@unsl.edu.ar; sergio.burdisso@idiap.ch

L. Cagnina
e-mail: lcagnina@unsl.edu.ar

M. Errecalde
e-mail: merreca@unsl.edu.ar

S. Burdisso
Idiap Research Institute, Rue Marconi 19, 1920 Martigny, Switzerland

L. Cagnina
Consejo Nacional de Investigaciones Científicas y Técnicas (CONICET), Buenos Aires, Argentina

M. Montes-y-Gómez
Instituto Nacional de Astrofísica, Óptica y Electrónica (INAOE), Puebla, Mexico
e-mail: mmontesg@inaoep.mx

F. Crestani et al. (eds.), *Early Detection of Mental Health Disorders by Social Media Monitoring*, Studies in Computational Intelligence 1018,
https://doi.org/10.1007/978-3-031-04431-1_7

1 Introduction

The term "mental health problem" comprises a broad spectrum of disorders that can be grouped into different categories, being "eating disorders" one of them [22]. Anorexia and bulimia are the most common eating disorders in childhood and adolescence years [7]. Both are characterized by an overvaluation of the weight and body shape such that even when people are underweight they try to avoid weight gain [8]. Anorexia is a severe psychiatric disorder with the highest mortality of all mental disorders [9] but can be worse in people facing a particular situation such as a pandemic. A recent survey showed that due to the COVID-19 pandemic, 62% of people in the U.S. with anorexia experienced a worsening of symptoms [20].

It is becoming increasingly common for people suffering from this kind of mental disease to share their own experience on social media, for instance, to seek support and containment. On the other hand, the increased use of social media and the advancement of computational technologies allow the extraction of valuable information to early prevent risky situations. In particular, early risk detection (ERD) on social media has become an important research area that is gaining increasing popularity [12–15] due to the potential impact it could have in people's lives—since early detection systems could help at-risk people to get the care and social support they need on time, before it is too late. This fostered the creation of the eRisk lab, hosted annually at the CLEF congress since 2017 [13], in which research teams from all over the globe can participate by creating different models to address specific ERD tasks.

Our team, UNSL, has participated in four of the five editions of the eRisk lab held to date. Throughout the different editions, we have participated using mainly two simple approaches, one based on a temporal document representation, called FTVT [6], and the other, on a novel text classifier that was specially designed for ERD scenarios, called SS3 [2]. Using these two approaches our team has obtained consistently competitive results in the different tasks proposed at each eRisk edition. For instance, among all participating teams, we achieve the best $ERDE_{50}$ value in the eRisk 2017's early depression detection task [5], the best $ERDE_5$ and precision in both early depression and anorexia detection tasks of the eRisk 2018 [6], the best $ERDE_5$ and $ERDE_{50}$, and the best overall ranking-based performance in both early anorexia and self-harm detection tasks of the eRisk 2019, and the best $F_{latency}$, F_1 and precision in the eRisk 2019's early self-harm detection task [3], and finally, the second-best $ERDE_5$ and $F_{latency}$ in the eRisk 2020's early self-harm detection task. Besides, using the SS3 classifier, we later obtained and published the best $ERDE_5$ and $ERDE_{50}$ reported values for the eRisk 2017 early depression detection task [2, 4] and the early depression and anorexia detection tasks of the eRisk 2018 [4].

This chapter describes how we addressed the early anorexia detection task. It is organized as follows: Sect. 2 introduces our two main approaches mentioned above, respectively, the FTVT representation and the SS3 classifier. Then, Sect. 3 describes in detail our participation in the two editions of this task, where details are given about how our models were implemented, trained, fine-tuned, and finally evaluated, as well as presenting and analyzing the obtained results. Finally, Sect. 4 summarizes the main conclusions and suggests possible future work.

2 Approaches

As with the other eRisk tasks, we used two different approaches to address the early anorexia detection task, one based on a document representation called FTVT, and the other, on a text classifier called SS3. Both FTVT and SS3, are introduced and described, respectively, in the following two sections.

2.1 Flexible Temporal Variation of Terms (FTVT)

As we described in the paper published on CLEF's eRisk 2018 track [6], the Flexible Temporal Variation of Terms (FTVT) is an improvement of the *temporal variation of terms* (TVT) document representation that we developed for the eRisk 2017 depression detection task [5]. The TVT representation is based on the *concise semantic analysis* (CSA) technique proposed by Li et al. [10]. CSA is a semantic analysis technique that interprets words in a space $\mathcal{C}$ of concepts that are close (or equal) to the category labels. For instance, if documents in the dataset are labeled with k different category labels, documents will be represented in a k-dimensional space. That space size is usually much smaller than standard BoW[23] representations which directly depend on the vocabulary size (usually much larger than the number of categories). CSA has been used in common text categorization tasks [10] and has been adapted to work in author profiling tasks under the name of *Second-Order Attributes* (SOA) [11].

More precisely, the TVT representation assumes we are dealing with chunk-based early risk detection scenarios as the ones originally proposed by Losada et al. [12]—and later used in the first two editions of the eRisk lab [13, 14]. That is, it assumes a corpus of documents written by p different individuals ($\{I_1, \ldots, I_p\}$). For each individual I_i ($i \in \{1, \ldots, p\}$), the complete chronological sequence of his/her d_i documents ($D_{I_i,1}, D_{I_i,2}, \ldots, D_{I_i,d_i}$) is split into n different "chunks", $C_{I_i,1}, C_{I_i,2}, \ldots, C_{I_i,n}$—therefore, $C_{I_i,1}$ contains the first $100/h\%$ of the documents of the individual I_i, chunk $C_{I_i,2}$ contains the second $100/h\%$, and so on. Then, models have to process those p individuals as p different sequences of n chunks and make a binary decision (as early as possible) on whether or not each individual might be a positive case of risk. Note that, as shown in Fig. 1a, using a standard CSA representation under this scenario will represent each individual I_i as a vector of only two concepts—since the decision is binary, there are only two category labels, *positive* (risk case) and *negative* (non-risk case). Instead, the TVT representation uses the additional temporal information available under this scenario to obtain an improved concept space. The underlying idea is that the variations of the terms (e.g. words)

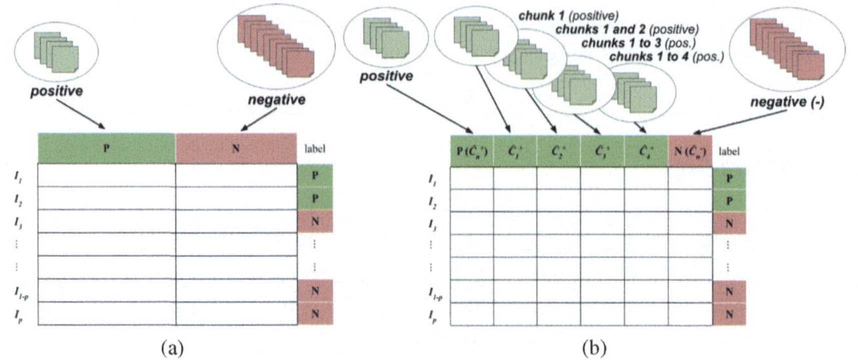

Fig. 1 Comparison of representations for early risk detection tasks: **a** Concise Semantic Analysis (CSA); **b** Temporal Variation of Terms (TVT) with $k = 4$

used in different sequential (temporal) stages can provide relevant information to the classification model. As a consequence, this representation enriches the documents of the minority *at-risk* class by including information of documents read in the first k chunks, as new CSA concepts in the original concept space. More precisely, in symbols, let $\hat{C}_j$ be the subset of the dataset containing only the first j chunks of each individual, $\hat{C}_j^+$ and $\hat{C}_j^-$ a partition of $\hat{C}_j$ in which $\hat{C}_j^+$ only contains the positive at-risk individuals and $\hat{C}_j^-$ the negative ones, then TVT uses the subsets $\hat{C}_1^+, \hat{C}_2^+, \ldots, \hat{C}_k^+$ as well as $\hat{C}_n^+$ (i.e. the complete positive dataset) as different concepts for the positive class and $\hat{C}_n^-$ (i.e. the complete negative dataset) for the negative class—as illustrated in Fig. 1b. Note that TVT not only enriches the original time-unaware representation with temporal information but also allows to address the unbalance of the minority class by augmenting it with this extra information. Preliminary results showed the potential of this representation, in comparison to CSA and BoW representations, to deal with ERD problems under this type of scenario [5]. Thus, when working with chunk-based early classification scenarios, as in the first two editions of the eRisk [13, 14], TVT naturally copes with both the sequential characteristics of ERD problems and also helps to deal with the class imbalance problem.

Finally, when we originally proposed this representation [5], the base CSA representation of the minority class was augmented by adding 4 extra dimensions. However, we then observed and empirically verified that, as expected, by varying this number, different performance was achieved depending on the specific o used for the ERDE_o measure to evaluate the results. Therefore, FTVT, the variant of TVT used in the present work, is simply a "flexible version" of the original TVT in which the user can specify the number k of chunks to be used to create the representation of the minority *at-risk* class. This number allows maximizing the model's performance according to the urgency level required for the specific ERD task (which is determined by the ERDE's threshold o). However, beyond this small distinction, TVT and FTVT are conceptually the same approaches.

2.2 *SS3 Text Classifier*

The SS3 text classifier is a novel classification model that we originally proposed in Burdisso et al. [2]. This model was specially designed and created with the goal of addressing early risk detection problems as naturally and integrally as possible. To achieve this, first, we noticed that these types of problems are especially challenging for conventional models because tackling them, as a whole, involves at least three key aspects: *sequence classification*, *early classification*, and also, given the sensitive nature of the problem, *model transparency and interpretability*. Then, we identified three key capabilities our model should have to tackle each of those three key aspects, respectively: *being able to work incrementally*, *provide support for early decision-making mechanisms*, and *having the ability to visually explain the reasons behind their predictions*. Finally, the SS3 text classifier was the result of our attempt to create a simple model that was able to integrate those three capabilities as a whole, naturally, by design. The following two sections briefly describe the model's training and the classification process, respectively.

2.2.1 Training

The SS3's training process is trivial since it only consists of building, for each given category, a dictionary to store word frequencies using all training documents of the given category. This simple training process allows the model to support online learning since when new training documents are available, instead of training again from scratch, the model only needs to update the dictionaries using the content of the new documents, making the training incremental.

Using the word frequencies stored in the dictionaries, the model computes a value for each word using a function, called gv,[1] to value words in relation to categories. This gv function can be computed "on demand" during classification or computed (and cached) as part of the training process. It takes a word w and a category c and returns a number, in the interval [0, 1], representing the degree of confidence with which w is believed to "be important" to c. Besides, since interpretability needs to be defined in a domain-specific way [18], we first defined what constituted interpretability by considering how people could explain to each other the reasoning processes behind a typical text classification tasks,[2] and then this gv function was designed to value words by trying to mimic that behavior –i.e. having gv to value words "the way people would intuitively do it". For instance, suppose categories are

[1] The name gv stands for "global value".

[2] As it turns out, for text classification, people would normally direct our attention only to certain "keywords" (filtering out all the rest) and explain why these words were important in their reasoning process.

$C = \{food, music, health, sports\}$, then, after training, SS3 would learn to assign values like:

$gv(\text{'}sushi\text{'}, food)$	$= 0.85;$	$gv(\text{'}the\text{'}, food)$	$= 0;$
$gv(\text{'}sushi\text{'}, music)$	$= 0.09;$	$gv(\text{'}the\text{'}, music)$	$= 0;$
$gv(\text{'}sushi\text{'}, health)$	$= 0.65;$	$gv(\text{'}the\text{'}, health)$	$= 0;$
$gv(\text{'}sushi\text{'}, sports)$	$= 0.02;$	$gv(\text{'}the\text{'}, sports)$	$= 0;$

To achieve this, the actual computation of gv is carried out by the product of three functions, lv, sg, and sn, respectively. In symbols:

$$gv(w, c) = lv_\sigma(w, c) \cdot sg_\lambda(w, c) \cdot sn_\rho(w, c) \tag{1}$$

The intuition captured by these functions can be briefly summarized as follows:

- $lv_\sigma(w, c)$ values a word based on the local frequency of w within c. As part of this process, the word distribution curve can be smoothed by a factor controlled by the hyperparameter σ.
- $sg_\lambda(w, c)$ captures the importance of w in relation to c. It is a sigmoid function that returns a value close to 1 when $lv(w, c)$ is "significantly greater" than $lv(w, c_i)$, for most of the other categories c_i; and a value close to 0 when, for all c_i, $lv(w, c_i)$ values are close to each other. The λ hyperparameter controls the "significantly greater" part, i.e. it allows to control how far $lv(w, c)$ must deviate from the median of all $lv(w, c_i)$ to be considered significant.
- $sn_\rho(w, c)$ decreases the final value in relation to the number of categories w is significant to. That is, the more categories c_i for which $sg_\lambda(w, c_i) \approx 1$, the smaller the $sn_\rho(w, c)$ value. The ρ hyperparameter controls how severe this sanction is.

As it is described in more detail by Burdisso et al. [2], the actual equation for each function was deduced by trying to capture a particular aspect/intuition involved in having gv assign a final value that, as mentioned above, matched our interpretability criteria. These equations are, respectively, the following[3]:

$$lv_\sigma(w, c) = \left(\frac{tf_{w,c}}{max\{tf_c\}}\right)^\sigma \tag{2}$$

where $tf_{w,c}$ denotes the frequency of w in c, $max\{tf_c\}$ the maximum frequency seen in c;

$$sg_\lambda(w, c) = \frac{1}{2} tanh\left(4\frac{(lv(w, c) - \widetilde{LV}_w)}{\lambda \cdot MAD_w} - 2\right) + \frac{1}{2} \tag{3}$$

where $LV_w = \{lv(w, c_i)|c_i \in C\}$, $\widetilde{LV}_w$ denotes the median of LV, $MAD_w = median(|lv(w, c_i) - \widetilde{LV}_w|)$ i.e. the *Median Absolute Deviation* of LV_w;

[3] Readers interested in knowing how these equations were determined are invited to read Sect. 3 of the original paper [2].

$$san_{\rho}(w,c) = \left(\frac{|C| - \left(\hat{C}_{wc} + 1\right)}{(|C| - 1)\left(\hat{C}_{wc} + 1\right)} \right)^{\rho} \tag{4}$$

where $|C|$ denotes the total number of categories and $\hat{C}_{wc}$ the accumulated "significance" of w across all the categories except c, in symbols:

$$\hat{C}_{wc} = \sum_{c_i \in C - \{c\}} sig_{\lambda}(w, c_i)$$

2.2.2 Classification

Before describing the overall classification process, we will introduce a vectorial version of the gv function since the classification process makes use of it. Namely, we will simply define $\overrightarrow{gv}$ as $\overrightarrow{gv}(w) = \langle gv(w, c_0), gv(w, c_1), \ldots, gv(w, c_k)\rangle$ where $c_i \in C$ and C is the set of all given categories. That is, $\overrightarrow{gv}$ takes a word and outputs a vector in which each component is the word's gv for each category c_i. Thus, for instance, given the previous example, we would have:

$\overrightarrow{gv}(\text{'}sushi\text{'}) = \langle 0.85, 0.09, 0.65, 0.02\rangle$;

$\overrightarrow{gv}(\text{'}the\text{'}) = \langle 0, 0, 0, 0\rangle$;

These vectors are called "confidence vectors" and, therefore, in the above example $\langle 0.85, 0.09, 0.65, 0.02\rangle$ is the *confidence vector* of the word "sushi" and $\langle 0, 0, 0, 0\rangle$ the *confidence vector* of "the".

As illustrated with an example in Fig. 2, the classification process can be thought of as a 2-phase process. In the first phase, the input is split into multiple blocks (e.g., paragraphs), then each block is in turn repeatedly divided into smaller units (e.g., sentences, words). Thus, the previously "flat" document is transformed into a hierarchy of blocks. In the second phase, the $\overrightarrow{gv}$ function is applied to each word to obtain the "level 0" *confidence vectors*, which then are reduced to "level 1" *confidence vectors* by means of a level 0 *summary operator*, $\oplus_0$.[4] This reduction process is recursively propagated up to higher-level blocks, using higher-level *summary operators*, $\oplus_j$, until a single *confidence vector*, $\overrightarrow{u}$, is generated for the whole input. Finally, the actual classification is performed based on the values of this single *confidence vector*, $\overrightarrow{u}$, using some policy—for example, selecting the category with the highest *confidence value*.

This process allows the model to possess the three desired capabilities: (a) keeping track of how the final vector $\overrightarrow{u}$ changes over time allows the model to *provide support for early decision-making mechanisms*, i.e. it allows deriving simple and clear rules to decide *when* the system should stop and make an early classification; (b) the model can visually explain the reasons behind the classification by painting, hierarchically, the different parts of the input in proportion to the values of the different *confidence*

[4] Any function $f : 2^{\mathbb{R}^n} \mapsto \mathbb{R}^n$ could be used as a *summary operator*. In this example, vector addition was used for $\oplus_1$ but not for $\oplus_0$ to highlight this fact.

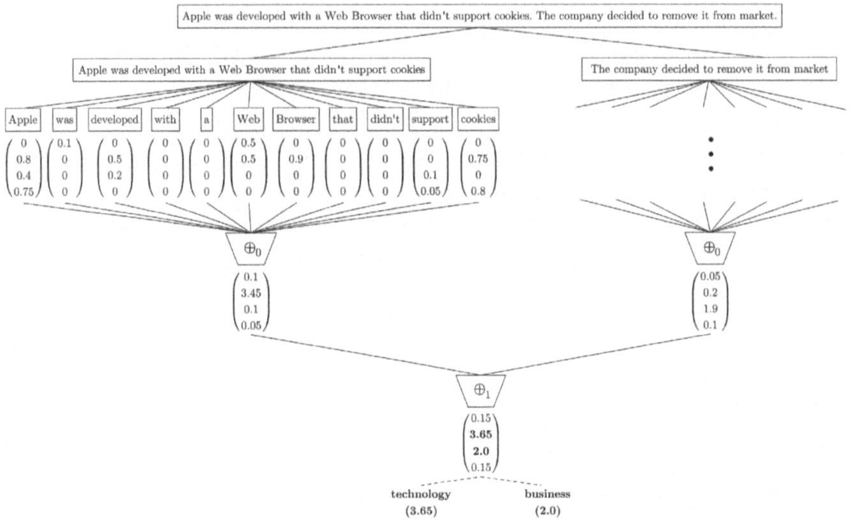

Fig. 2 Classification process for a hypothetical example document "Apple was developed with a Web Browser that didn't support cookies. The company decided to remove it from market". In the first stage, this document is split into two sentences (for instance, by using the dot as a delimiter) and then each sentence is split into single words. In the second stage, *global values* are computed for every word to generate the first set of *confidence vectors*. Then, all these word vectors are reduced by the $\oplus_0$ operator to sentence vectors, $\langle 0.1, 3.45, 0.1, 0.05\rangle$ and $\langle 0.05, 0.2, 1.9, 0.1\rangle$ for the first and second sentence respectively. After that, these two sentence vectors are reduced by another operator ($\oplus_1$, which in this case is the addition operator) to a single *confidence vector* for the entire document, $\langle 0.15, 3.65, 2.0, 0.15\rangle$. Finally, a policy is applied to this vector to make the classification—which in this example was to select *technology*, the category with the highest value, and also *business* because its value was "close enough" to *technology*'s

vectors in the hierarchy[5]; (c) finally, this process also allows the model to work incrementally, so long as the *summary operator* for the highest level can be computed incrementally. For instance, suppose that later, a new sentence is appended to the example shown in Fig. 2. Since $\oplus_1$ is the vector addition, instead of processing the whole document again, the already computed vector, $\langle 0.15, 3.65, 2.0, 0.15\rangle$, is simply updated by adding the new sentence *confidence vector* to it.

[5] A live demo is provided at http://tworld.io/ss3where the interested readers can try out the model online. Along with the classification result, the demo provides an interactive visual explanation as the one suggested here. We believe explanations like these are vital when models' predictions could affect people's lives since it allows human experts to inspect the reasons behind the classifications and validate them [Las accessed date: April 2021].

3 Participation and Results

In this section, we show the details of our participation addressing the eRisk's early detection of anorexia tasks. We first describe the experimental settings, then we present the results obtained after the evaluation stage. Our team participated in the two editions of this task, eRisk 2018 [6] and 2019 [3]. Since the evaluation was performed differently in the two editions,[6] this section is organized in two main subsections, one for each one.

3.1 Early Detection of Anorexia—2018 Edition

The 2018 edition had the participation of 9 different research teams and a total of 34 models were submitted. As described in more detail in our eRisk paper [6], we participated with five models, three of them made use of the FTVT representation (referred as to UNSLA, UNSLB, and UNSLC) and the other two (UNSLD and UNSLE), used the SS3 classifier.

The three models using the FTVT representation used the same early classification policy which was based on the probability p assigned by the classifiers. More precisely, as soon as the probability exceeded some given threshold θ (i.e. $p \geq \theta$), the subject was classified as positive (at risk). Since we also participated in the early depression detection task of this eRisk edition, to obtain more confident statistics, we used only the depression training set for setting the parameters of our models because it was the largest. Thus, in order to find the best values for this threshold θ, as well as the other parameters, we performed a *stratified 5-fold cross-validation* on the depression training set and then we carried out two grid searches, one minimizing the $ERDE_5$ measure, and the other the $ERDE_{50}$. In addition to optimizing the probability threshold θ, the grid search also evaluated different values for the FTVT's n parameter (number of chunks used to enrich the representation of the positive class), as well as different classification models. Namely, we considered values ranging from 0 to 5 for the n parameter, the values 0.6, 0.7, 0.8 and 0.9 for the threshold θ, and different classification models such as Logistic Regression (LR), Support Vector Machine (SVM), and Naive Bayes (NB)—these models were coded in Python 2.7 using the implementation provided by the *Scikit-learn* package with the default parameters. Finally, from the results obtained after the grid searches we selected the following 3 models for participating:

- *UNSLA*: an SVM classifier using the FTVT representation with $n = 0$ and a probability threshold $\theta = 0.8$. This model was selected because it obtained the best $ERDE_5$ of 13.58 compared to the second-best model which achieved 13.68. Note

[6] For instance, in the first edition [13] the release of the evaluation data was chunk-by-chunk whereas, in the second edition [14], user content was released post by post. Additionally, a new set of evaluation metrics was used.

that, from Sect. 2.1, this $n = 0$ means that no enrichment of the positive class is performed in the FTVT representation, and thus, the actual representation is identical to the standard CSA representation.
- *UNSLB*: a Logistic Regression classifier using the FTVT representation with $n = 2$ and a probability threshold $\theta = 0.6$. This model was selected because it obtained the best balance between $ERDE_5$ and $ERDE_{50}$.
- *UNSLC*: an SVM classifier using the FTVT representation with $n = 4$ and a probability threshold $\theta = 0.7$. This model was selected because it obtained the best $ERDE_{50}$.

As mentioned at the beginning of this section, the remaining 2 models, UNSLD and UNSLE, did not use the FTVT representation and instead used the SS3 classifier. In particular, these two models used a version of the SS3 classifier in which the vector addition was used as the *summary operator*, $\oplus_j$, for all the hierarchy levels and, as a consequence, the classification process was simplified to the following word summation:

$$\overrightarrow{u} = \sum_{w \in S} \overrightarrow{gv}(w) \tag{5}$$

where S is the subject's writing history. Note that, in this particular task, $\overrightarrow{u}$ is a vector with two components, one for the positive *at-risk* class (anorexic) and the other for the negative one. The early classification policy used to classify a subject as at-risk was performed by analyzing how $\overrightarrow{u}$ changed over time (i.e. over "chunks"). More precisely, subjects were classified as positive when the accumulated positive confidence value exceeded the negative one, as shown in Fig. 3. Regarding the hyperparameter values, they were manually selected using a subset of the training set as a validation set, from which we obtained the following 2 model configurations for participating:

- *UNSLD*: SS3 classifier with $\sigma = 0.5$, $\rho = 1$ and $\lambda = 3$.
- *UNSLE*: SS3 classifier with the same hyperparameter configuration as UNSLD but with $\lambda = 7$.

Since a word's value has to be 7 ($\lambda = 7$) times greater than the median to be considered by UNSLE, we expected this model to yield a higher precision than UNSLD with the risk of having a lower recall. Similarly, by having $\lambda = 3$, UNSLD was meant to consider a wider range of words as being "important", thus, we expected this model to have a higher recall compared to UNSLE.

Finally, we trained our 5 models using the entire training set available for this task and proceeded to the evaluation stage in which they were evaluated along with all the other 29 participant models. The results obtained by our 5 models, after the evaluation stage, are shown in Table 1. As we can see, UNSLB obtained the best $ERDE_5$ (11.40%) and UNSLD the best precision (0.91) value among all participant models. It is worth mentioning, again, that the parameters for the models using the FTVT representation were not specially selected for the anorexia task but for the depression task and yet, they obtained good results, especially UNSLB and UNSLC.

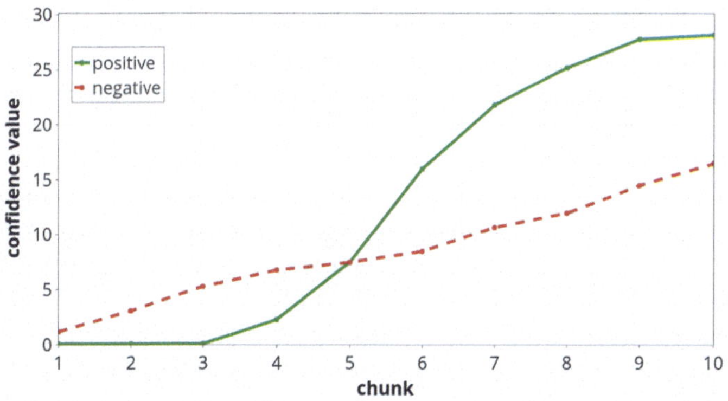

Fig. 3 Subject 9579's confidence vector $\overrightarrow{u}$ variation over time (chunks). This plot shows how the positive and negative values stored in $\overrightarrow{u}$ changed as more chunks were processed for this subject. For instance, only after processing the 3rd chunk, the positive confidence started to grow, probably because this subject was talking about topics not related to anorexia up until that point. Finally, after the 5th chunk, the positive confidence outweighed the negative one and the subject is classified as "anorexic"

Table 1 Results obtained by our five models on the eRisk 2018 early anorexia detection task. For comparison, the models that obtained the best results for the other 7 participating teams are also included

Model	$ERDE_5$ (%)	$ERDE_{50}$ (%)	R	P	F_1
UNSLA	12.48	12.00	0.10	0.57	0.17
UNSLB	**11.40**	7.82	0.51	0.75	0.61
UNSLC	11.61	7.82	0.51	0.75	0.61
UNSLD	12.93	9.85	0.71	**0.91**	0.79
UNSLE	12.93	10.13	0.63	0.90	0.74
FHDO-BCSGD	12.15	**5.96**	**0.88**	0.75	0.81
FHDO-BCSGE	11.98	6.61	0.83	0.87	**0.85**
PEIMEXB	12.41	7.79	0.73	0.57	0.64
RKMVERIA	12.17	8.63	0.56	0.82	0.67
LIIRB	13.05	10.33	0.73	0.79	0.76
LIIRA	12.78	10.47	0.63	0.81	0.71
TBSA	13.65	11.14	0.76	0.60	0.67
UPFA	13.18	11.34	0.71	0.74	0.72
UPFD	12.93	12.30	0.46	0.86	0.60
TUA1C	13.53	12.57	0.32	0.42	0.36
LIRMMB	14.45	12.62	0.71	0.41	0.52
LIRMMA	13.65	13.04	0.56	0.52	0.54

UNSLA did not obtain competitive results and its performance was the lowest among all participating models. This suggests that, in fact, the "temporal enrichment" performed by the FTVT representation does have a considerable positive impact on the classifier performance.[7]

Regarding the two models using the SS3 classifier, as we expected, UNSLE obtained a recall lower than UNSLD's since it considers fewer words as being important—only words whose values are 7 times greater than the median. However, against our expectation, UNSLE's precision was also lower than UNSLD's—we were expecting a higher precision given that words were more strictly selected. This suggests that $\lambda = 3$ represents a good balance between recall and precision, and that increasing its value further, i.e. being more strict at selecting words, only yields a lower recall. Among our 5 models, both SS3 models achieved a better performance than the 3 FTVT models in terms of the standard (timeless) measures but were considerably less efficient in terms of the ERDE measures. However, we later discovered that we could have also obtained a better performance in terms of the ERDE measures with the SS3 classifier if we had used the same hyperparameter configuration as the one used in the chunk-based experimental scenario for the early depression detection task in the SS3's original paper [2]. More precisely, as we published later [4], an SS3 classifier with $\lambda = \rho = 1$ and $\sigma = 0.45$ would have outperformed all three FTVT-based models by achieving a better performance in term of standard measures (0.71, 0.77 and 0.66 for F_1, precision and recall, respectively) as well as in terms of both ERDE measures—obtaining the best $ERDE_5$ value (11.31%) and the second-best $ERDE_{50}$ value (6.26%) among all participating models.

Finally, it is interesting to mention that the FHDO-BCSGD model was a Convolutional Neural Network (CNN) with an architecture consisting of 100 filters with 2 feature maps, and a max-pooling layer followed by 4 fully connected layers. In addition, the input of this network consisted of 6 million different word embeddings (fastText) manually trained using a dataset of 1.7 billion Reddit comments specifically built for this task [21]. On the other hand, FHDO-BCSGE consisted of a late fusion ensemble of other FHDO-BCSG's models, namely, an ensemble of two CNN models (one of which is FHDO-BCSGD) with a model that, in turn, is an ensemble of 4 Logistic Regressions with different BoW representations augmented with hand-crafted domain-specific metadata [21]. The complexity of these models contrasts with the simplicity of ours which, besides using simpler classifiers, did not make use of any external resources besides the available training data. For instance, UNSLD consisted only of a simple SS3 classifier[8] and yet its performance in terms of standard measures (F_1, precision and recall) were comparable to the more complex FHDO-BCSG's models described above—i.e. despite its simplicity, this SS3 model not only achieved the best precision (0.91) among the participating models but also

[7] Note that, unlike UNSLB and UNSLC, UNSLA used FTVT with $n = 0$ and, therefore, the actual representation was identical to a standard CSA representation—with no temporal chunk-based enrichment of the positive class.

[8] Which simply consisted of a summation of word values learned from the available training data (Eq. 5).

obtained an F_1 value (0.79) that was only outperformed by the considerably more complex FHDO-BCSG's models (0.81 and 0.85).

3.2 Early Detection of Anorexia—2019 Edition

As described in more detail in the overview of the 2019 edition of the eRisk [15], the task was intended as a continuation of the previous edition, so even though a new test set was built, the training set was formed by joining the 2018 Edition's training and test sets. As indicated at the beginning of this section, the evaluation methodology was different from the previous one since users were no longer processed using the chunk-by-chunk approach. Instead, they were processed in a more realistic way, one post (writing) at a time. Also, performance evaluation was improved since, in addition to reporting the time taken for each team to complete the task, two different types of metrics were used. The first type was focused on early classification decisions, and the second on rankings of users by risk level (estimated by the models). More precisely, in addition to the ERDE measure, this edition also incorporated the $F_{latency}$ [19] measure as an extra decision-based metric. Regarding the ranking-based metrics, to create the rankings for evaluating each model, after processing each user post, models were asked to respond with a score representing the risk level estimated for each user up to that moment. Then, for each participating model, the ranking was created by ordering the users using the given score. Finally, the quality of the rankings was evaluated using two standard IR metrics, $P@k$, and $NDCG@k$. Specifically, models were evaluated in terms of $P@10$, $NDCG@10$, and $NDCG@100$ for 4 different rankings, the one obtained after processing, respectively, 1, 100, 500, and 1000 user posts.

The 2019 edition had the participation of 13 different research teams and a total of 50 models were submitted. As described in more detail in our eRisk paper [3], in this edition we also participated with five models. However, due to this edition replacing the chunk-based release of users data by a more realistic post-by-post one, unlike in the previous edition, none of our five models used the FTVT representation and, instead, all of them were implemented using the SS3 classifier. This decision was motivated by the promising results previously obtained with SS3 [2, 4] as well as by the fact that, unlike the FTVT representation that requires the input data being released using the chunk-by-chunk approach, SS3 was designed to naturally work over text streams and, as a consequence, it can naturally process data incrementally regardless of the specific approach being used to release it—e.g. chunk-by-chunk, post-by-post, word-by-word, and so on.

In this edition we again made use of the same simple version of the SS3 classifier as in the 2018 edition (Eq. 5) and the same simple early classification policy—i.e. subjects were classified as positive as soon as the accumulated positive confidence value exceeded the negative one. However, this time we did use the hyperparameter configuration with which, as mentioned in the previous section, we could have obtained the best ERDE values in the 2018 edition—i.e. we used $\lambda = \rho = 1$ and

$\sigma = 0.45$ for our five SS3 models. We decided to use this configuration for all five models because in previous experiments they showed to be very effective and robust in terms of the ERDE measures [2, 4].[9] Finally, since we used the same classifier with the same hyperparameter configuration for our five models, the main difference among them was given by the amount of data used for the training and whether the model took into account only words or also bigrams, as described below:

- *UNSL#0*: the model was trained only with a subset of the total training data available for this edition. Particularly, the training was performed using only the data equivalent to the training set of the 2018 edition. The idea behind this model was to evaluate the consistency and robustness of results obtained in that edition.
- *UNSL#1*: this model was the same as the previous one but allowing SS3 to also recognize word bigrams—i.e. SS3 learned to compute $gv(w_0, c)$ as well as $gv(w_0w_1, c)$ for each w_0, w_1 seen during training. This variant was driven by good preliminary results obtained by SS3 using variable-length word n-grams with data from previous eRisk editions [4].
- *UNSL#2*: this model was, again, the same as UNSL#0 but this time, the training was performed using all available data for this edition—i.e. joining training set and test sets from the 2018 edition.
- *UNSL#3*: this model was the same as UNSL#2 but, as with UNSL#1, allowing SS3 to also recognize word bigrams.
- *UNSL#4*: this model was a slightly modified version of the UNSL#2 model in which, during the classification process, only words with a *global value* greater than 0.3 were taken into account—i.e. SS3 assigned $gv(w, c_i) = 0$ to all w and c_i such that $gv(w, c_i) \leq 0.3$.[10] With this variant, we tried to measure what impact words with a low *global value* have on classification performance. That is, with this model we intended to address questions such as: "How sensitive is the model to the noise that could be caused by a large number of words with low *global value*?" or "Could it be the case that because of words with low *global value* the early classification policy condition could be incorrectly triggered due to the noise accumulated by processing them?".

Besides, since in this edition, as described above, models were also asked to provide a score representing the risk level estimated for each user, we used the user *confidence vector*, $\overrightarrow{u}$ in Eq. 5, to calculate this score simply as the difference between the positive and negative *confidence value*, that is:

$$\text{score} = \overrightarrow{u}[positive] - \overrightarrow{u}[negative] \quad (6)$$

[9] This hyperparameter configuration was originally discovered with the eRisk 2017 early depression detection dataset by applying a grid search to minimize the ERDE_{50} metric with the training set using a 4-fold cross-validation [2].

[10] Using the training data, starting from 0 and incrementally, different values were tested from which 0.3 was finally selected for obtaining the best ERDE_{50}.

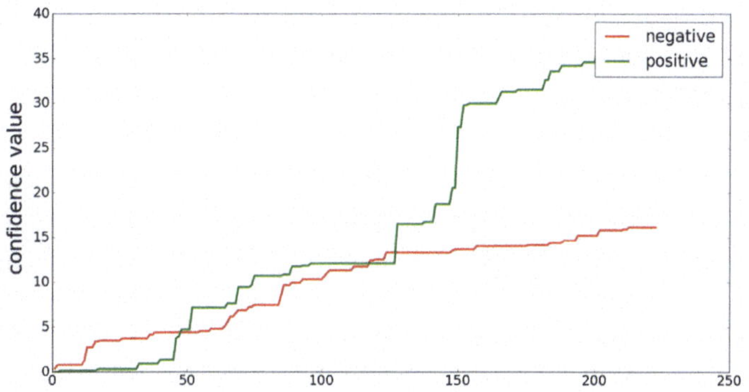

(a)

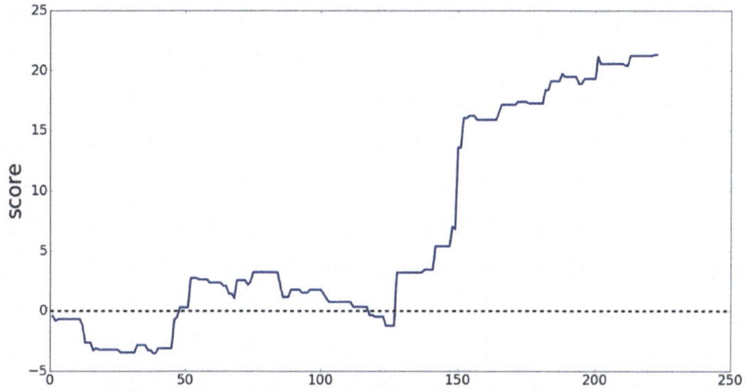

(b)

Fig. 4 Values for one of the actual users (subject 968) from the test set used for this task. **a** Variation of our model's positive and negative *confidence value* over time (post by post) for this user. **b** Variation of our model's estimated score over time for this user. Note that this user was classified as at-risk after processing around 50 of his/her posts, i.e. as positive as soon as the positive value exceeded the negative one or, equivalently, when the score became a positive number

As illustrated with an example in Fig. 4, this simple subtraction allows the two positive and negative confidence values to be represented, at any point in time, by a single and unified confidence value that no longer represents the confidence value for each class, but rather, a "decision-making" confidence value that represents the risk level estimated by the model used to classify and detect at-risk users.

Finally, after training our models we proceeded to the evaluation stage along with all the other 45 participant models, in which models had to connect to the remote server to receive user posts and to send their decisions along with the estimated risk level. The main results obtained with our 5 models are described below, grouped according to the type of metric used to measure performance:

Table 2 Results obtained for the early classification decision-based performance measures (sorted by $ERDE_{50}$). For comparison, the models that obtained the best results for the other 12 participating teams are also included

Model	$ERDE_5$ (%)	$ERDE_{50}^{\blacktriangle}$ (%)	$F_{latency}$	R	P	F_1
UNSL#4	6.14	**2.96**	0.46	0.92	0.31	0.47
UNSL#2	5.56	3.34	0.50	0.86	0.36	0.51
UNSL#3	5.59	3.48	0.49	0.85	0.35	0.50
UNSL#0	**5.53**	3.92	0.55	0.78	0.42	0.55
UNSL#1	5.68	4.10	0.55	0.75	0.43	0.55
CLaC#1	5.73	3.12	0.69	0.82	0.61	0.70
BiTeM#1	5.89	3.40	0.54	0.70	0.44	0.54
CLaC#4	6.25	3.42	**0.69**	0.79	0.64	**0.71**
UDE#0	8.48	3.87	0.58	0.74	0.51	0.61
UDE#1	7.48	3.94	0.53	0.73	0.44	0.55
INAOE-CIMAT#0	9.29	3.98	0.62	0.78	0.56	0.66
LTL-INAOE#1	7.74	4.19	0.55	0.75	0.47	0.58
INAOE-CIMAT#3	9.17	4.75	0.63	0.68	0.67	0.68
SINAI#2	9.04	4.89	0.30	0.95	0.18	0.30
INAOE-CIMAT#4	9.12	5.07	0.61	0.63	0.69	0.66
lirmm#0	9.13	5.14	0.63	0.63	0.74	0.68
lirmm#1	9.10	5.51	0.62	0.60	**0.77**	0.68
UppsalaNLP#4	5.73	5.66	0.41	0.42	0.40	0.41
BioInfo@UAVR#0	5.84	5.77	0.37	0.44	0.32	0.37
lirmm#3	9.08	6.62	0.48	0.42	0.74	0.54
SSN-NLP#3	7.61	6.86	0.33	0.26	0.48	0.34
HULAT#0	10.84	8.14	0.16	0.30	0.11	0.17
UDE#2	12.52	8.21	0.53	0.68	0.13	0.22
Fazl#2	17.11	11.22	0.14	**1**	0.09	0.16
Fazl#1	17.11	13.91	0.11	**1**	0.09	0.16

- **Early classification decision-based performance**: Table 2 shows the results obtained for the decision-based performance metrics. It can be observed that UNSL#0 obtained the best $ERDE_5$ and UNSL#4 the best $ERDE_{50}$ among all participating models. However, among our models, UNSL#4 was also the model with the lowest $F_{latency}$, which suggest that ignoring the words with low *global value* may contribute to improving performance in terms of the ERDE measure but at the cost of a worse performance in terms of the $F_{latency}$ measure.[11] The models

[11] This is probably caused by the final model heavily prioritizing recall over precision, affecting their harmonic mean which ultimately affected the $F_{latency}$. For instance, among our 5 models, UNSL#4 obtained the best recall (0.92) but the lowest precision value (0.31).

UNSL#2 and #3, trained with the entire training set, obtained a better performance in terms of the $ERDE_{50}$ measure compared to their two counterparts, UNSL#0 and #1, trained only with the training set corresponding to the previous edition. However, the performance of the former in terms of the $F_{latency}$ measure was lower compared to the latter, this is probably due to the fact that the selected hyperparameter configuration was meant to fit the model to the training data according to the $ERDE_{50}$ measure, not the $F_{latency}$—the $F_{latency}$ measure is based on the standard F_1 measure, as such, it favors models that assign equal importance to both recall and precision, whereas the ERDE measure models that prioritize recall over precision.[12] Unlike the results previously reported in the literature [4], in this particular task the use of word bigrams led to a slight loss of performance since the performance of the two models using word n-grams (UNSL#1 and #3) was slightly lower than their counterparts without n-grams (respectively, UNSL#0 and #2). Perhaps the fact that here, unlike in the reported results, users were processed one post at a time and not using a chunk-based approach—where even the most "hasty" models had to process at least one entire chunk before being able to make a decision. Another cause could be the fact that n-grams, although having superior semantic qualities, also suffer from inferior statistical qualities[13] which, depending on the data being used, could negatively affect performance. Finally, regarding the $F_{latency}$ measure, we did not achieve the best performance. More precisely, our best $F_{latency}$ values, obtained by UNSL#0 and #1, were 0.14 points below the best, 0.69, obtained by CLaC#4. This was mainly due to the fact that, as we mentioned above, our 5 models used the same hyperparameter configuration, originally selected to optimize the ERDE measure. Nevertheless, our best $F_{latency}$ value (0.55) was considerably above the average (0.38), and ranked 11th among the 50 participating models.

- **Performance in terms of execution time**: Table 3 shows, for each team, details on the total time used to complete the task. As can be seen, the time taken to complete the task differs widely from team to team, varying from a few to a large number of hours—one team even took as long as about a month. However, to have a more precise view of how efficient the models of each team were, not only the total time taken to complete the task must be considered, but also the total number of posts processed in that time, and the number of models used to carry it out. For example, in terms of processing speed, BiTeM does not seem as efficient as UNSL, since although the former completed the task in only 4 h, it only processed the first 11 posts from each user, while the latter, although completing the task in 23 h, it processed all 2000 posts from each user. Likewise, although BioInfo@UAVR took 14 h to classify all users with a single model, UNSL had to do it with 5 of them, which required not only 5 times more processing load but also

[12] The $ERDE_o$ measure is calculated with the cost of false positives (*cfp*) being considerably lower than that of false negatives (*cfn*). Note that giving more importance to recall than to precision is reasonable since, in early risk detection tasks, every single undetected (positive) user is a life at risk.

[13] The probability with which a particular sequence of words occurs will never be greater than the probability of each individual word.

Table 3 Details of the participating teams: team name, number of models (#*models*), number of user posts processed (#*posts*), time taken to complete the task and to process each post ($\frac{total\ time}{\#posts \times \#models}$)

			Time	
Team	#models	#posts	Total	Per post
UNSL⋆	5	2000	23h	**8s**
UppsalaNLP	5	2000	2 days + 7h	20s
BioInfo@UAVR	1	2000	14h	25s
UDE	3	2000	5 days + 3h	1m + 12s
lirmm	5	2024	8 days + 15h	1m + 12s
INAOE-CIMAT	4	2000	8 days + 2h	1m + 30s
HULAT	5	83	18h	2m + 36s
Fazl	3	2001	21 days + 15h	5m + 12s
BiTeM	4	11	4h	5m + 30s
LTL-INAOE	2	2001	17 days + 23h	6m + 30s
SINAI	3	317	10 days + 7h	15m + 36s
CLaC	5	109	11 days + 16h	31m
SSN-NLP	5	9	6 days + 22h	3h + 42m

5 times more requests sent to the server.[14] For this reason, Table 3 also includes an estimate of the time taken by each team's model to process each post, which was obtained by normalizing the total time relative to the number of models used and the total number of posts processed. Using this normalized time, it can be seen that UNSL models were the fastest, having processed each post in approximately 8 seconds[15] each—in other words, 2000 posts from each user processed with 5 models in 23 h. It is worth mentioning that our models were the fastest not because of superior computing capabilities,[16] but because the SS3 model was designed to be able to work incrementally, processing the input sequence in $O(n)$ time with respect to n, the length of the sequence [2]. This contrasts with other teams, such as CLaC [16], INAOE-CIMAT [1] or lirmm [17], which, although performed better in terms of the $F_{latency}$ measure, were considerably slower, taking them days to complete the same task. For example, the 5 CLaC [16] models were SVM

[14] For each of the users 2000 posts, not only was it necessary to send a request to the server to obtain the post, but also 5 more requests to send the response of each model. Therefore, for teams with 5 models like UNSL, completing the task required sending a total of $2000 + 2000 * 5 = 12000$ requests to the server. Therefore, if the connection latency was, for instance, 3 s, approximately 10 h of the total time would be consumed only by communication.

[15] Much of these 8 s corresponded to communication latency, since they include the latency of receiving the post, processing time, and the latency of sending the response.

[16] We coded our script in plain Python 2.7 and only using built-in functions and data structures; no external library was used (such as *NumPy*). Additionally, to run our script we used one of the author's laptop which had standard technical specifications (Intel Core i5, 8GB of DDR4 RAM, etc.).

classifiers that used neural features as input. More precisely, these features were extract from an ensemble approach that employs several attention-based neural sub-models, one such models (CLaC#1) obtained the best $F_{latency}$ value among all participating models. Nevertheless, these models were 232 times slower than UNSL's simple SS3 models, since CLaC took 11 days and 16 h to complete the task, having processed only 109 posts in total—which indicates that these models were computationally/algorithmically less efficient.

- **Ranking-based performance**: Table 4 shows the results obtained for the ranking-based performance metrics. It can be seen that our 5 models obtained, in the 4 rankings, the best values for the $P@10$ and $NDCG@10$ measures. Additionally, we also obtained the best $NDCG@100$ values for the rankings obtained after processing 1 and 100 posts, and the second and third best ones, respectively, after processing 500 and 1000 posts. Unlike with the decision-based metrics, here there was no noticeable difference in performance between the two SS3 models using word n-grams (UNSL#1 and #3) and their counterparts (respectively, UNSL#0 and #2). Between the models trained with the entire training set (UNSL#2, #3 and #4) and those trained only with the training set corresponding to the previous edition (UNSL#0 and #1), there was also no noticeable difference in terms of the $P@10$ and $NDCG@10$ measures, however, the former were considerably better in terms of the $NDCG@100$ measure. In other words, the three models that were trained with all available data, as expected, improved their ability to estimate the risk level of users—for example, the top-100 ranking of users ordered by the score given by UNSL#0, after processing the first 100 posts, was 77% perfect[17] (i.e. $NDCG@100 = 0.77$), whereas the one obtained by its counterpart, UNSL#2, was 83% perfect (i.e. $NDCG@100 = 0.83$).

	(after 500 post)			(after 1000 post)		
Model	P@10	NDCG@10	NDCG@100	P@10	NDCG@10	NDCG@100
UNSL#0	**1**	**1**	0.79	**1**	**1**	0.79
UNSL#1	**1**	**1**	0.79	**1**	**1**	0.79
UNSL#2	**1**	**1**	0.83	**1**	**1**	*0.84*
UNSL#3	**1**	**1**	0.84	**1**	**1**	*0.84*
UNSL#4	**1**	**1**	*.85*	0.9	0.94	*0.84*
UDE#1	**1**	**1**	**0.87**	**1**	**1**	**0.88**
UDE#0	0.9	0.93	*.85*	0.9	0.94	0.86
LTL-INAOE#0	0.9	0.92	0.73	0.7	0.78	0.65
Fazl#1	0.7	0.78	0.67	0.7	0.78	0.68
UppsalaNLP#4	0.8	0.75	0.52	0.8	0.75	0.52
BioInfo@UAVR#0	0.6	0.59	0.47	0.6	0.59	0.47

In general terms, it can be observed that, among all the participating models, the risk level estimated by our five SS3 models were the most consistent throughout the 4 rankings, having achieved the best values even when the ranking was generated after reading only the first post of each user. For example, it is interesting to note that, regardless of whether they were trained with the entire training set or not, or whether word n-grams were taken into account or not, all SS3 models were

[17] In this task, a perfect ranking is a ranking where all 73 at-risk users are located in the first 73 positions.

Table 4 Ranking-based evaluation results for the 4 reported rankings, respectively, the ranking obtained after processing 1, 100, 500, and 1000 posts. For comparison, the models that obtained the best results from the other 12 participating teams are also included

Model	(After 1 post)			(After 100 posts)		
	P@10	NDCG@10	NDCG@100	P@10	NDCG@10	NDCG@100
UNSL#0	**0.8**	***0.82***	0.54	**1**	**1**	0.77
UNSL#1	**0.8**	***0.82***	0.54	**1**	**1**	0.77
UNSL#2	**0.8**	***0.82***	***0.55***	**1**	**1**	0.83
UNSL#3	**0.8**	***0.82***	0.53	**1**	**1**	0.83
UNSL#4	**0.8**	***0.82***	0.52	0.9	0.94	***0.85***
LTL-INAOE#0	**0.8**	0.75	0.34	**1**	**1**	0.76
UDE#1	0.6	0.75	0.54	0.9	0.94	0.81
UppsalaNLP#4	0.8	0.75	0.52	0.8	0.75	0.52
BiTeM#1	0.8	0.75	0.47	–	–	–
SSN-NLP#3	0.6	0.64	0.3	–	–	–
BioInfo@UAVR#0	0.6	0.59	0.47	0.6	0.59	0.47
BiTeM#0	0.6	0.44	0.52	–	–	–
HULAT#0	0.3	0.33	0.18	–	–	–
Fazl#1	0.3	0.29	0.26	0.6	0.6	0.59
UDE#0	0.2	0.12	0.11	0.9	0.92	0.81
SINAI#0	0.2	0.12	0.11	–	–	–
CLaC#0	0.1	0.1	0.05	0.8	0.86	0.28
CLaC#1	0.1	0.1	0.04	0.3	0.45	0.16

able to construct a top-10 ranking of at-risk users which was 82% perfect (i.e. $NDCG@10 = 0.82$) after processing only the first post from each user. This indicates that our models, despite their simplicity, are capable of estimating the risk level of users with considerable efficiency, even when only a few posts have been processed.[18] This contrasts with other more complex models that, although performed better in terms of the $F_{latency}$ measure, were not as efficient in estimating risk levels—even when some took days to complete the task. For instance, although CLaC#1 obtained the best $F_{latency}$ value, ranking-based results show that its ability to estimate the risk level of the users was the lowest among all the participating models. Finally, it is important to mention that the ranking-based evaluation results obtained by our models imply two relevant points: (a) the score generated by SS3 (see Eq. 6) is estimating the risk level of the subjects correctly, and (b) the fact that user risk level is being estimated correctly implies that our models have room for improvement in terms of decision-based metrics (ERDE, $F_{latency}$, precision, and recall) by using better early classification policies.[19] This last point is not

[18] Which would explain why our models obtained the best ERDE values despite having classified all at-risk users, on average, after having processed only their first 2 posts.

[19] That is, if our models were not able to obtain better classification results, it was not due to a poor estimation of the risk level of the users, but due to the policy used to decide *when* to classify them based on that estimation.

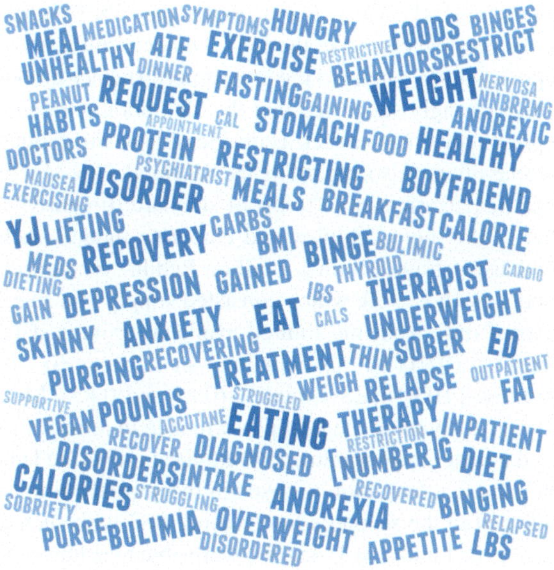

Fig. 5 Word cloud of the top-100 words selected by *global value* learned by the SS3 model (UNSL#2) from the training set available for this task (words are sized by actual value)

minor, since it allows identifying possible lines of work to extend and improve our models, as will be discussed in the next and final section. Note that point (a) indicates us that the *global value* learned by the model, given by Eq. 1, is correctly capturing the degree of importance of each word—which could also be asserted from a more qualitative point of view in Fig. 5.

4 Conclusion and Future Work

In this chapter, we described the participation of our research team in the eRisk addressing the two editions of the early anorexia detection task. In the first edition, we used two main approaches, one based on a time-aware chunk-based document representation, called FTVT, and the other, on a novel text classifier that was specially designed for early risk detection scenarios, called SS3. In the second edition, given that evaluation data was released more realistically as a stream of (user) posts and not using the chunk-based approach, FTVT was no longer appropriate and, consequently, we addressed the task by focusing only on approaches based on the SS3 classifier.

Regarding the results obtained after the evaluation stage, in the first edition, we achieved the best $ERDE_5$ and the best precision values among all participant models, respectively, with one of our FTVT-based model and one of our SS3 models. It was interesting to note that the models using the FTVT representation performed well in terms of ERDE measures, even although the hyperparameter configuration, such as the FTVT n parameter, was not specially selected for this task (but rather for the depression task). We also noticed that the FTVT model with no temporal enrichment of the positive class, i.e. the FTVT model with $n = 0$ equivalent to a standard CSA representation, obtained the lowest performance among all the participating models which strongly suggested that the "temporal enrichment" performed by the FTVT representation has, in fact, a considerable positive impact on the final performance of the classifiers. Also, regarding the SS3 model used for this edition, it is worth noticing that the performance in terms of standard (timeless) measures were comparable to that of the more complex and elaborate models such as the FHDO-BCSG CNN models pre-trained with 1.7 billion Reddit comments [21]. More precisely, our SS3 model (with $\lambda = 3$), which consisted simply of a summation of word values (Eq. 5) learned only from the limited available training data, not only achieved the best precision (0.91) but also obtained an F_1 value (0.79) that was only outperformed by those FHDO-BCSG models (0.81 and 0.85). Moreover, this SS3 model could also have obtained the best performance in terms of the ERDE measures if we had used a better hyperparameter configuration, as we later discovered [4]—which was the same configuration we used in the second edition. Finally, regarding the results obtained in the second edition, using SS3 with such hyperparameter configuration ($\lambda = \rho = 1$ and $\sigma = 0.45$), we were able to achieve the best values for both $ERDE_5$ and $ERDE_{50}$ showing that this hyperparameter setting is robust in terms of this measure. Moreover, our models were the fastest in processing time and achieved remarkable results in terms of the ranking-based metrics, obtaining the best $P@10$ and $NDCG@10$ values, consistently, in all four rankings, and the best $NDCG@100$ values for the rankings after processing 1 and 100 posts—and the second and third best $NDCG@100$, respectively, for the rankings after 500 and 1000 posts. In general terms, the results suggest that, despite its simplicity, the SS3 classifier could be considerably competent when dealing with these types of scenarios. Results also suggest that this classifier possess certain robustness since, having used the same hyperparameter configuration and regardless of the data used to train it or whether word n-grams were taken into account or not, the performance of all five SS3 models was consistent across the three different dimensions used to measure it: execution time, users risk level estimation, and early classification performance.

Finally, for future work, we plan to explore better hyperparameter configurations to improve the performance of our models in terms of the $F_{latency}$ measure—for which we were unable to obtain the best result. More importantly, based on the promising ranking-based evaluation results suggesting that user risk level were properly estimated, we will also explore and design better early classification policies since the simple policy that we used proved to be "too hasty"—as we described earlier, all at-risk users were classified, on average, after having processed only their first 2 posts. For example, we believe that a more elaborated policy able to delay the decision until the estimated risk level is high enough, or the use of global information such as taking into account the current estimated risk level of all users to make the decision, could greatly improve the early classification performance.

References

1. Aragón, M. E., López-Monroy, A. P.,& Montes-y Gómez, M. (2019). INAOE-CIMAT at eRisk 2019: Detecting signs of anorexia using fine-grained emotions. In *Working Notes of CLEF, CEUR Workshop Proceedings*, Lugano, Switzerland.
2. Burdisso, S. G., Errecalde, M., and Montes-y Gómez, M. A text classification framework for simple and effective early depression detection over social media streams. Expert Systems with Applications 133 (2019), 182–197.
3. Burdisso, S. G., Errecalde, M., & Montes-y Gómez, M. (2019). UNSL at eRisk 2019: a unified approach for anorexia, self-harm and depression detection in social media. In *Working Notes of CLEF 2019, CEUR Workshop Proceedings*, Lugano, Switzerland.
4. Burdisso, S. G., Errecalde, M., & Montes-y Gómez, M. (2020). τ-SS3: A text classifier with dynamic n-grams for early risk detection over text streams. *Pattern Recognition Letters, 138,* 130–137.
5. Errecalde, M. L., Villegas, M. P., Funez, D. G., Ucelay, M. J. G., & Cagnina, L. C. (2017). Temporal variation of terms as concept space for early risk prediction. In *Working Notes of CLEF 2018, CEUR Workshop Proceedings*, Dublin, Ireland.
6. Funez, D. G., Ucelay, M. J. G., Villegas, M. P., Burdisso, S. G., Cagnina, L. C., Montes-y Gómez, M., & Errecalde, M. L. (2018). UNSL's participation at eRisk 2018 lab. In *Working Notes of CLEF 2018, CEUR Workshop Proceedings*, Avignon, France.
7. Gonzalez, A., Clarke, S., & Kohn, M. (2007). Eating disorders in adolescents. *Australian Family Physician, 36,* 8.
8. Hay, P. (2020). Current approach to eating disorders: a clinical update. *Internal Medicine Journal, 50,* 24–29.
9. Kakhi, S., and McCann, J. Anorexia nervosa: diagnosis, risk factors and evidence-based treatments. Progress in Neurology and Psychiatry 20 (2016), 24–29.
10. Li, Z., Xiong, Z., Zhang, Y., Liu, C., and Li, K. Fast text categorization using concise semantic analysis. Pattern Recognition Letters 32, 3 (2011), 441–448.
11. López-Monroy, A. P., Montes-y Gómez, M., Escalante, H. J., Villasenor-Pineda, L., and Stamatatos, E. Discriminative subprofile-specific representations for author profiling in social media. Knowledge-Based Systems 89 (2015), 134–147.
12. Losada, D. E., & Crestani, F. (2016). A test collection for research on depression and language use. In N. Fuhr, P. Quaresma, T. Gonçalves, B. Larsen, K. Balog, C. Macdonald, L. Cappellato & N. Ferro (Eds.),*Experimental IR Meets Multilinguality, Multimodality, and Interaction* (Cham, 2016) (pp. 28–39). Springer International Publishing.
13. Losada, D. E., Crestani, F., & Parapar, J. (2017). eRisk 2017: CLEF lab on early risk prediction on the internet: Experimental foundations. In G. J. Jones, S. Lawless, J. Gonzalo, L. Kelly, L. Goeuriot, T. Mandl, L. Cappellato, & N. Ferro, (Eds.), *Experimental IR Meets Multilinguality, Multimodality, and Interaction* (Cham, 2017) (pp. 346–360). Springer International Publishing.
14. Losada, D. E., Crestani, F., & Parapar, J. (2018). Overview of eRisk: Early risk prediction on the internet. In P. Bellot, C. Trabelsi, J. Mothe, F. Murtagh, J. Y. Nie, L. Soulier, E. SanJuan, L. Cappellato & N. Ferro, (Eds.), *Experimental IR Meets Multilinguality, Multimodality, and Interaction* (Cham, 2018) (pp. 343–361). Springer International Publishing.
15. Losada, D. E., Crestani, F., and Parapar, J. (2019). Overview of eRisk 2019 early risk prediction on the internet. In F. Crestani, M. Braschler, J. Savoy, A. Rauber, H. Müller, D. E. Losada, G. Heinatz Bürki, L. Cappellato & N. Ferro (Eds.), *Experimental IR Meets Multilinguality, Multimodality, and Interaction* (Cham, 2019) (pp. 340–357). Springer International Publishing.
16. Mohammadi, E., Amini, H., & Kosseim, L. (2019). Quick and (maybe not so) easy detection of anorexia in social media posts. In *Working Notes of CLEF 2019, CEUR Workshop Proceedings*, Lugano, Switzerland.
17. Ragheb, W., Azé, J., Bringay, S., & Servajean, M. (2019). Attentive multi-stage learning for early risk detection of signs of anorexia and self-harm on social media. In *Working Notes of CLEF 2019, CEUR Workshop Proceedings*, Lugano, Switzerland.

18. Rudin, C. Stop explaining black box machine learning models for high stakes decisions and use interpretable models instead. Nature Machine Intelligence 1, 5 (2019), 206–215.
19. Sadeque, F., Xu, D., & Bethard, S. (2018). Measuring the latency of depression detection in social media. In *Proceedings of the Eleventh ACM International Conference on Web Search and Data Mining* (pp. 495–503).
20. Termorshuizen, J., Watson, H., & Thornton, LM, et al. (2020). Early impact of COVID-19 on individuals with self-reported eating disorders: A survey of 1,000 individuals in the United States and the Netherlands. *International Journal of Eating Disorders, 53*, 1780–1790.
21. Trotzek, M., Koitka, S., & Friedrich, C. M. (2018). Word embeddings and linguistic metadata at the CLEF 2018 tasks for early detection of depression and anorexia. In *Working Notes of CLEF 2018, CEUR Workshop Proceedings*, Avignon, France.
22. Vikram, P. (2005). *Gender in Mental Health Research.* Gender and Health Research Series: World Health Organization.
23. Zhang, Y., Jin, R., & Zhou, Z.-H. (2010). Understanding bag-of-words model: A statistical framework. *International Journal of Machine Learning and Cybernetics, 1*(1–4), 43–52.

Early Risk Detection of Self-Harm Using BERT-Based Transformers

Rodrigo Martínez-Castaño, Amal Htait, Leif Azzopardi, and Yashar Moshfeghi

Abstract In the past few years, individuals choose increasingly to share online about themselves, which reflect greatly about their personality and self-image. In particular, individuals with mental health issues tend to discuss or mention such issues online, in an obvious or concealed way. Thus, analysing individuals' online posts for mental health, became critical for an early detection and fast intervention. This chapter presents our efforts towards detecting mental health issues by focusing on the task: *Early Detection of Signs of Self-Harm*. Core to how we approached this problem was the use of BERT-based classifiers which were trained specifically for each task. Additional investigations of the efficiency of this method in detecting mental health issues are also presented with the following tasks: *Early Detection of Signs of Anorexia* and *Early Detection of Signs of Depression*. Our results indicate that this approach delivers high performance across a series of measures, particularly for self-harm and anorexia, where our classifiers obtained the best performance for precision, F1, latency-weighted F1, and ERDE at 5 and 50. This work suggests that BERT-based classifiers, when trained appropriately, can accurately infer which social media users are at risk of self-harming, with precision up to 91.3 and 83.9% for anorexia. Given these promising results, it will be interesting to further refine the training regime, classifier and early detection scoring mechanism, as well as apply the same approach to other related tasks (e.g., pathological gambling, suicide).

R. Martínez-Castaño (✉)
Centro Singular de Investigación en Tecnoloxías Intelixentes (CiTIUS), Universidade de Santiago de Compostela, Galicia, Spain
e-mail: rodrigo.martinez@usc.es

A. Htait · L. Azzopardi · Y. Moshfeghi
Department of Computer and Information Sciences, University of Strathclyde, Glasgow, UK
e-mail: amal.htait@strath.ac.uk

L. Azzopardi
e-mail: leif.azzopardi@strath.ac.uk

Y. Moshfeghi
e-mail: yashar.moshfeghi@strath.ac.uk

F. Crestani et al. (eds.), *Early Detection of Mental Health Disorders by Social Media Monitoring*, Studies in Computational Intelligence 1018,
https://doi.org/10.1007/978-3-031-04431-1_8

1 Introduction

People might think that mental illness is rare, only happens to others and that it will never affect them. Yet several studies indicated that mental illnesses are very common [23], and early intervention is critical to prevent and reduce its progress. Since major mental illnesses are rarely unanticipated, early detection could be life-saving before an illness appears in its full-blown form. A new source of information is found in social media posts, where individuals choose increasingly to share about themselves, reflecting about their personality, self-image and mental state through words they use that indicate their psychological states. Therefore, individuals with mental health issues could be identified through an early detection of mental illness within their online posts. In this work we focus on self-harm, which is the infliction of pain or injury onto oneself [20]. Self-harm is not considered a mental illness by itself, but it is a behavior that indicates the presence of severe mental illnesses such as depression, eating disorders and anxiety. Self-harm is often practiced in secret and on easy-to-hide body parts, making early detection difficult, therefore delaying intervention and treatment. However, self-harm is often shared publicly in social media. In this chapter, we present our work in detecting mental health issues by focusing on the early detection of signs of self-harm by triggering alerts when early traces of committing self-harm are detected in online posts.

The main goal of this chapter is to explore the potential of BERT-based classifiers coupled with a novel scoring mechanism for the early detection of self-harm. Further more, this chapter examine the extension and enrichment effect of the training datasets on the system's efficiency. In addition, and for a further examination of the method's efficiency in the detection of different mental health issues, we expand the experiments with the early detection of signs of anorexia[1] and depression.

This chapter is structured as follows. In Sect. 2 we provide an overview of the main approaches used to detect signs of self-harm in addition to the approaches presented in previous editions of the eRisk workshop[2] of CLEF.[3] In Sect. 3 we describe our general approach for the tasks by using BERT-based models for sentence classification. In Sect. 4 we explain how the classifiers were trained and applied. Section 4.4 covers the analysis of our results, where our approach performs the best across a number of metrics for Self-Harm. Section 5 concerns additional trials in an effort to assess the ability of the proposed method in detecting signs of anorexia and signs of depression. Finally, in Sect. 6 we summarise the contributions of this chapter.

[1] An emotional disorder characterised by an obsessive desire to lose weight by refusing to eat.

[2] https://early.irlab.org/.

[3] http://www.clef-initiative.eu/.

2 Related Work

Analyzing mental health-related discourse and language usage in social media is getting an increasing attention from researchers [4, 24], and the specific subject of self-harm had been highlighted on in various efforts investigating approaches for detecting the self-harm risk of mental health forum online posts. The early related work in this subject mainly used variations of linear classifiers with feature engineering. For example, in the work of [5], the authors used lexicons as a feature in their supervised classifier that identifies posts showing signs of self-harm, with various other features including psycho-linguistic and topic modeling features. To abandon the feature engineering process, researchers exploited the deep learning approaches, such as CNN (Convolutional Neural Network), that learns documents representations by considering only their textual content [18, 26].

In 2019, the workshop eRisk [14] introduced a new task concerning the early detection of self-harm signs with the participation of 8 teams. The best performing team was UNSL [3] with their text classifier SS3 [2], where their system was extremely fast at making classification decisions but slightly modest in the effectiveness of these decisions. As a continuation of eRisk 2019, eRisk 2020 [15] hosted 12 participants including our team iLab [16]. Our BERT-based classifiers were able to achieve the best performance in terms of Precision, F1, ERDE measures and latency-weighted F1.

3 Approach

A breakthrough in the use of machine learning for Natural Language Processing (NLP) appeared with the generative pre-training of language models on a diverse corpus of unlabelled text, such as ELMo [21], BERT [8], OpenAI GPT [22], XLM [10], and RoBERTa [11]. Such a technique demonstrated large gains on a variety of NLP tasks (e.g., sequence or token classification, question answering, semantic similarity assessment, document classification). In particular, BERT (Bidirectional Encoder Representations from Transformers) [7, 8], the model by Google AI, proved to be one of the most powerful tools for text classification [9, 17, 19]. BERT is based on the Transformer architecture [25] and it was trained for both masked word prediction and next sentence prediction at the same time. As input, BERT takes two concatenated segments of text which are delimited with special tokens and whose length respects a defined maximum. The model was pre-trained on a huge dataset of unlabelled text. It is typically used within a text classifier for sentence tokenisation and text representation. A standard BERT classifier is presented in Fig. 1 where a sentence is tokenised, represented in embeddings and then classified. The results are normalised between 0 and 1 using the softmax function, representing the probability of the *input* sentence to belong to a certain class (e.g., the probability of the sentence to be written by a self-harmer).

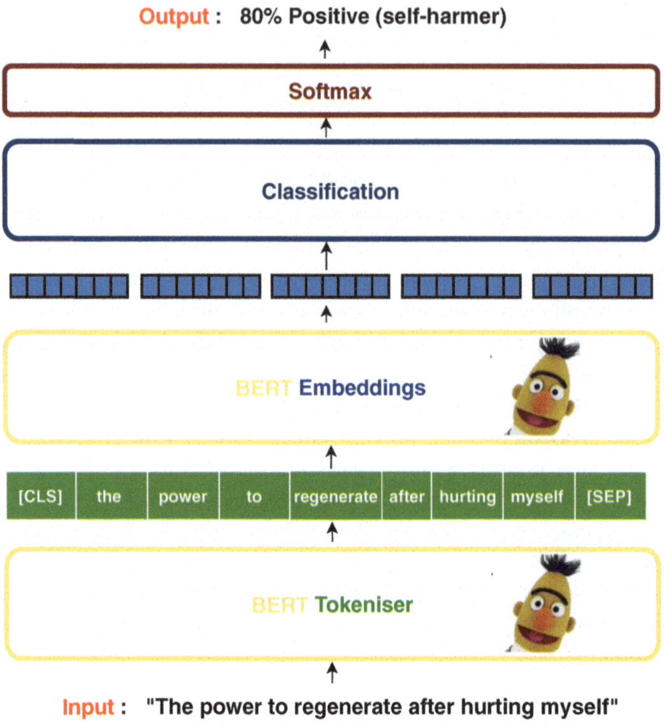

Fig. 1 BERT-based Classification Architecture

As for RoBERTa [11] (a replication study of BERT pre-training by Facebook AI), it shares a similar architecture with BERT but with a different pre-training approach. RoBERTa was trained over ten times more data, the next sentence prediction objective was removed, and the masked word prediction task was improved with the introduction of a dynamic masking pattern applied to the training data. In another attempt to improve the language model, Facebook AI presented XLM-RoBERTa [6] with the pre-training of *multilingual* language models. This new improvement led to significant performance gains in text classification.

In this work, a variety of pre-trained language models were tested: BERT, DistillBERT, RoBERTa (base), and XLM-RoBERTa (base), among others. However, the best performance was achieved when using XLM-RoBERTa on our training data. In particular, we used Ernie,[4] a Python library for sentence classification built on top of Hugging Face Transformers,[5] the main library that implements state-of-the-art general-purpose Transformer-based architectures.

[4] Github: https://github.com/labteral/ernie/.

[5] Github: https://github.com/huggingface/transformers/.

Most of the pre-trained language models, including XLM-RoBERTa, have a maximum input length of 512 tokens. In our work, we experimented with input sentences of sizes between 32 and 128 tokens due to GPU memory restrictions. The best results were achieved with an input size of 128 tokens. Note that Reddit posts are usually shorter than 128 tokens. Therefore, using an input size larger than 128 would not substantially increase performance, but it would significantly increase the required computational resources. In the few cases where the Reddit posts were longer, we split them based on punctuation marks in an attempt to respect the context of the writings posted by the users. When training the classifiers, the weights of the pre-trained base models (e.g., XLM-RoBERTa) are updated, in addition to the classification head.

4 Experiments

For our work in detecting signs of self-harm within online posts, a tagged set of users and their posts to Reddit[6] groups was provided for training purposes. The different methods were benchmarked using a system that simulates a real-time scenario introduced in [14]. The posts from the users of the test dataset are served in rounds, one post at a time (simulating their live posting to the Reddit groups). Then, The task aim to provide a decision about each user given their posts, and to do so as early as possible (i.e., with the fewest posts). For the evaluation, the correctness of the prediction (i.e., whether the user will cause self-harm or not) is not the only factor taken into account, but also the delay taken to emit the alerts. Clearly, the sooner a person who is likely to self-harm is identified the sooner the intervention can be provided.

We fine-tuned a number of different language models based on the original BERT architecture with a classification head to predict whether a sentence was written by a subject that *self-harms or not*. Those models are the base to predict if a user is likely to be the victim of self-harm by triggering an alert given a stream of texts. All of our final models were based on XLM-RoBERTa, which demonstrated better performance for this task.

4.1 Provided Training Data

The first group of data collections used to train our models is composed of the latest available original datasets provided by eRisk CLEF workshop organisers: 2020 for Self-Harm [15]. We split the users of the training datasets into two chunks for training (80%) and validation (20%). We created a variant of the training chunk in which only

[6] https://reddit.com/.

the first texts for each user of the positive class were taken into account. Specifically, the average number of texts of the positive class.

4.2 Created Training Data

The second group of datasets used for training our models was collected from the Pushshift Reddit Dataset [1] through its public API,[7] which exposes a repository with a constantly updated and almost complete dataset of all the public Reddit data. We downloaded all the available submissions and comments written to the most popular subreddit about self-harm (r/selfharm). From those posts, we extracted 42,839 authors. In addition, we collected all of the posts in any other subreddit for those authors (SELFHARM- USERS- TEXTS dataset). Then, we obtained an equivalent amount of random users from which we also extracted all their posts (RANDOM- USERS- TEXTS dataset). We filtered the obtained datasets in several ways. First, we checked that there were no user collisions between the two collections. After identifying some of the main self-harm related subreddits (r/selfharm, r/Cutters, r/MadeOfStyrofoam, r/SelfHarmScars, r/StopSelfHarm, r/CPTSD and r/SuicideWatch), we removed the users from RANDOM- USERS- TEXTS having at least one post in any of them. All the users with more than 5,000 submissions were removed since those with an extremely high number of posts seem more likely to be bots. Besides, the vast majority of the users had posted fewer times so we presumed to have more chances to profile the average user below that threshold. We also pruned the less active users under 50 submissions. The number of sentences was expanded by splitting the users' texts that were too long for the parameters we utilised in our models. Otherwise, the sentences would be truncated during training, potentially losing valuable information. We split the large posts into groups of contiguous sentences of approximately the maximum length in tokens utilised in our models and following the punctuation marks hierarchy (e.g., prioritising the splits on full stops over commas). As commented before, a maximum length of 128 tokens was set so the models could be fine-tuned in commercial GPUs.

As a result, we created several datasets mainly derived from SELFHARM- USERS- TEXTS and RANDOM- USERS- TEXTS for training our model candidates as it is shown in Fig. 2. These datasets are presented in Table 1, and explained below:

- A manually created dataset:
  - REAL- SELFHARMERS- TEXTS: This dataset was created with the aim of obtaining a bigger but similar dataset to the one provided by the eRisk organisers. We manually tagged 354 users as real self-harmers from the users of the SELFHARM- USERS- TEXTS dataset. Then, we filtered the last 1,000 submissions and comments for every user. We also pruned the writing sequences just before their first writing at r/selfharm. After that, we filtered the users with at least 10 writings

[7] https://pushshift.io/api-parameters/.

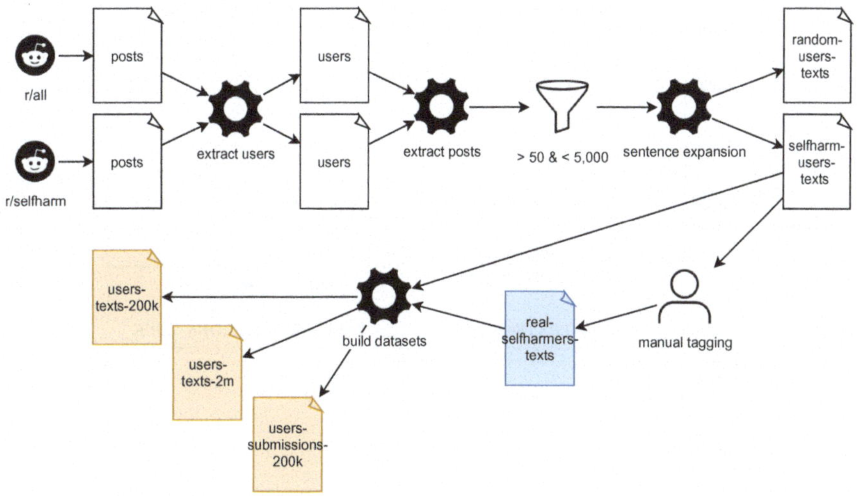

Fig. 2 The workflow of building the created training data for the detection of signs of Self-Harm

remaining, ending up with a total of 120 real self-harmers. For the negative class, we took a sample of random users from the dataset RANDOM- USERS- TEXTS in the same proportion as in the provided training data: $\sim$ 7.3 random users per self-harmer.

- Datasets automatically generated from SELFHARM- USERS- TEXTS and RANDOM- USERS- TEXTS after removing the users from REAL- SELFHARMERS- TEXTS. In Fig. 3, we show the distribution of posts per user for the original datasets (SELFHARM- USERS- TEXTS and RANDOM- USERS- TEXTS) and the derived ones utilised to train the final classifiers:
  - USERS- TEXTS- 200K: This dataset was generated by random sampling $200K$ writings from both SELFHARM- USERS- TEXTS (as self-harmers) and RANDOM- USERS- TEXTS (as non self-harmers), with 100 K from each dataset. Note that we experimented by replicating last years' task with different sizes of sampling such as 2, 20, 100, 300, 400 and 500 K writings, but the best results were achieved with a sampling size of $200K$ writings.
  - USERS- TEXTS- 2 M: This dataset is a variant of USERS- TEXTS- 200 K; a balanced dataset with ten times more sentences, totalling 2 M writings. Note that, during our experimentation replicating last years' task, using a training set larger than $200K$ did not improve the results except for the $ERDE_5$ metric with the 2 M writings.
  - USERS- SUBMISSIONS- 200 k: This dataset was generated in a similar procedure as USERS- TEXTS- 200 k, with 200K randomly sampled writings, but with the difference of avoiding comments. Therefore, sampling users' submissions exclusively.

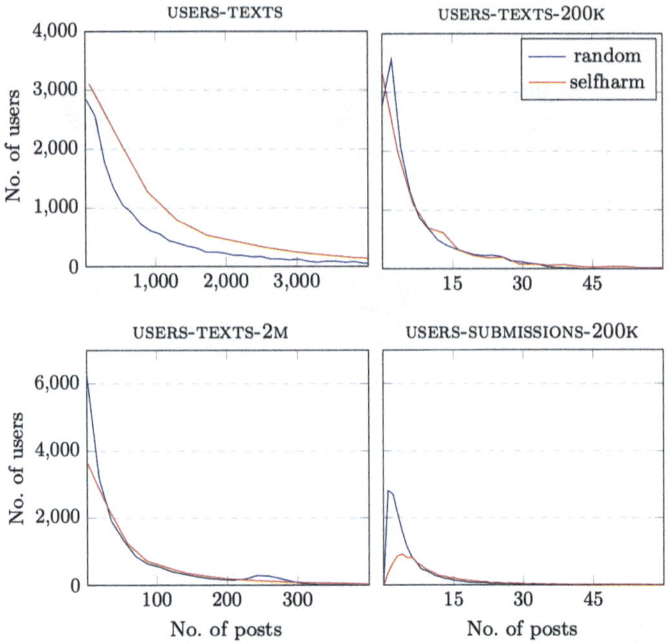

Fig. 3 Distribution of the number of posts per user in the datasets SELFHARM- USERS- TEXTS, RANDOM- USERS- TEXTS and the derived datasets from them

Table 1 Some statistics of the datasets used to train the classifiers

Dataset	Class	Users	Subreddits	Sentences	Years
REAL-SELFHARMERS-TEXTS	Selfharm	120	1, 346	8, 943	2013–2020
	Random	875	5, 585	87, 260	2009–2020
USERS-TEXTS- 200 K	Selfharm	9, 487	9, 797	107, 277	2006–2020
	Random	14, 280	9, 793	107, 152	2006–2020
USERS-TEXTS- 2 M	Selfharm	10, 454	26, 931	1, 075, 476	2006–2020
	Random	17, 548	26, 409	1, 076, 707	2005–2020
USERS-SUBMISSIONS-200 K	Selfharm	10, 319	13, 681	131, 233	2006–2020
	Random	15, 937	14, 913	128, 064	2005–2020

4.3 Method

For this work, we created three models:

- The first one (LR- ERISK) acted as the baseline. An L1 regularised Logistic Regression classifier built with the training data provided by the eRisk organisers for each task. Similar to the baseline used in [12]. The parameters of the model were set by running a 10-fold cross-validation on the 80% of the training data. The parameters of the user classifier were adjusted with the other 20% of the training data.
- The second model (XLMRB- ERISK) was trained by fine-tuning the XLM-RoBERTa language model (since it behaved better than other variants we tried such as BERT, DistillBERT, XLNet, etc.) with the variant of the provided training data with only the first texts for the users of the positive class. Also, the parameters of the classifier were adjusted with the other 20% of the training data.
- The third model (XLMRB- RANDOM) was also trained again by fine-tuning the XLM-RoBERTa language model, but this time with the variant of the created training data (see Sect. 4.2).

We established for the XLM-RoBERTa models a maximum length of tokens as 128 per sentence, a training rate of $2e-5$ and a validation size of the 20%.

The parameters were adjusted for each model in all variants by finding their optimal values for F1 and the eRisk related metrics: latency-weighted F1, $ERDE_5$ and $ERDE_{50}$ (see Sect. 4.4) with the validation set (20% of the provided training set). An exception in parameters extraction occurred with the XLMRB- RANDOM classifier, where we used the created REAL- SELFHARMERS- TEXTS dataset for that purpose. An example of parameters adjustment is presented in Fig. 4 where it can be observed that the best value for latency-weighted F1 with any θ is obtained when waiting for at least 10–12 texts for XLMRB- RANDOM- SELFHARM- 200 K. The model with the best performance for each target metric is then chosen, and the selected parameters for each variant can be observed in Table 2.

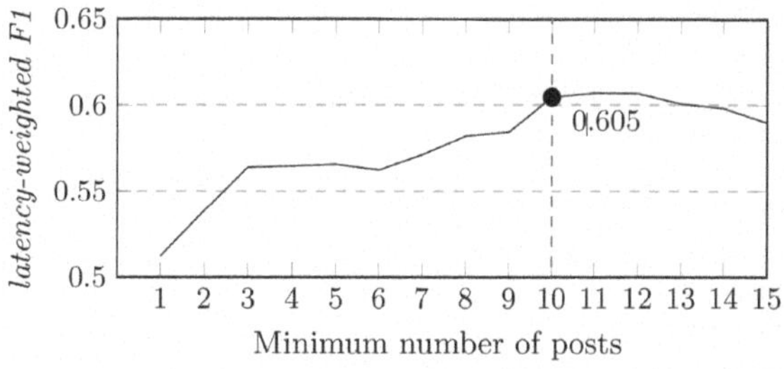

Fig. 4 Latency-weighted F1 when varying the minimum number of texts to trigger an alert. Model XLMRB- RANDOM- SELFHARM- 200 K with the REAL- SELFHARMERS- TEXTS dataset. A maximum of 50 posts are taken into account

Table 2 Combinations of models and parameters for early risk detection of self-harm. For parameters extraction we used 20% of the provided training data as the validation set with LR- ERISK and XLMRB- ERISK. For XLMRB- RANDOM we used REAL- SELFHARMERS- TEXTS

Run	Model	Target metric	θ	Min. posts	Max. posts
0	LR- ERISK- SELFHARM	*latency-weighted F1*	0.970	10	50
1	LR- ERISK- SELFHARM	*ERDE_5*	0.370	2	5
2	LR- ERISK- SELFHARM	*ERDE_50*	0.050	45	45
3	LR- ERISK- SELFHARM	*F1*	0.790	100	100
0	XLMRB- ERISK- SELFHARM	*latency-weighted F1*	0.030	10	50
1	XLMRB- ERISK- SELFHARM	*ERDE_5*	0.015	2	5
2	XLMRB- ERISK- SELFHARM	*ERDE_50*	0.015	45	45
3	XLMRB- ERISK- SELFHARM	*F1*	0.020	100	100
0	XLMRB- RANDOM- SELFHARM- 200K	*latency-weighted F1*	0.750	10	50
1	XLMRB- RANDOM- SELFHARM- 2M	*latency-weighted F1*	0.760	10	50
2	XLMRB- RANDOM- SELFHARM- 2M	*ERDE_5*	0.690	2	5
3	XLMRB- RANDOM- SELFHARM- SUB- 200K	*ERDE_50*	0.640	45	45
4	XLMRB- RANDOM- SELFHARM- 200K	*F1*	0.680	100	100

In order to predict if a user has or has not risk of self-harm, we averaged the predicted probability of the known writings for every user. We omitted the prediction of sentences with less than 10 tokens for the models fine-tuned on top of XLMR-ROBERTA- BASE as we concluded that the performance on smaller sentences is poor. We defined several parameters to determine if the system should trigger an alert given a list of known user's texts: the minimum average probability threshold (θ), the minimum number of texts necessary to trigger an alert, and the maximum number of texts that the system will take into account to make its decisions on the subjects. Given a growing list of texts from a user, the system will trigger an alert if the average probability of the known texts for that user is equal or greater than θ, the number of known texts is greater or equal to the minimum, and lower or equal to the maximum.

4.4 Results

After running our models on the different test datasets, we present the results in Table 3 with the performance of our runs for early risk detection of self-harm, and where the best scores among all the variants are highlighted in bold.

Our team's performance with the XLMRB- RANDOM- SELFHARM- 200 K classifier was the best for each of the key metrics compared to the other teams in 2020. Given our training schedule which tried to maximise the performance for each metric per run, we can see that no specific run was the best across all the metrics, but rather there is a trade-off between metrics. For example, Run 1 obtains a precision score of 0.913, but has the lowest recall, while Run 4 obtains the highest F1, but not the best precision or recall. Of most interest is the performance on the eRisk-specific metrics, where our runs obtained notably the best results. With Run 0 we obtained a latency-weighted F1 of 0.66, where the second-best result was obtained by the team UNSL with their run 1 at 0.61. For $ERDE_5$, Run 2 scored 0.134, whereas the second-best team was again UNSL with their run 1 at 0.172 (where lower is better). For $ERDE_{50}$, our Run 3 obtained a score of 0.071, whereas all the other runs ranged between 0.11 to 0.25.

In addition, we present the posts with the highest probability of risk of self-harm, by each used model, in Table 4. The presented posts reveal certain characteristics to the different models employed on the different tasks. First, the majority of the posts classified as users with high risks of self-harm by the Logistic regression model (LR-ERISK) are very short sentences and mostly include a specific expression or term such as *feel*. As for the BERT-based methods, the classification is more accurate toward the specific mental health issue. In addition, the classified posts include much more complex expressions describing the mental illness.

Table 3 The performance for each run for early detection of signs of self-harm. Note that for each bolded metric our run gave the overall highest performance, including other teams

Run	P	R	F1	ERDE 5	ERDE 50	Latency TP	Speed	Latency-Weighted F1
LR- ERISK- SELFHARM								
0	0.658	0.260	0.372	0.253	0.190	10	0.965	0.358
1	0.271	0.817	0.407	0.202	0.178	2	0.996	0.404
2	0.274	**0.971**	0.427	0.402	0.167	45	0.830	0.353
3	0.600	0.548	0.573	0.268	0.268	100	0.632	0.360
XLMRB- ERISK- SELFHARM								
0	0.833	0.481	0.610	0.251	0.133	10	0.965	0.588
1	0.457	0.769	0.573	**0.126**	0.112	2	0.996	0.571
2	0.592	0.808	0.683	0.280	0.082	45	0.830	0.567
3	0.802	0.625	0.703	0.255	0.255	100	0.632	0.444
XLMRB- RANDOM- SELFHARM- 200 K								
0	0.833	0.577	0.682	0.252	0.111	10	0.965	**0.658**
1	**0.913**	0.404	0.560	0.248	0.149	10	0.965	0.540
2	0.544	0.654	0.594	0.134	0.118	2	0.996	0.592
3	0.564	0.885	0.689	0.287	**0.071**	45	0.830	0.572
4	0.828	0.692	**0.754**	0.255	0.255	100	0.632	0.476
UNSL								
1	0.618	0.606	0.612	0.172	0.124	2	0.996	0.609

5 Additional Experiments

The proposed BERT-based method combined with an enrichment of training data has shown to be effective in predicting early signs of self-harm. In this section, we ask the question: *will it be as effective in detecting other forms of mental health problems?* To answer that question we expanded the previous experiments with new ones concerning the early detection of signs of anorexia and signs of depression.

5.1 Provided Training Data (Anorexia and Depression)

The first group of data collections used to train our models is also provided by eRisk CLEF workshop organisers: 2019 for Anorexia [14] and 2018 for Depression [13]. We apply the same previous procedure of splitting the users of the training datasets into two parts for training (80%) and validation (20%) (see Sect. 4.1).

Table 4 The posts with highest probability of risk of self-harm by each of the employed models

Rank	Posts
LR- ERISK- SELFHARM	
1	Abby I feel you
2	Feel the Eel
3	Tumblr. Just because I don't have one
4	Libleft should be Tumblr
5	I feel you
6	I feel serious pity for you
7	I would feel honored
8	r/tumblr are comrades
9	I feel violated
10	Many feel the same
XLMRB- ERISK- SELFHARM	
1	I want to cut again. I miss it. I've been free for 6 months, almost 7. I want to do it again. I just miss the feeling. Nothing is really wrong [...]
2	I hate the feeling anti-depressants give me. I feel that every part of my brain is telling me to be anxious and be depressed [...]
3	Hmm I keep relapsing in anorexia and self harm (cutting), never had the energy to stop my depression and anxiety [...]
4	Having a Crush. I feel I've gotten a crush only because it's like a coping mechanism. Recently I've been incredibly anxious and depressed [...]
5	How to stopping self harm. So I've been hurting myself for a long time a couple of years now and I've been trying hard for these last couple of months to stop [...]
6	[...] Not with drugs or help or therapy. I hardened myself to my thoughts and feelings, knowing that my depression couldn't be fixed [...]
7	I have clinical depression, which makes me overestimate my failures. I know I'm being irrational, but I just hate myself for getting even a single question wrong
8	The future. all I do is worry about the future. I don't know what college I want to attend yet, or what I want to major in [...]
9	my life is okay at the moment but my head is still constantly throwing bad thoughts at me. i feel like a piece of shit constantly even though i know I'm not [...]
10	if i wasn't living with my partner i'd be cutting myself to shreds and starving myself. now i just b/p and starve if i can [...]

(continued)

Table 4 (continued)

Rank	Posts
XLMRB- RANDOM- SELFHARM- 200 K	
1	I want to cut again. I miss it. I've been free for 6 months, almost 7 [...]
2	I just know I'll eventually do it. It's like a matter of time. I'm so afraid. All I can do is scream and stomp. Overdosing scares me the most [...]
3	Hmm I keep relapsing in anorexia and self harm (cutting), never had the energy to stop my depression and anxiety [...]
4	How to stopping self harm. So I've been hurting myself for a long time a couple of years now and I've been trying hard for these last couple of months to stop [...]
5	I forbade myself from cutting on my wrists, and for me the tention is unbearable. I have one scar on my wrist [...]
6	I am on medication, three types and Xanax too to help with anxiety attacks. I can tell that it helps but I'm still struggling a lot [...]
7	I'm currently doing IOP after doing inpatient, residential, and php a bunch of times. I'm seeing my therapist in a few days so hopefully that helps [...]
8	Been on it for a year and a half and I'm going through exactly this. I'm 21 and have been on different depression bullshit meds since 13 [...]
9	I'm pretty sure people will be better of without me. Like I want to commit suicide but that means I'll escape the pain that is my life [...]
10	I'm scared and need help. So tonight I self harmed for the first time. I burned myself pretty badly all over my forearms [...]

5.2 Created Training Data (Anorexia and Depression)

The second group of datasets used for training our models, for both anorexia and depression signs detection, was also collected from the Pushshift Reddit Dataset (see Sect. 4.2). For anorexia, we downloaded all the available submissions and comments written to the most popular and open subreddits about anorexia (r/AnorexiaNervosa, r/AnorexiaRecovery). We performed the same action for depression (r/depression, r/depression_help). From the posts, as in Sect. 4.2, we extracted the unique authors and their submissions and comments. For the negative class, we reused the RANDOM-USERS- TEXTS dataset. We followed the same steps as in Sect. 4.2 in avoiding collisions between the positive and the negative datasets, and in removing the users from RANDOM- USERS- TEXTS that had been published in some of the main directly related subreddits. In the case of anorexia, we considered the related subreddits to be: r/anorexia, r/AnorexiaRecovery, r/AnorexiaNervosa, r/Ednos, r/BingeEating Disorder, r/fat-logic, r/fuckeatingdisorders, r/eating_disorders, r/EatingDisorders, r/bulimia, and r/edsupport. For depression: r/depression, r/depres-sion_help, r/AnxietyDepressi-on, and r/depressionregimens. For these two tasks, since we already had the provided test collections in our hands, we used the timestamps of the posts to avoid any collision between the provided datasets (anonymised) and ours. For the positive class, we pruned the collections to the last 500 posts before their first interaction in any of the directly related subreddits for each mental health disorder. From the remaining data, we created a balanced dataset for anorexia and depression with 200 K posts randomly sampled.

5.3 Method (Anorexia and Depression)

Following the same method as in Sect. 4.3, the parameters were adjusted for each model in all variants by finding their optimal values. The model with the best performance for each target metric is then chosen, and the selected parameters for each variant can be observed in Tables 5 and 6.

5.4 Results (Anorexia and Depression)

In a similar way as in Sect. 4.4, we obtained the best results for the main metrics for anorexia: precision (0.839, Run 3), F1 (0.77, Run 3), $ERDE_{50}$ (0.022, Run 2) and latency-weighted F1 (0.69, Run 0) were obtained with the classifier XLMRB-ERISK- ANOREXIA. Note that we matched the latency-weighted F1 score with the team CLaC's run 4. The best result for $ERDE_5$ was obtained by our classifier XLMRB-RANDOM- ANOREXIA- 200K with the Run 2 at 0.036. Finally, for depression, the obtained results were notably worse than the ones for the other two tasks. However,

Table 5 Combinations of models and parameters for early risk detection of anorexia. For parameters extraction we used 20% of the provided training data as the validation set

Run	Model	Target metric	θ	Min. posts	Max. posts
0	LR- ERISK- ANOREXIA	*latency-weighted F1*	0.315	10	50
1	LR- ERISK- ANOREXIA	*ERDE_5*	0.370	2	5
2	LR- ERISK- ANOREXIA	*ERDE_50*	0.240	45	45
3	LR- ERISK- ANOREXIA	*F1*	0.450	100	100
0	XLMRB- ERISK- ANOREXIA	*latency-weighted F1*	0.260	10	50
1	XLMRB- ERISK- ANOREXIA	*ERDE_5*	0.210	2	5
2	XLMRB- ERISK- ANOREXIA	*ERDE_50*	0.135	45	45
3	XLMRB- ERISK- ANOREXIA	*F1*	0.200	100	100
0	XLMRB- RANDOM- ANOREXIA- 200K	*latency-weighted F1*	0.835	10	50
1	XLMRB- RANDOM- ANOREXIA- 200K	*ERDE_5*	0.720	2	5
2	XLMRB- RANDOM- ANOREXIA- 200K	*ERDE_50*	0.690	45	45
3	XLMRB- RANDOM- ANOREXIA- 200K	*F1*	0.680	100	100

we obtained the best scores for precision with the XLMRB- RANDOM- DEPRESSION- 200K classifier (0.702, Run 0), and ERDE_5 (0.064, Run 1), and ERDE_{50} (0.047, Run 2) with the XLMRB- ERISK- DEPRESSION classifier. The best result for F1 was obtained by the team FHDO-BCSG with their run B at 0.64. The results of running our models on the different test datasets are presented in Tables 7 and 8. To conclude, and to answer the question: *Will the proposed method be as effective in detecting other forms of mental health problems?*, the proposed method performed very well in detecting signs of anorexia, but did not perform as well in detecting signs of depression since we obtained some of the best scores (precision, ERDE metrics), but the overall performance was noticeably worse compared to the other tasks.

We present the posts with the highest probability of risks by each used model as follows: For detecting signs of anorexia, they are shown in Table 9. And for detecting signs of depression, the top posts with highest probability are shown in Table 10.

Table 6 Combinations of models and parameters for early risk detection of depression. For parameters extraction we used 20% of the provided training data as the validation set

Run	Model	Target metric	θ	Min. posts	Max. posts
0	LR- ERISK-DEPRESSION	*latency-weighted F1*	0.375	10	50
1	LR- ERISK-DEPRESSION	*ERDE_5*	0.205	2	5
2	LR- ERISK-DEPRESSION	*ERDE_50*	0.080	45	45
3	LR- ERISK-DEPRESSION	*F1*	0.310	100	100
0	XLMRB- ERISK-DEPRESSION	*latency-weighted F1*	0.098	10	50
1	XLMRB- ERISK-DEPRESSION	*ERDE_5*	0.074	2	5
2	XLMRB- ERISK-DEPRESSION	*ERDE_50*	0.039	45	45
3	XLMRB- ERISK-DEPRESSION	*F1*	0.068	100	100
0	XLMRB- RANDOM-DEPRESSION- 200K	*latency-weighted F1*	0.910	10	50
1	XLMRB- RANDOM-DEPRESSION- 200K	*ERDE_5*	0.650	2	5
2	XLMRB- RANDOM-DEPRESSION- 200K	*ERDE_50*	0.958	45	45
3	XLMRB- RANDOM-DEPRESSION- 200K	*F1*	0.962	100	100

Again, the tables show that the majority of posts classified as positive (showing signs of anorexia or depression) by the logistic regression model (LR-ERISK) are very short sentences and mostly include a specific expression or term such as *anxiety* and *depression*, contrarily to the BERT-based methods where the classification is more accurate and detect better the specific mental health issue.

Table 7 The performance for each run for early detection of signs of anorexia. Note that for each bolded metric our run gave the highest performance, including other teams

Run	P	R	F1	ERDE 5	ERDE 50	Latency TP	Speed	Latency-Weighted F1
LR- ERISK- ANOREXIA								
0	0.526	0.562	0.543	0.093	0.043	10	0.965	0.522
1	0.439	0.247	0.316	0.073	0.070	2	0.996	0.313
2	0.360	0.808	0.498	0.101	0.030	45	0.830	0.411
3	0.712	0.712	0.712	0.092	0.092	100	0.632	0.448
XLMRB- ERISK- ANOREXIA								
0	0.766	0.671	0.715	0.091	0.031	10	0.965	**0.690**
1	0.526	0.685	0.595	0.038	0.033	2	0.996	0.593
2	0.659	0.795	0.720	0.093	**0.022**	45	0.830	0.598
3	**0.839**	0.712	**0.770**	0.091	0.091	100	0.632	0.487
XLMRB- RANDOM- ANOREXIA- 200K								
0	0.702	0.548	0.615	0.091	0.042	10	0.965	0.594
1	0.302	0.849	0.446	**0.036**	0.029	2	0.996	0.444
2	0.591	0.712	0.646	0.094	0.030	45	0.830	0.536
3	0.621	0.740	0.675	0.093	0.093	100	0.632	0.427
LIRMM								
1	0.77	0.60	0.68	0.091	0.055	21	0.92	0.62
CLAC								
4	0.64	0.79	0.71	0.063	0.034	7	0.98	**0.69**
UNSL								
0	0.42	0.78	0.55	0.055	0.039	2	1	0.55
4	0.31	0.92	0.47	0.061	0.030	3	0.99	0.46

6 Summary

In this chapter, we have described how we employed a BERT-based classifier for the early detection of signs of self-harm using the provided datasets by the CLEF eRisk Track, in addition to a number of datasets which we created for that work. In the experiments, the classifier (XLMRB- RANDOM- SELFHARM) performed best as the result of two main factors, first, the impact that BERT-based models have been making in improving many tasks in the natural language process domain, and second, a key difference that we applied in this work which is the way we trained the model. We extended our work to examine the method's efficiency in the detection of other mental health issues with the early detection of signs of anorexia and depression. In the case of anorexia, we managed to improve most of the main metrics by using the provided dataset: precision, F1, both ERDE metrics and we matched the best result for

Table 8 The performance for each run for early detection of signs of depression. Note that for each bolded metric our run gave the highest performance, including other teams

Run	P	R	F1	ERDE 5	ERDE 50	Latency TP	Speed	Latency-Weighted F1
LR- ERISK- DEPRESSION								
0	0.531	0.215	0.306	0.098	0.077	10	0.965	0.294
1	0.346	0.228	0.275	0.081	0.078	2	0.996	0.273
2	0.157	0.823	0.264	0.137	0.060	45	0.830	0.218
3	0.538	0.633	0.581	0.101	0.101	100	0.632	0.365
XLMRB- ERISK- DEPRESSION								
0	0.569	0.468	0.514	0.099	0.055	10	0.965	0.496
1	0.325	0.468	0.383	**0.064**	0.060	2	0.996	0.382
2	0.258	0.722	0.380	0.116	**0.047**	45	0.830	0.315
3	0.559	0.481	0.517	0.100	0.100	100	0.632	0.327
XLMRB- RANDOM- DEPRESSION- 200K								
0	**0.702**	0.772	0.199	0.151	0.078	10	0.965	0.192
1	0.098	0.975	0.178	0.090	0.086	2	0.996	0.177
2	0.150	0.595	0.239	0.128	0.071	45	0.830	0.199
3	0.166	0.595	0.260	0.124	0.124	100	0.632	0.164
FHDO- BCSG								
B	0.64	0.65	**0.64**	0.095	0.064	–	–	–
RKMVERI								
C	0.67	0.38	0.48	0.098	0.091	–	–	–
UNSL								
A	0.48	0.32	0.38	0.088	0.074	–	–	–

latency-weighted F1. For depression, we obtained some of the best scores (precision, ERDE metrics), but the overall performance was noticeably worse compared to the other tasks.

Acknowledgements The first author would like to thank the following funding bodies for their support: FEDER/Ministerio de Ciencia, Innovación y Universidades, Agencia Estatal de Investigación/Project (RTI2018-093336-B-C21), Consellería de Educación, Universidade e Formación Profesional and the European Regional Development Fund (ERDF) (accreditation 2019-2022 ED431G-2019/04, ED431C 2018/29, ED431C 2018/19).
The second and third authors would like to thank the UKRI's EPSRC Project *Cumulative Revelations in Personal Data* (Grant Number: EP/R033897/1) for their support. We would also like to thank David Losada for arranging this collaboration.

Table 9 The posts with highest probability of risk of anorexia by each of the employed models

Rank	Posts
LR- ERISK- ANOREXIA	
1	Optimus Rhyme—Anxiety [Nerdcore]
2	Fuuuuuuuuck anxiety
3	Some weight behind that scorpion
4	I think so. I alays worry about it though, as it's a pretty cheap scale. I have anxiety that any higher weight is correct and any lower weight is a mistake
5	Oh my anxiety!
6	How much are you eating at your goal weight?
7	That's called anxiety
8	OP, this really screams eating disorder to me, and not binge eating like a lot of people are saying but more anorexia or anorexia with binging and purging. [...]
9	I would have so much anxiety in that line
10	this gave me anxiety
XLMRB- ERISK- ANOREXIA	
1	I made friends and started drinking and finally feel like a real college student. My life is pretty exciting now! I'm finally having some body confidence and feel less [...]
2	I'm really sad to hear your girlfriend is struggling so much. But you're amazing for supporting her and asking for advice. Dating/living with/even being friends with someone with an active eating disorder is incredibly emotionally taxing at the best of times, so make sure you're looking after you too [...]
3	Thank you so much and congrats on your recovery!! I can totally relate. I'm 17 years old, and have suffered with disordered eating and body image issues since age 11 [...]
4	I'm sitting here crying like a baby at this. It's so horrifying to think how easily my eating disorder could stick with me forever. I don't want to be anorexic [...]
5	That's how I felt getting diagnosed with my eating disorder. Having a doctor verify my anorexia was nothing short of surreal, yet I'm still paranoid I'm faking it and that I don't have it anymore [...]
6	Awesome! Eating disorders are a total bitch, and you are clearly doing an amazing job of beating yours!!!
7	Be patient with yourself. Self-compassion is nicer than relentless, harsh critique. Food is not a moral choice, but rather a right and a necessity for everyone. Eating disorders thoughts are simply thoughts [...]
8	From my experience with relapsing because of those "I could have one and start over again tomorrow thoughts," I know that I'm telling myself a lie. Once I started, I never stopped at one, and I very rarely started sobriety over again the next day [...]
9	I thought mine was fungal, but honestly it's probably hormones and stress. A few years ago I was really dealing with an eating disorder that threw my hormones for a loop and they've kind of been up and down ever since then [...]
10	Yeah, I can definitely understand you there! My scale always goes up 5–7lbs after a binge [...]

(continued)

Table 9 (continued)

Rank	Posts
XLMRB- RANDOM- ANOREXIA- 200K	
1	Wow, the 12th house is the house of the unknown and the unseen. So a stellium there could mean that you are a very very very secretive person. You act one way in [...]
2	[TOMT] [Song] When I was a kid (early 1990s) my family had a cassette of children's songs. One song's lyrics went, "He's my new guy, he's a cool guy. Instead of [...]
3	I was playing laser tag with some friends when I was like 8/9 and I hadnt properly tied my shoes and couldnt be bothered doing it because I knew I wouldnt be [...]
4	I haven't, I'm too scared to try them or pretty much any product that has more than like 2 ingredients because my skin is so sensitive and crazy prone to closed [...]
5	Need a quick answer on Wifi Pineapple. Bought this thing a while ago and trying to play with it the first time. Read the instuctions and reconfigured my lan for the [...]
6	Be a parent! Teach the child that there are hardships in this world that many can't avoid. Let them know that things will be hard, but you will be there to support [...]
7	I'm mostly doing the clips trying to create the sounds that are in my head without spending hours on something that doesn't sound right. I do the same thing when [...]
8	A couple were having sex. The girl said "Put a finger in there". The guy does and she asks "Does it fit?" He says "Yeah" "Put 2 fingers, does it fit?" "Yes it [...]
9	I'm a child for saying that you obviously have no idea what oppression is? Way to prove ny point, kid. Oppression is being beaten and killed for being different [...]
10	Remember Roy—Titans: Rebirth #1 Discussion. So, this subreddit, although named r/GreenArrow it's not just about the Emerald Archer, but about his family [...]

Table 10 The posts with highest probability of risk of depression by each of the employed models

Rank	Posts
LR- ERISK- DEPRESSION	
1	Depression
2	Some might be Postpartum depression
3	Yeah i have depression too
4	Everyone's depression is the same depression but the stress everyone has is far from the same
5	How not to talk to someone with depression
6	If depression had a face
7	How do you deal with depression?
8	I also dropped out not because of depression but other reasons. But depression is hell
9	Depression special
10	What was the feel? WHAT WAS THE FEEL?!?!

(continued)

Table 10 (continued)

Rank	Posts
XLMRB- ERISK- DEPRESSION	
1	Depression is an actual illness, not an event or state of mind. Depression is definitely a real illness [...]
2	[...] But don't expect someone with depression to just change their own life because of yours or others advice [...]
3	Have you brought these feelings up to your therapist? I would also let your boyfriend know how you're feeling, if you haven't already. I struggle with anxiety as well, and self talk helps me [...]
4	Food wasn't my only issue. I had gone from a straight A student to almost failing out of my second year of uni. I had severe depression and social phobia [...]
5	Hey I'm going through the same thing, [...] I finished 70 straight weeks of chemo in January and have been suffering from terrible depression ever since [...]
6	I absolutely agree with you on this. My depression (previous to last week) mostly manifested in me being a little b**** to everyone around me for a hot moment [...]
7	I know the pain of that kind of depression and thinking, I've been there. I want you to know you are not the worthless person you feel you are, that's the depression driving your thoughts [...]
8	I know it is irrational, selfish and plain stupid. I know that I am ill and it is the depression that makes me feel like this. I know life can be wonderful, but even if I don't value mine there are many things that I can do to help others [...]
9	High Functioning Depression. I don't know too many people like me, who are diagnosed with depression anxiety but are very high functioning individuals [...]
10	How 2 seduce, while having depression. Ok so for a while now I have been having an issue handling girls and depression [...]
XLMRB- RANDOM- DEPRESSION- 200K	
1	LBC currently discussing male suicide right now. One of the UKs better talk radio stations are discussing it right now and I thought some of you may be interested. www.lbc.co.uk or DAB or 97.3FM
2	Of course it's likely!!!! Life might be all over our galaxy. It's too bad we're killing all the life on this one
3	Really? Is it? I love these dogs but don't double down on a false narrative. Not everyone should own these dogs. They are wonderful animals in the right hands
4	The heart wants what the heart wants. That's actually the title. It used to be Granger Things Have Happened
5	I've always wanted to enter a photography contest with a very close in shot of my nuts. It is rolling sand dunes? Perhaps a picture of somewhere overseas? Nope. It's a ballsack
6	Mistakes like this tend to be valued by collectors. If people care about the album, it'll increase value. This was a mistake in pressing; whomever was running the press loaded the wrong labels
7	I hate gun control. I hate lack of gun control. I am a centrist extremist. Nobody is safe
8	Monolithic architecture. It certainly is a hell hole fo real doe. I don't want to be there or anywhere in view of it
9	There is also a difference between repairing a road and repaving entire stretches. Too many want new or assume new will be 'the' solution. Replacing is not repairing
10	I actually think Pence may be out of the loop. Pence will give us the shitty policies without the crazy. Bannon would be gone

References

1. Baumgartner, J., Zannettou, S., Keegan, B., Squire, M., & Blackburn, J. (2020). The pushshift reddit dataset. *In Proceedings of the International AAAI Conference on Web and Social Media, 14*, 830–839.
2. Burdisso, S. G., Errecalde, M., & Montes-y Gómez, M. (2019). A text classification framework for simple and effective early depression detection over social media streams. *Expert Systems with Applications, 133*, 182–197.
3. Burdisso, S. G., Errecalde, M., & Montes-y Gómez, M. (2019). Unsl at erisk 2019: a unified approach for anorexia, self-harm and depression detection in social media. In *CLEF (Working Notes)*.
4. Chancellor, S., & De Choudhury, M. (2020). Methods in predictive techniques for mental health status on social media: A critical review. *NPJ Digital Medicine, 3*(1), 1–11.
5. Cohan, A., Young, S., & Goharian, N. (2016). Triaging mental health forum posts. In *Proceedings of the Third Workshop on Computational Linguistics and Clinical Psychology* (pp. 143–147).
6. Conneau, A., Khandelwal, K., Goyal, N., Chaudhary, V., Wenzek, G., Guzmán, F., Grave, É., Ott, M., Zettlemoyer, L., & Stoyanov, V. (2020). Unsupervised cross-lingual representation learning at scale. In *Proceedings of the 58th Annual Meeting of the Association for Computational Linguistics* (pp. 8440–8451).
7. Devlin, J., & Chang, M.-W. (2018). Open sourcing bert: State-of-the-art pre-training for natural language processing. Retrieved April 22, 2021, from http://aiweb.techfak.uni-bielefeld.de/content/bworld-robot-control-software/.
8. Devlin, J., Chang, M.-W., Lee, K., & Toutanova, K. (2018). *Bert: Pre-training of deep bidirectional transformers for language understanding*. arXiv:1810.04805.
9. Gao, Z., Feng, A., Song, X., & Wu, X. (2019). Target-dependent sentiment classification with bert. *IEEE Access, 7*, 154290–154299.
10. Lample, G., & Conneau, A. (2019). *Cross-lingual language model pretraining*. arXiv:1901.07291.
11. Liu, Y., Ott, M., Goyal, N., Du, J., Joshi, M., Chen, D., Levy, O., Lewis, M., Zettlemoyer, L., & Stoyanov, V. (2019). *Roberta: A robustly optimized bert pretraining approach*. arXiv:1907.11692.
12. Losada, D. E., & Crestani, F. (2016). A test collection for research on depression and language use. In *International Conference of the Cross-Language Evaluation Forum for European Languages* (pp. 28–39). Springer.
13. Losada, D. E., Crestani, F., & Parapar, J. (2018). Overview of eRisk 2018: Early risk prediction on the internet (extended lab overview). *CEUR Workshop Proceedings, 2125*.
14. Losada, D. E., Crestani, F., & Parapar, J. (2019). Overview of eRisk 2019 early risk prediction on the internet. *Lecture Notes in Computer Science (including subseries Lecture Notes in Artificial Intelligence and Lecture Notes in Bioinformatics) 11696 LNCS*, September 2019 (pp. 340–357).
15. Losada, D. E., Crestani, F., & Parapar, J. (2020). Overview of eRisk 2020: early risk prediction on the internet. In *Experimental IR Meets Multilinguality, Multimodality, and Interaction Proceedings of the Eleventh International Conference of the CLEF Association (CLEF 2020)*.
16. Martínez-Castaño, R., Htait, A., Azzopardi, L., & Moshfeghi, Y. (2020). Early risk detection of self-harm and depression severity using bert-based transformers: Ilab at clef erisk 2020. *Early Risk Prediction on the Internet*.
17. Nikolov, A., & Radivchev, V. (2019). Nikolov-radivchev at semeval-2019 task 6: Offensive tweet classification with bert and ensembles. In *Proceedings of the 13th International Workshop on Semantic Evaluation* (pp. 691–695).
18. Obeid, J. S., Dahne, J., Christensen, S., Howard, S., Crawford, T., Frey, L. J., Stecker, T., & Bunnell, B. E. (2020). Identifying and predicting intentional self-harm in electronic health record clinical notes: Deep learning approach. *JMIR Medical Informatics, 8*(7), e17784.

19. Parikh, P., Abburi, H., Badjatiya, P., Krishnan, R., Chhaya, N., Gupta, M., & Varma, V. Multi-label categorization of accounts of sexism using a neural framework. In *EMNLP/IJCNLP, (1)* (2019).
20. Pater, J., & Mynatt, E. (2017). Defining digital self-harm. In *Proceedings of the 2017 ACM Conference on Computer Supported Cooperative Work and Social Computing* (pp. 1501–1513).
21. Peters, M., Neumann, M., Iyyer, M., Gardner, M., Clark, C., Lee, K., & Zettlemoyer, L. (2018). Deep contextualized word representations. In *Proceedings of the 2018 Conference of the North American Chapter of the Association for Computational Linguistics: Human Language Technologies, Volume 1 (Long Papers)* (pp. 2227–2237).
22. Radford, A., Narasimhan, K., Salimans, T., & Sutskever, I. (2018). Improving language understanding by generative pre-training. Retrieved April 22, 2021, from https://s3-us-west-2.amazonaws.com/openai-assets/research-covers/language-unsupervised/language_understanding_paper.pdf.
23. Satcher, D. (2000). Mental health: A report of the surgeon general-executive summary. *Professional Psychology: Research and Practice, 31*(1), 5.
24. Skaik, R., & Inkpen, D. (2020). Using social media for mental health surveillance: A review. *ACM Computing Surveys (CSUR), 53*(6), 1–31.
25. Vaswani, A., Shazeer, N., Parmar, N., Uszkoreit, J., Jones, L., Gomez, A. N., Kaiser, Ł., & Polosukhin, I. (2017). Attention is all you need. In *Advances in Neural Information Processing Systems* (pp. 5998–6008).
26. Yates, A., Cohan, A., & Goharian, N. (2017). Depression and self-harm risk assessment in online forums. arxiv:1709.01848.

Detecting Traces of Self-harm on Reddit Through Emotional Patterns

Mario Ezra Aragón, A. Pastor López-Monroy, Luis C. González, and Manuel Montes-y-Gómez

Abstract Currently, self-harm is considered one of the leading causes of death by suicide in young people. Timely detection of self-inflicted injury is important to help people before the illness gets worse, minimizing disabilities and returning them to their normal life. A popular way for people to share information is using social media platforms, where they tend to share topics related to work issues and personal matters. In fact, people suffering from mental disorders tend to share information about their concerns looking for some advice, support, or just because they want to relieve suffering. This creates an excellent opportunity to, for example, automatically detect users that have a suicidal intention and refer them as soon as possible to seek professional help. In this chapter, we describe a new text representation named Bag of Sub-Emotions (BoSE), which considers fine-grained emotions as the key information for the detection of users suffering from self-harm. We also present some extensions to BoSE aimed to better model and capture the emotional changes expressed by social media users through their posts. The proposed approach showed competitive performance in comparison to other methods evaluated in the eRisk collections but providing an easier understanding and interpretability of results.

M. E. Aragón (✉) · M. Montes-y-Gómez
National Institute of Astrophysics Optics and Electronics, Puebla, Mexico
e-mail: mearagon@inaoep.mx

M. Montes-y-Gómez
e-mail: mmontesg@inaoep.mx

A. P. López-Monroy
Mathematics Research Center, Guanajuato, Mexico
e-mail: pastor.lopez@cimat.mx

L. C. González
School of Engineering, Autonomous University of Chihuahua, Chihuahua, Mexico
e-mail: lcgonzalez@uach.mx

F. Crestani et al. (eds.), *Early Detection of Mental Health Disorders by Social Media Monitoring*, Studies in Computational Intelligence 1018,
https://doi.org/10.1007/978-3-031-04431-1_9

1 Introduction

Self-harm is defined as the direct and intentional injuring of one's body; in extreme cases with the intent to commit suicide [16]. People that commit self-harm commonly use a sharp object to make cuts in their skin. This practice includes other acts such as burning, hitting body parts, ingestion of toxic substances, or scratching.

On the other hand, for an important part of the world population, social life goes beyond their surroundings or immediate environment, that is, it takes place in a virtual world created by social media platforms like Facebook, Twitter, Reddit, or similar platforms. Social media has become a vital link for many people that live far from their loved ones, like family and friends. This reality presents a great opportunity to understand *what* and *how* we communicate.

Analyzing digital communication presents an advantage due to the potential amount of available information that could be explored. Social media corpora are often employed in the evaluation of automated methods that identify authors' characteristics, motives, and even inclinations. In this line of thought, it would be interesting to benefit from the social media corpora's features to develop and evaluate automated tools to help identify people in risk situations. Particularly, this study focuses on detecting traces of self-harm signs in users' comments. By detecting self-harm we could provide an auxiliary tool to extend the analysis to important mental disorders, since self-harm is a common symptom of people suffering depression, anxiety, or anorexia.

In 2020, for the second year in a row, eRisk@CLEF proposed a task on "Early Detection of Signs of Self-Harm", where several teams competed in detecting social media users, specifically from Reddit, that present signs of committing self-harm [19]. To this end, participants were invited to process the post history of the users as pieces of evidence and make predictions as early as possible. There were 12 teams participating on this challenge, our team, INAOE-CIMAT, competed via an approach based on recognizing that a given emotion could have several shades, which in this study we call sub-emotions. One of our premises is that emotions expressed by users could be helpful to differentiate between users who commit self-harm and those who do not (control group).

We proposed a representation called Bag of Sub-Emotions (BoSE), which is based on the use of fine-grained emotions, sub-groups of emotions that capture specific emotional topics on posts [2]. In a single quote, we can say that our representation consists of replacing the users' posts with a string of sub-emotions. We created this representation using a clustering algorithm over a lexical resource of (common) emotions. Then, we generated a histogram of these new fine-grained emotions. Our proposal is inspired by two main hypotheses. The first hypothesis is that words assigned to (common) emotions cannot capture subtle emotional differences. We argue and show that these differences provide important insights into the mental health condition of users. Our second hypothesis is that people with a mental health problem tend to express greater emotional variability than a healthy person. Our main goal is to capture these differences and variability with our proposed approach.

In this chapter, besides presenting in detail our approach, we extend our previous work using BoSE not only to capture the presence of sub-emotions but also to model their changes over time by using a representation called Δ-BoSE. Furthermore, we integrate popular neural network architectures with the aim to learn the relations between the embeddings of the sub-emotions and the users that present signs of self-harm. Results are very interesting, since they suggest that the presence and variability of emotions allow to highlight important information about social media users suffering from self-harm.

The remainder of this chapter is as follows: Sect. 2 presents some related work for the self-harm detection task and early predictions. Section 3 describes our inspiration for working with emotions. Section 4 introduces the creation of the sub-emotions. Section 5 presents how we model the sub-emotions. Section 6 shows our approach for learning sequential information from the sub-emotions. In Sect. 7 we present our approaches using deep learning and sub-emotions. Lastly, Sect. 8 depicts our conclusions.

2 Related Work

In the last few years, the study of public mental health through social media has increased in the research community. This is mainly due to the fact that these media provide a source of support for those who suffer from a mental health disorder, like for example, sense of community, relatedness and understanding [10, 11]. Recent works related to the detection of self-harm in social media have focused on the analysis of the post content [24, 25]. Some of them consider different kinds of word-based features, such as word n-grams, and employ traditional classification algorithms. Unfortunately, there is usually a high overlap in the vocabulary of users with and without self-harm, which causes a moderate performance. Other works focused on the use of deep neural models implementing attention mechanisms. For example, in [22], the authors implemented a method aimed to model the temporal mood variation through an attention network, and in [13], the authors proposed an attentive model combined with sentiment and topic analysis to detect suicidal ideation. The results obtained showed the potential of using an attention mechanism, since it contributes to improve the performance shown by other deep neural models.

From a different perspective, emotions have been studied in the fields of Psychology and Neuroscience [8]. In them, emotions have been defined as an important aspect of human nature, and it has been established their relationship with the expression of language, and consequently, their relationship with the manifestation of some mental disorders [9]. In particular, a study in psychiatry found that self-harm is associated with an emotion regulation function and trait emotion dysregulation [1]. Drawing from these ideas, we proposed to use a finer concept of emotions, that we previously presented in [2], although for a different task, detection of depression. In

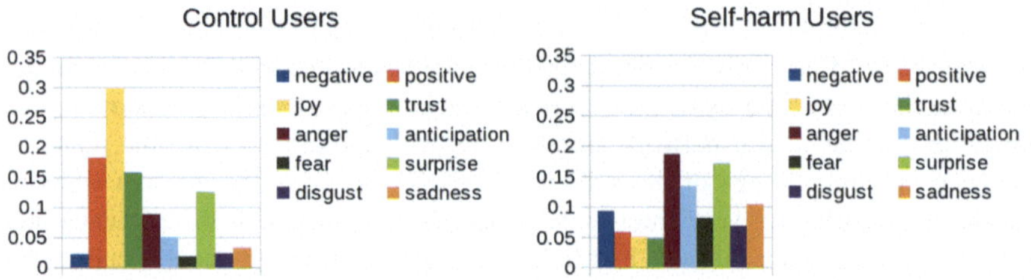

Fig. 1 Distribution of emotions at the eRisk 2020 collection, self-harm task

this chapter, we continue exploring the use of sub-emotions. This time, we consider emotional changes and the potential of this representation with deep neural networks for self-harm detection.

3 From Sentiments to Emotions

The inspiration behind our work started in the sentiment analysis task for social media corpora. Sentiment analysis is the process of detecting positive and negative sentiments in text. A well known strategy consists on counting the number of occurrences of positive, negative and neutral words in texts [14], or on measuring how similar are their words to some reference negative and positive words [12]. Analyzing sentiments has shown interesting results, since it has been found that negative comments are more abundant in people with a declared mental health disorder than in comments generated from a control group, which loosely we can call *healthy users* [9, 21]. Moving a step forward, in a recent work [26], the authors proposed the use of emotions to identify depression in Twitter users. That study openly exposed the potential of using discrete emotions as features, instead of only using linguistic features, and broad sentiment categories to represent them. The analysis of emotions showed promising results, improving the detection of depressed users in comparison with only using sentiments and word frequency.

Motivated by the results reported in [26], we decided to apply a similar methodology to analyze the distribution of emotions in the posts of users suffering from self-harm. For this analysis, we used a lexical resource of eight emotions and two sentiments [20] (which is explained in more detail in the next subsection). We first counted the number of words associated with each emotion, and then computed their average value for all users. Figure 1 presents the distribution of emotions corresponding to the users from the eRisk 2020 dataset. Broadly, it shows that control and no-control users tend to express different emotions through their posts. In particular, people suffering from self-harm use more negative words than control users, whereas the later express joy and trust more frequently than the former.

4 Can Emotions Have Shades? A Sub-emotion Based Representation

In the previous sub-section we explained why emotions are important for the detection of users with a mental health disorder. However, we did not mention an important limitation for it: when we consider the words assigned to coarse emotions in lexicons, we can not capture subtle emotional differences. For example, the lexicon associated with the anger emotion includes words such as *furious*, *angry* and *upset* that represent different degrees of anger, however, they are all tagged with the same emotion, that is, at the same level (in this case, anger). We argue that these differences provide important insights into the mental health condition of users.

Inspired by this intuition, we decided to evaluate emotions, or more precisely, fine-grained emotions as a representation to successfully identify Reddit's users that commit self-harm. We believe that the analysis of the expression of these kind of emotions is suitable to reveal symptoms or insights of people that have some psychological distress.

Our proposed method for the detection of self-harm consists of the representation of the user's post history based on their expressed fine-grained emotions. The first step in order to construct these representations is to generate groups of fine-grained emotions (referred to as *sub-emotions* from here on). For this, we used the EmoLEX lexicon [20], and selected each general emotion that belongs to it. EmoLEX is a lexical resource that indicates the relation of words to eight different emotions: Anger, Fear, Anticipation, Trust, Surprise, Sadness, Joy, and Disgust, and two sentiments: Negative and Positive.[1] To construct EmoLEX, its authors manually annotated the words to indicate if they express one or more of the after mentioned emotions. This lexical resource is available in 40 different languages. Once we have the sub-emotions, we masked the user's posts using the sub-emotions labels instead of the original words. In the following sections, we describe in detail each step of this procedure.

4.1 Generating Sub-emotions

To generate the sub-emotions we follow the next process:

1. Use a set of words associated with emotions in the EmoLEX lexicon. In the lexicon, there are some words associated with more than one emotion. We formally represent this set of emotions as $E = \{E_1, E_2, \ldots, E_{10}\}$, where $E_i = \{t_1, \ldots, t_n\}$ is the set of words associated to emotion E_i.
2. Compute an embedding vector for each word that the EmoLEX lexicon resource contains. For this, we used Wikipedia pre-trained sub-word embeddings of size

[1] In the rest of the chapter we refer to these sentiments as emotions as well.

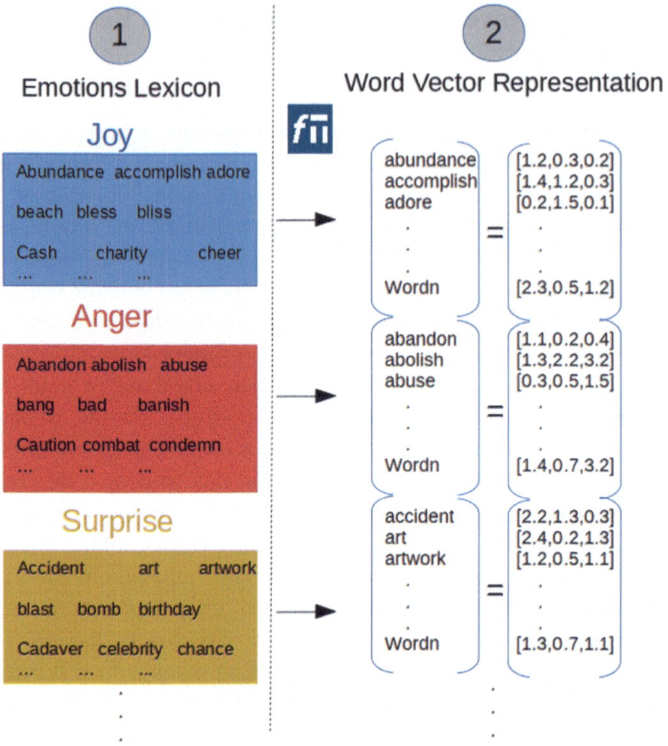

Fig. 2 Compute word embedding vectors for each word in the EmoLEX lexicon. For simplicity, in the Figure we only use three emotions, but this process was applied to the eight emotions and two sentiments considered

300 from FastText [7]. It is important to mention that for this step we could use any other type of word embeddings. We depict these first two steps in Fig. 2.

3. Form groups of sub-emotions. For this, for each emotion, we clustered the words using the *Affinity Propagation (AP)* algorithm. This method is a graph-based clustering algorithm similar to k-means, but that does not require the number of clusters to be specified in advance. An additional advantage of this algorithm is that it finds examples of members of the input set, and use them as representatives of the clusters [23]. After the clustering, each centroid represents a different sub-emotion.
4. Save for each emotion a set of sub-emotions, $E_i = \{S_1, \ldots, S_k\}$, where each S_j is a subset of the words from E_i. This whole process creates a super set $\mathbb{S}$ with all computed sub-emotions. In Fig. 3 we present these last two steps.

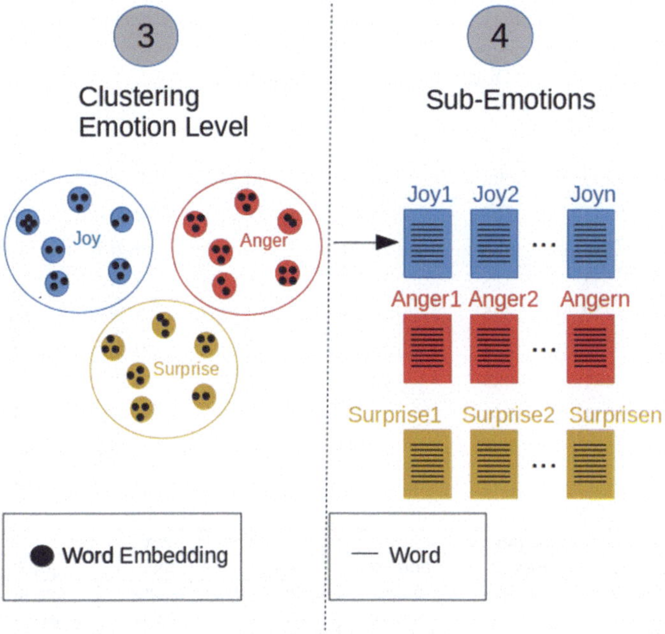

Fig. 3 Sub-emotions obtained with the affinity propagation algorithm for each emotion. Each sub-emotion represents a group of words with the same label

4.2 Analysis of the Novel Sub-emotions

For a complete picture of how the vocabulary in the EmoLEX lexicon is distributed among emotions, as well as how it is distributed across the created sub-emotions by the affinity propagation (AP) algorithm, in Table 1 we present some statistics of the lexicon. We indicate the number of words and clusters (i.e., sub-emotions) per broad emotion, as well as the average and standard deviation of their internal cohesion (μCoh and σCoh, respectively). The internal cohesion is a metric used to calculate how similar an object is to its own cluster; a value closer to 1 indicates high similarity and a value closer to -1 indicates very low similarity. We obtain this metric by measuring the cosine similarity of each word with respect to the others in its same cluster.

Some interesting aspects to note from Table 1 are the following. First, the size of the vocabularies associated with each broad emotion is large, as well as diverse, since the number of clusters obtained per emotion is also large. However, it can be seen that the average number of words per cluster (μW) is similar for all emotions, which indicates that the AP algorithm could find a similar distribution of words in the clusters even for emotions with large vocabularies. Second, the cohesion values indicate that although not all the sub-emotions generated present high cohesion, in

Table 1 Size of the vocabulary for each emotion presented in the lexical resources, and number of generated clusters (Cls)

Coarse emotion stats		Discovered sub-emotions stats				
Emotion	Vocabulary	Cls	μ W	σ **W**	μ Coh	σ Coh
Anger	6035	444	13.60	16.53	0.2932	0.1588
Anticip	5837	393	14.77	20.53	0.2910	0.1549
Disgust	5285	367	14.4	21.29	0.2812	0.1601
Fear	7178	488	14.70	23.36	0.2983	0.1455
Joy	4357	318	13.70	21.25	0.2928	0.1638
Sadness	5837	395	14.78	20.48	0.2911	0.1549
Surprise	3711	274	13.54	28.68	0.2874	0.1626
Trust	5481	383	14.31	21.59	0.2993	0.1609
Positive	11021	740	14.89	24.53	0.2967	0.1466
Negative	12508	818	15.29	23.75	0.2867	0.1417

Anger			**Joy**		
anger1	***anger2***	***anger3***	***joy1***	***joy2***	***joy3***
abomination	growl	battle	accomplish	bounty	charity
fiend	growling	combat	achieve	cash	foundation
inhuman	thundering	fight	gain	money	trust
abominable	snarl	battler	reach	reward	humanitarian
unholy	snort	fists	goal	wealth	charitable
Surprise			**Disgust**		
surprise1	***surprise2***	***surprise3***	***disgust1***	***disgust2***	***disgust3***
accident	art	magician	accusation	criminal	cholera
crash	museum	wizard	suspicion	homicide	epidemic
disaster	artwork	magician	complaint	delinquency	malaria
incident	gallery	illusionist	accuse	crime	aids
collision	visual	sorcerer	slander	enforcement	polio

Fig. 4 Examples of words grouped in different sub-emotions

all cases there are groups with an important degree of cohesion, which help capturing very specific topics.

It is important to note that some high-cohesive sub-emotions provide an easy understanding and interpretability. For example, the obtained sub-groups of words separate each coarse emotion in different related topics, which in turn capture more specific emotions expressed by users in their posts. In Fig. 4, we present some examples of the groups of words that represent the sub-emotions. It is important to mention that these groups were automatically obtained using this approach. Note that words with similar contexts tend to group together. For example, for the emotion **Anger** one group expresses topics related to fighting and battles, and for another group, we can appreciate topics related to loud noises or growls. In another example, the **Surprise** emotion has one group that is related to accidents and disasters, whereas

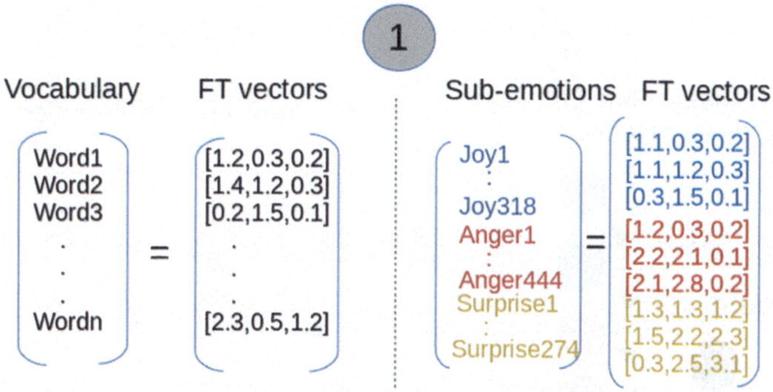

Fig. 5 Determination of the the vocabulary words and sub-emotions vectors

other groups have words that are related to art and museums, and magic and illusion, respectively.

4.3 *Converting Text to Sub-emotions Sequences*

Our general procedure is to concatenate all the individual posts of each user and create a single document for each one. Then, we mask all users' documents replacing their words with the label of the closest sub-emotion. The following points describe in detail our approach:

1. Compute prototypical sub-emotion vectors by averaging the word embeddings in each cluster. We use the labels of these prototypes to count each word in the text as an occurrence of each sub-emotion. We also compute the word vector for each word in the vocabulary of the users. Figure 5 depicts this step.
2. Measure for each word t in the vocabulary its cosine similarity with all sub-emotions vectors S.
3. Replaced the word t by a label $\tau(t)$ related to its closest sub-emotion.[2] That is, $\tau(t) = S_j : \max_{\forall S_j \in \mathbb{S}} sim(\mathbf{t}, \mathbf{S_j})$. We present these two steps in Fig. 6.
4. Mask the words from the post history with their corresponding sub-emotion. After this step, documents are sequences of sub-emotions instead of sequences of words. We present this final step in Fig. 7.

To illustrate this process consider the following two example sentences:

1. `Two days ago I found out my girlfriend cheated on me and we broke up while I was coming down it was the worst day of my`

[2] We assigned the labels selecting the name of the emotion followed by the sequential number. For example, for anger, the labels were assigned as anger1, anger2, ...,angerK. Where K is the number of clusters in that emotion.

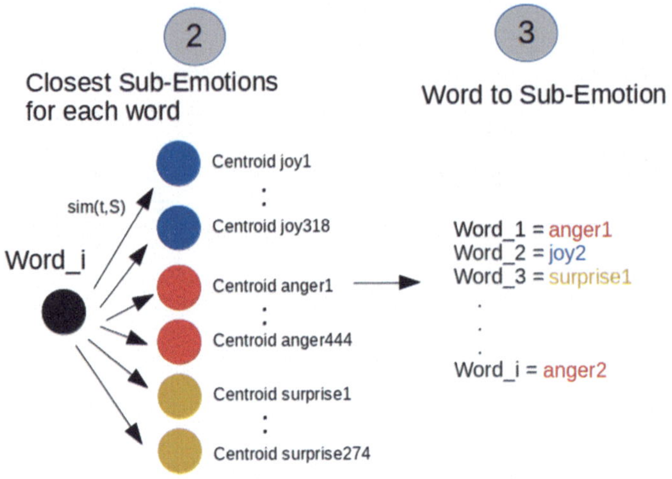

Fig. 6 Replace each word in the vocabulary with its closest sub-emotion

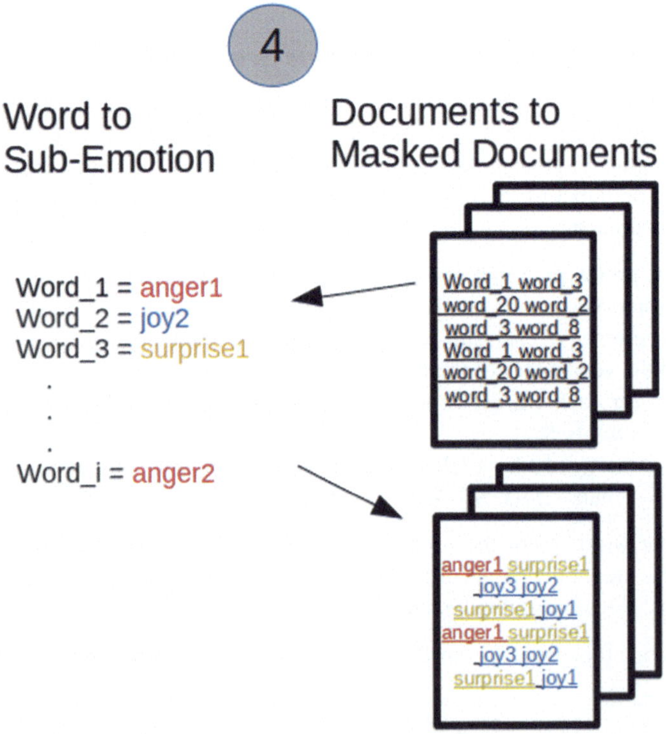

Fig. 7 Masking the users' documents, replacing word sequences for sequences of sub-emotions

life I tried to buy a gun to kill myself with but the guy never showed up (thankfully).
2. I guess my point is comedowns suck especially if your life is collapsing around you.

These sentences will be masked as:

1. disgust3 trust12 surprise18 joy6 joy4 trust27 surprise18 positive12 disgust6 anticipation22 anticipation16 joy6 surprise18 disgust19 surprise24 disgust9 joy6 joy6 anticipation22 surprise24 anger9 joy6 joy6 disgust19 surprise9 joy6 surprise18 sadness1 joy6 trust27 positive2 trust2 joy6 anger8 positive2 surprise7 positive9 anger9 trust15 joy6 anticipation1 joy16 surprise3 surprise24 trust12 joy16 trust23
2. joy6 surprise18 surprise18 anger9 anger9 negative28 disgust23 joy4 surprise18 positive9 sadness1 anger9 disgust19 anger9 positive9

From these examples, it is possible to appreciate how different contexts are captured by different sub-emotions. It is important to mention that we replaced the whole vocabulary of all users including stopwords, for their closest sub-emotions. Our decision to keep stopwords was completely experimental, we performed experiments removing them before masking the texts, but consistently we got slightly lower performances. We believe some stopwords add important information to the model for interpreting their surrounding words.

5 Using BoSE to Identify Self-harm

In this section, we present the subemotion-based representation, the so-called Bag of Sub-Emotions (BoSE), which allows us to model the presence of the sub-emotions through the users' posts.

5.1 BoSE Definition

Once we masked the documents, the next step is to build the BoSE representation by using histograms of sub-emotions. For this, we represent each document d as a vector of weights associated with sub-emotions. Represented in a formal way we have:

$$\mathbf{d} = \langle w_1, \ldots, w_m \rangle \tag{1}$$

where m is the total number of generated sub-emotions, and $0 \leq w_i \leq 1$ represents the relevance of sub-emotion S_i to the document d. This weight is computed in a *tf-idf* fashion as:

$$w_i = freq(S_i, d) \cdot \log\left(\frac{|\mathcal{D}|}{\#_{\mathcal{D}}(S_i)}\right) \tag{2}$$

where $freq(S_i, d)$ represents a function that denotes the frequency of the sub-emotion S_i in the document d, $|\mathcal{D}|$ is the number of documents in the whole collection, and $\#_{\mathcal{D}}(S_i)$ is a function denoting the number of documents containing the sub-emotion S_i. With this information, we determine how relevant that sub-emotion is in the entire training set. Observe that this representation only considereds the presence of individual sub-emotions in the documents. Therefore, we call it **BoSE-unigrams**. In the case when we consider the presence of sequences of sub-emotions, we named the representation as **BoSE-ngrams**.

5.2 BoSE at eRisk 2020

The eRisk 2020 T1 task (Early Detection of Signs of Self-Harm) was a continuation of the eRisk 2019 T2 task, having the same title [18]. This task consisted of detecting traces of self-harm in users of Reddit as early as possible. The purpose is to observe these traces while the users' posts are sequentially processed. For this, a server iteratively provided users' writings in chronological order. For each user, systems should respond with a positive or negative prediction, that is, they should indicate if each user presents or not signs of committing self-harm. After sending the predictions, the server continued with the next set of writings for each user.

Similar to the previous edition, the collection used in the eRisk 2020 shared task on self-harm detection contains two categories of users: self-harm and control. Table 2 reports the main statistics of the train and test collections for this task.

For our participation in this task, we used the BoSE representation, previously detailed in Sect. 5. To start with the round of experiments, we first trained and evaluated our model using the 2019 eRisk dataset. These evaluations helped us select the best parameters before sending our predictions. The 2019 dataset contains two categories of users: control and self-harm. For the experiment, we used the users' whole post history and performed cross-validation. We considered the F1 over the positive class as evaluation measure.

Table 2 Self-harm data sets used for experimentation. (NC = No Control, C = Control)

Data set	Training		Test	
	NC	C	NC	C
Users	41	299	104	319
Avg. num. posts	169.0	546.8	112.4	285.6
Avg num. words per post	24.8	18.8	21.4	11.9

Table 3 F1 results over the positive class in the 2019 training dataset

Method	F1-positive class	Training set
BoSE	0.52	Self-harm
BoSE	0.53	Depression and self-harm
BoSE+BoW	0.44	Self-harm
BoSE+BoW	**0.58**	Depression and self-harm

In order to improve predictions, we also attempted to take advantage of the relationship that exists between self-harm and depression. For this, we used the 2018 depression dataset in conjunction with the 2019 self-harm dataset during the training of our model. In addition, we enriched the BoSE representation with a simple BOW, aiming to capture some specific words related to self-harm. In Table 3 we present the obtained results for these experiments. The results suggest that the combination of these two extensions to BoSE helped to improve the detection of users committing self-harm.

Trying to understand what our model captures, as well as the reason for the usefulness of the depression data, we carried out an analysis of the most relevant words of each dataset. In Table 4, we present five of the most relevant words obtained by using the chi^2 test for each task. We observe that the model captures some differences between self-harm and depression. For depression, the most relevant words are more related to emotional problems, and for self-harm, the words are more related to physical damage. However, there is also a relevant subset of words shared by the two tasks.

A relevant question that appeared at this point was: *Are there specific sub-emotions related to self-harm?* In order to answer this question we need to analyze what sub-emotions BoSE captured. In Table 5 we show some of the top relevant sub-emotions (according to the chi^2 distribution), as well as some examples of the words that correspond to these sub-emotions in the self-harm task. Some topics are related to negative aspects, like hate, criticism, or refuse. An interesting sub-emotion captured automatically by our model is the negative sub-emotion related to young people, since people that commit self-harm usually are teenagers or closer to that age.

Table 4 Words with high chi2 distribution for each dataset

Depression
Mental, therapy, treatment, medication and addiction
Self-harm
Scars, mania, skin, obsessions and compulsion
Shared words
Anxiety, antidepressants, depressed, concern and lonely

Table 5 Examples of relevant sub-emotions for self-harm detection

Self-harm	
Anger11	Unsociable, crowd, mischievous
Anger108	Traumatic, trauma, traumatize
Anticip104	Attack, offensive , harass
Anticip10	Hurting, refused, anxious, afraid
Disgust17	Condemn, criticise, refuse, repudiate
Disgust32	Breakdown, fight, crushed, abandoned
Fear5	Dreadful, hate, bad, nasty
Fear114	Aggression, hostile, discord
Joy14	Life, time, moment
Joy104	Effort, chance, opportune
Negative18	Adolescence, teen, juvenile
Negative115	Conceal, hide, concealment
Positive110	Protect, safeguard, protection
Positive19	Helpful, information, relevant
Surprise20	Distress, embarrassment, shame
Surprise108	Oddness, quirkiness, strangeness
Trust22	Impatient, desire, anxious
Trust20	Ambition, desire, wanted

Once the model is trained, for generating the predictions over the test set we evaluated the following strategies to make the classification more robust:

1. Run 0: it considered only the training set from the previous edition, and employed the BoSE representation. A user was classified as committing self-harm if his/her probability of belonging to the positive class was higher than 0.60 in two consecutive predictions.
2. Run 1: it is similar to Run 0, but the model was trained using the depression data set from the eRisk 2018 task.
3. Run 2: It combined a BoW representation with BoSE and trained the classification model using the self-harm and depression datasets together.
4. Run 3: It is similar to Run 2, except that the training was done using the self-harm dataset.
5. Run 4: It employed the BoW and BoSE representations trained with the depression and self-harm datasets; a positive prediction was generated when its probability was higher than 0.55.

Table 6 shows the results obtained by the five strategies over the 2020 test partition. It can be observed that the third strategy (Run 3) was the one that obtained the best results. It consisted of the usage of BoSE and BoW trained only over the self-harm dataset. In this strategy, a user was identified as committing self-harm if the probability of the positive class was higher than 0.60 in two consecutive pre-

Table 6 Results over the positive class in the 2020 test data set

Method	F1	ERDE5	ERDE50	Latency TP	Latency-weighted F1	Training set
Run 0	0.524	0.203	0.145	4	0.518	Self-harm
Run 1	0.523	0.193	0.144	4	0.517	Depression and self-harm
Run 2	0.520	0.207	0.160	5	0.512	Depression and self-harm
Run 3	**0.601**	0.174	0.119	3	**0.596**	Self-harm
Run 4	0.526	0.198	0.160	4	0.519	Depression and self-harm

dictions. This indicates the temporal emotional stability of the user. We noticed that this approach also obtains the best ERDE score, which implies a good prediction with relatively less information. The usage of both representations, BoSE and BoW, suggests that not only the emotional information but also the presence of certain words (associated with certain topics) are important for the detection of people who commit self-harm.

To offer more context about these results, Fig. 8 compares our approach against all other participants at eRisk 2020. The first two columns show the boxplots corresponding to all F1 and Latency-weighted F1 results. The green **X** mark represents

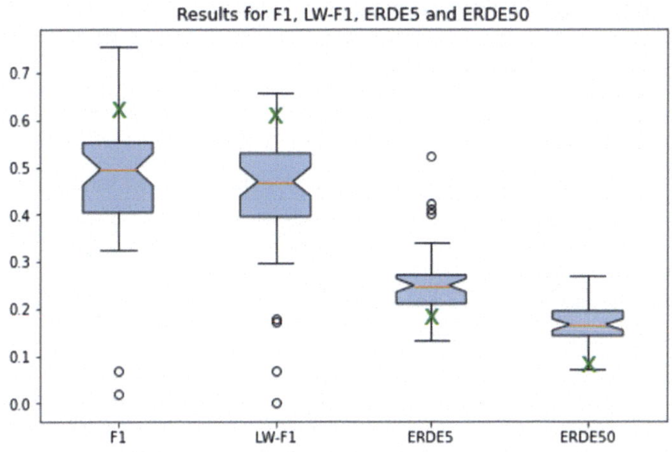

Fig. 8 Boxplot for the results in F1, Latency-weighted F1, ERDE5, and ERDE50 in the 2020 self-harm test dataset. Where the green X mark represents our obtained results

the position of our results. Note that our results are in the highest quartile for both indicators. In the last two columns of the figure, we present two boxplots for all participants in accordance to the ERDE5 and ERDE50 evaluation metrics. It is worth mentioning that ERDE is an error measure, which means that the lower its value, the better the performance. Thus, our results for these metrics are also positioned in the best quartile, implying a competitive prediction with relatively less information in comparison with other participants.

5.3 BoSE for Whole Post's History

The main goal of this experiment is to analyze the performance of BoSE using the whole post history of the users, instead of an early approach. We introduce the next baselines to contrast all the results. Inspired by [26], we implemented a slightly different approach. For this approach, we applied a similar strategy as BoSE, but instead of sub-emotions, we masked the words with their closest coarse emotion. This approach is named as Bag-of-Emotions (BoE). We also considered a traditional Bag-of-Words (BoW) representation, and similar to BoSE, we incorporated the words with the highest relevance according to the chi^2 distribution. For both representations, we used the word unigrams and n-grams. For BoW, we added an extra experiment using char-grams of length 3. For all these experiments, we consider the F_1 score, precision, and recall over the positive class. Table 7 presents the results over the positive class for this evaluation. From this comparison, we observe that BoSE outperforms all baseline results in terms of F_1 and recall, offering the next remarks:

1. BoSE outperformed the BOW representation in both F_1 and recall. These results indicate that considering emotional information is more relevant for the detection of self-harm than only considering the use of words.
2. The use of sub-emotions as features improves the results from a representation that only considers coarse emotions.

Table 7 F_1, Precision and Recall results over the positive class in the self-harm data set

Method	F1	Precision	Recall
BoW	0.50	**0.95**	0.34
n-grams	0.52	**0.95**	0.36
3-grams	0.53	0.74	0.42
BoE	0.43	0.45	0.40
BoSE	**0.62**	0.78	**0.51**

6 Learning Sequential Information from Sub-emotions

Sequential information is valuable to discover discriminative patterns in natural language processing tasks. This information in terms of emotions and sub-emotions can be interpreted as finding emotional variability and regularities among the posts of users. Unfortunately, this information is not naturally captured by approaches based on bag of terms or concepts, such as the previously described BoE/BoSE strategies, which lose the order of the occurrence of emotions. In this section we describe different sequential strategies adapted to take advantage of our proposed ideas to model emotions and sub-emotions. In Sect. 6.1 we introduce **Δ-BoSE** [4], where we extract new features based on statistical values to capture the emotional variability through the sequence at chunk level. This strategy allow us to exploit our proposed ideas for emotions and sub-emotions by a wide range of traditional classifiers such as SVMs. Then, in Sect. 7, we go a step further by using deep learning techniques to model the emotional variability by means of adapting convolutional and recurrent neural networks with attention in order to find patterns at local and global levels of the masked text.

6.1 Δ-BoSE

The main idea of **Δ-BoSE** is that users express their emotions in a different way, and that this could reveal a valuable pattern to improve their identification. In other words, users that present signs of self-harm tend to expose greater emotional variability than a healthy person. Following this hypothesis, we propose a new representation to capture this variability in the emotions by extracting statistical features. We named this representation **Δ-BoSE**. The following steps describe the construction of Δ-BoSE; Fig. 9 graphically shows this process.

1. Process the post history of each user using a chunk by chunk framework similar to the eRisk competition. Therefore, consider from now on that we have n chunks of text for each user.
2. Compute for each chunk the BoSE representation as described in Sect. 5.1, then consider the sequence of chunks as a sequence of documents represented with BoSE.
3. For each chunk represented under BoSE, expand the representation of each m dimension (sub-emotion) by a vector of n values $\mathbf{S_i} = \langle w_{i,1}, \ldots, w_{i,n} \rangle$, where $w_{i,j}$ indicates the weight of sub-emotion S_i in the chunk j as determined by Formula (2).
4. Transform each sub-emotion vector $\mathbf{S_i}$ into a vector $\Delta\mathbf{S_i}$ that models the temporal variability of the sub-emotions. For this, we represent each sub-emotion by a $\Delta-$vector of the following eight statistical values that capture its changes through the n-chunks sequence: mean(μ), sum($\sum$), max-value(max), min-value(min), standard deviation(σ), variance(σ^2), average($\bar{x}$), and median($\tilde{x}$). With this sta-

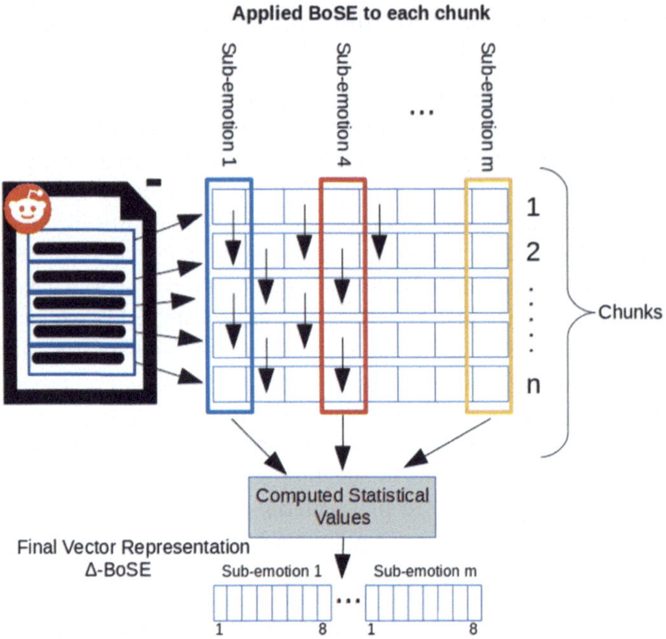

Fig. 9 Construction of the Δ-BoSE representation. First, BoSE is obtained for each part of the document; then, statistical values are computed for each sub-emotion creating a new vector representation

tistical values we create a new vector $\Delta \mathbf{S_i} = \langle \mu, \sum, max, min, \sigma, \sigma^2, \bar{x}, \tilde{x} \rangle$ that represents the changes of the sub-emotion S_i in the post history of the user.

5. Concatenate the Δ-vectors from all sub-emotions in one single vector of size $8 \times m$, where m is the number of sub-emotions (see Fig. 9).

One of the main benefits of Δ-BoSE representation is that it makes possible to observe the emotional change in users. The latter significantly improves the interpretability of the model, which becomes highly relevant in medical domains. To appreciate this, in Fig. 10 we compared the occurrences of certain sub-emotions over time and selected some of the top sub-emotions based on their chi-squared value. These signals indicate the average value of the occurrence of the sub-emotions in all users from each group. It is worth to note that the self-harm group presents higher changes through time than those in the control group. This could be interpreted as that self-harm users have high emotional variability and it could be further analyzed through emotion-based representations. Finally, our experimental evaluation in Table 8 shows that, although Δ-BoSE is sightly below the performance of BoSE, it offers better interpretability and is still better than baselines.

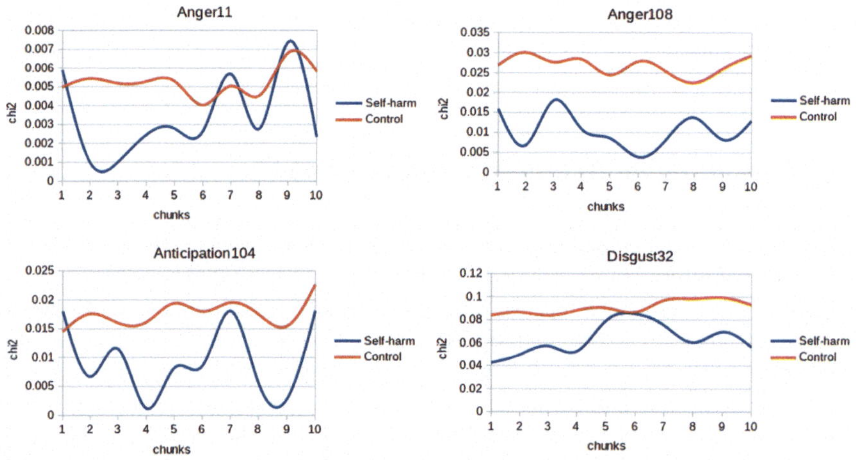

Fig. 10 Comparison of the emotional signals between control and self-harm groups. X-axis represents the chunks (time span) and Y-axis represents the average value of the sub-emotion at each chunk

Table 8 F_1, Precision and Recall results over the positive class in the self-harm data set

Method	F1	Precision	Recall
BoSE	**0.62**	**0.78**	**0.51**
Δ-BoSE	0.58	0.72	0.48

7 Deep Learning for Extracting Sequential Emotion Patterns

To this point we have only used our proposed sub-emotions (Sect. 4.1) to build representations using the framework of *bag of features*, which consist in building emotion vectors that are fed into standard classifiers. However, there are some sequential patterns that will be hardly captured in this *bag of emotions*. This is because the occurrence order of the emotions is lost once they are codified into the representation. In spite that some sequential information can be captured by extracting sub-emotion n-grams or by using Δ-BoSE, there are better approaches to capture long dependencies and complex patterns among sequences of user emotions [3].

In this section we show how to adapt deep neural networks to take advantage of their capacity to automatically learn sequential patterns. The key idea is to see the documents as sequences of sub-emotion vectors associated to each word. This step is similar to what we described in Sect. 4.3 and is showed in Fig. 7, where we treated the document as a sequence of sub-emotion labels. The representation of documents as a sequence of sub-emotion vectors, allow us to fed them into Convolutional and Recurrent Neural Networks with Attention just as if they were processing standard sequences of word embeddings. The advantage is that we can capture emotional patterns at local and global levels at the same time to better model users that could commit self-harm.

7.1 Convolutional Neural Network and BoSE

Now that we have our embeddings for the sub-emotions, we want to take advantage of the contextual information presented. For this purpose, our next experiments consist of the usage of neural networks. More specifically a Convolutional Neural Network (CNN). A CNN is an algorithm designed to recognized patterns. These patterns are numbers contained in a vector, in our case, sub-emotion embeddings. The CNN is a neural network that applies convolutional layers to local features. These convolutional layers, also named kernels or filters, can transform the large input data into local features. We use these filters, multiply its values element-wise with the original matrix, then sum them up. A full convolution consists of sliding the filter over the whole matrix and to the convolutional operation for each element.

For our problem, we explain this process in Fig. 11 and through the following steps:

1. Represent each sub-emotion with an embedding vector. This embedding vector corresponds to the centroid obtained when we cluster the sub-emotions.
2. Use a convolutional neural network architecture for feature extraction of the sub-emotions inspired in [15]. We represent this step in Fig. 11 with the filters in blue and red.
3. Obtain different feature maps for each region and concatenate them together to form a single feature vector. This can be interpreted as summarizing the local information to find patterns.
4. Apply a sigmoid to classify the vector.

The intuition about this network is to see the post history as a sequence of sub-emotion embeddings. We look for the convolution taking one or two sub-emotions at once since our filter sizes are 1 and 2. In this process, we choose the maximum value of the result from each filter vector. We can think of filter sizes as unigrams and bigrams, since they are finding patterns at this level of neighborhood.

The purpose of the following experiment is to know if using the sub-emotion embeddings allow to obtain better results than the regular word embeddings and our previously BoSE representation. Table 9 presents the results of this experiment. We observe that using BoSE with a CNN obtains a better performance that traditional embeddings in terms of $F1$ score and recall, whereas using only BoSE obtains a better precision.

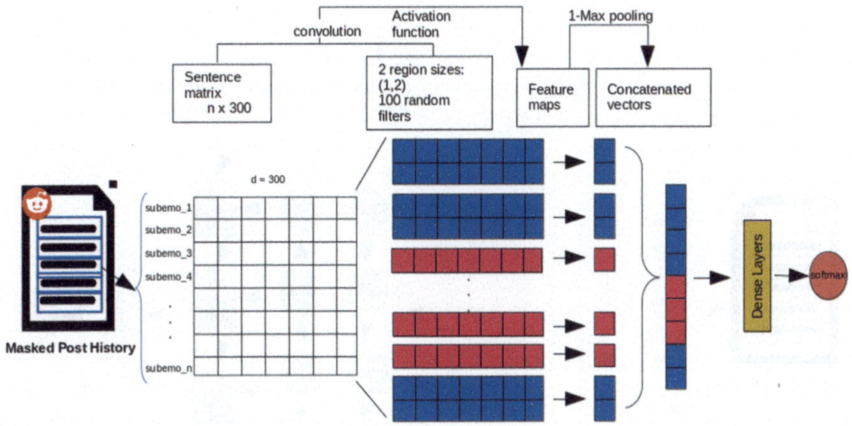

Fig. 11 Diagram of the Convolutional Neural Network Model. We used 100 random filters of size 1 and 2 to extract the local features

Table 9 F_1, Precision and Recall results over the positive class in the self-harm data set

Method	F1	Precision	Recall
CNN-glove	0.57	0.54	**0.59**
CNN-word2vec	0.56	0.54	0.58
BoSE	0.62	**0.78**	0.51
CNN-BoSE	**0.65**	0.73	**0.59**

7.2 Recurrent Neural Network and BoSE

Recurrent Neural Networks (RNN) are neural networks that are ideal for sequential information such as text. In our scenario the idea is to capture sequential patterns of sub-emotions expressed by users, which can be achieved because the RNN has a feedback loop that allows to inspect longer dependencies among sub-emotions. The proposed strategy based on RNNs process an input sequence sub-emotion by sub-emotion instead of word by word, which helps to preserve the information about past sub-emotions on the sequence. This information flows through the hidden states and affects the decisions without revealing all learned. RNNs are dynamic systems, but they present a problem maintaining the relation of long sequences. Because the backpropagated gradient shrink at each time step and after many steps vanish [17]. To alleviate this problem, we use a special type of RNN, with explicit memory named Gated Recurrent Unit (GRU). GRUs use two gates named update gate and reset gate. These gates are two vectors that help to decide the amount of information that should be pass to the output.

For this experiment, we used the sub-emotions embeddings and used as input for a BiDirectional GRU. GRU helps us to remember previous information learning the

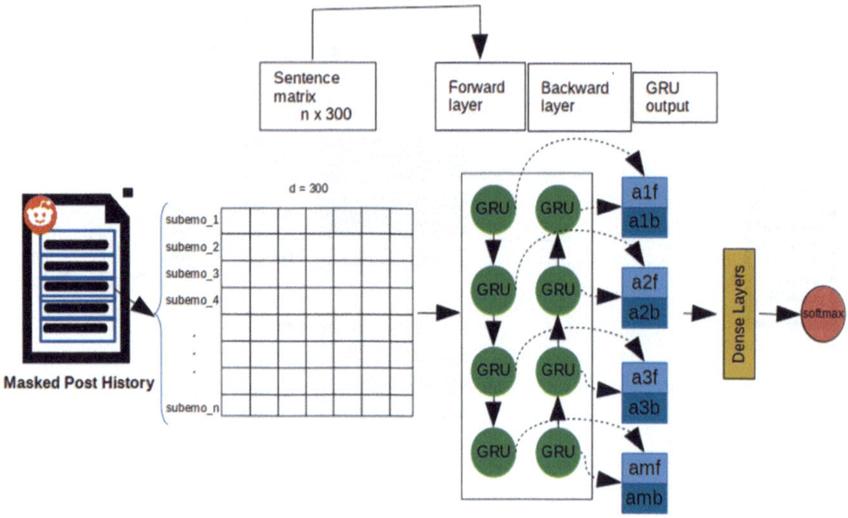

Fig. 12 Diagram of the Recurrent Neural Network Model. We used a bi-GRU network and combining the outputs before the decision making

Table 10 F_1, Precision and Recall results over the positive class in the self-harm data set

Method	F1	Precision	Recall
RNN-glove	0.57	0.54	**0.59**
RNN-word2vec	0.57	0.62	0.53
BoSE	0.62	**0.78**	0.51
RNN-BoSE	**0.64**	0.70	**0.59**

sequential structure of the sub-emotions. Furthermore, the BiDirectional GRU keeps the contextual information in both directions. We present this process in Fig. 12. Similar to the CNN experiment, we wanted to know if our sub-emotion embeddings obtain better results than regular word embeddings and BoSE representation. Table 10 presents the results of this experiment. We observe that using BoSE with a RNN again obtains a better performance that traditional embeddings in terms of $F1$ score and recall. Again using only BoSE obtains a better precision. This result shows that this strategy has high confidence when saying that a user has traces of self-harm, but struggles in finding all the users with these symptoms.

7.3 *Adding Attention to the Sub-emotions*

Although GRUs can capture the long-range dependencies in sequences of words, the information of the whole sequence is forced to be encoded into the fixed size hidden vector. Determining the size of the hidden vector is not trivial, and sometimes when an input sequence exceeds the average length it could not be well codified. Another problem is that we can not give more importance to some of the input sub-emotions depending on the context. Then, the following question arises: *Is there a way we can keep all the relevant information of the input sentence?*

First, we need to remember the intuition behind previous representations. In BoSE, we used a conventional method like tf-idf with a count vectorizer. This method finds features from the users' post by doing a keyword extraction. Some words (sub-emotion) are more helpful in determining the class of the posts than others. However, when we use this method, we lost the sequential structure of the text. With the GRU network, while we can learn from the sequence structure, we lose the ability to give different weights to the more important words. Then, *could we combine both of them?* The answer is yes, the authors in [5] came up with a simple but elegant idea. They suggested considering all the input words in the context but also add relative importance to each word. This idea is called "Attention".

The attention mechanisms are parts of the networks that separately weight the hidden states each time the network process an input item (sub-emotion vector), instead of only using the final RNN hidden-state to encode the whole sequence [6]. The advantage of having a mechanism (attention) to see how the recurrent hidden states are evolving after each input sub-emotion, is that it makes easier to find higher level patterns among input sub-emotions and highlight only those hidden states that contribute more to the representation.

In this experiment, we added the ability to give higher weight to more important sub-emotions using an attention mechanism. This mechanism extracts sub-emotions that are important in the sentence and add the information of those sub-emotions. Then, we multiplied each sub-emotion score with their GRU output obtaining a weight according to their importance. In Fig. 13 we present this whole process. We also experimented with a CNN before the GRU and the attention layer to capture local features before the sequence learning. We present this process in Fig. 14.

For this experiment our goal was to corroborate whether adding attention improves the results of our aforementioned approaches. Table 11 presents the results of this experiment. We observe that using BoSE with attention mechanism obtains a better performance that normal FT embeddings. Again using only BoSE obtains a better precision.

Table 11 F_1, Precision and Recall results over the positive class in the self-harm data set

Method	F1	Precision	Recall
RNN-Attention	0.58	0.56	0.60
BoSE	0.62	**0.78**	0.51
RNN-Attention-BoSE	**0.66**	0.72	0.62
CNNRNN-Attention-BoSE	**0.66**	0.64	**0.69**

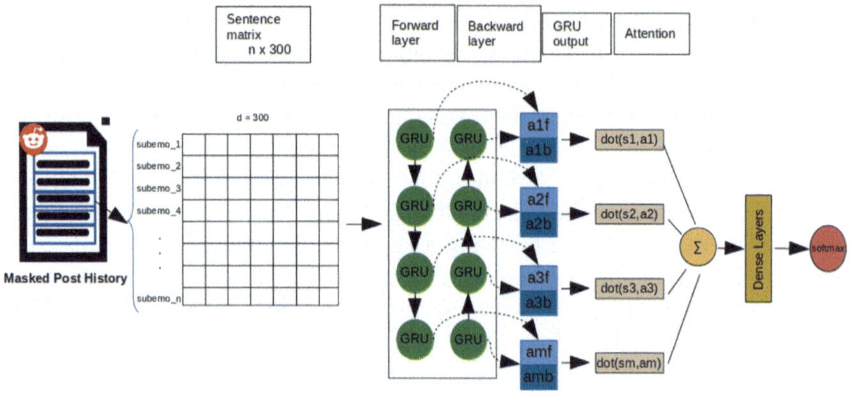

Fig. 13 Diagram of our bi-GRU model with Attention. We add the attention after the concatenation of both the forward and backward output

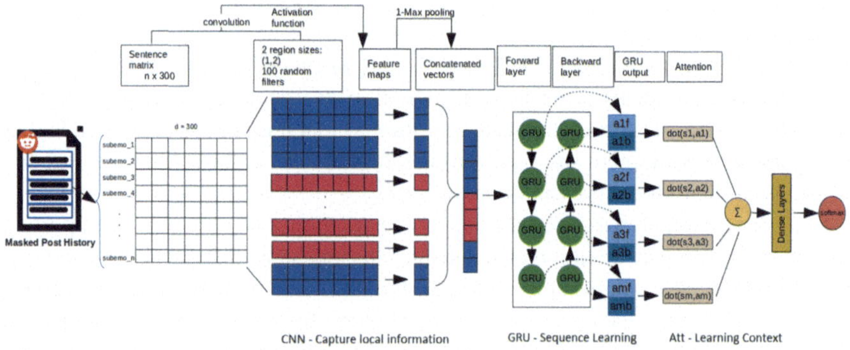

Fig. 14 Diagram of our bi-GRU model wit Attention and a CNN network. We add a CNN before the bi-GRU to extract local features and add this information for the sequence learning

For a further analysis of these results, Fig. 15 presents a boxplot of the F_1, precision and recall scores of all participants. The green **X** represents the results of the CNNRNN-Attention-BoSE approach. We can appreciate that our results are in the highest quartile (except for recall), indicating that the representation of the contexts and changes of fine-grained emotions obtains promising results in self-harm detection.

Analysis of the results. For the analysis, we want to know what the attention model captures. For this, we extracted the weights given to each sub-emotion on different sequences. We selected examples of sequences with a high probability of being positive cases of self-harm and extracted the weights assigned to them. In Fig. 16, we present some examples of these sequences. The shading represents the weight given to the sub-emotion, a darker shade means a higher weight. We can appreciate in these examples that the weight of each sub-emotion depends on their surrounding context. For example, if we analyze the sub-emotion "anticipation16"

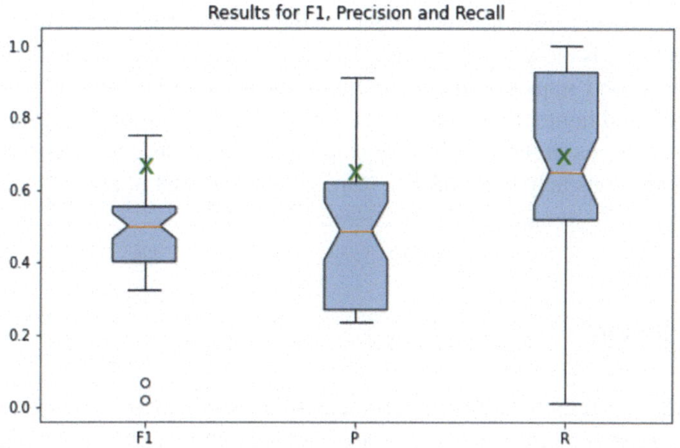

Fig. 15 Boxplot for the results in F1, Precision and Recall over the 2020 self-harm test data set. Where the green X mark represents our obtained results

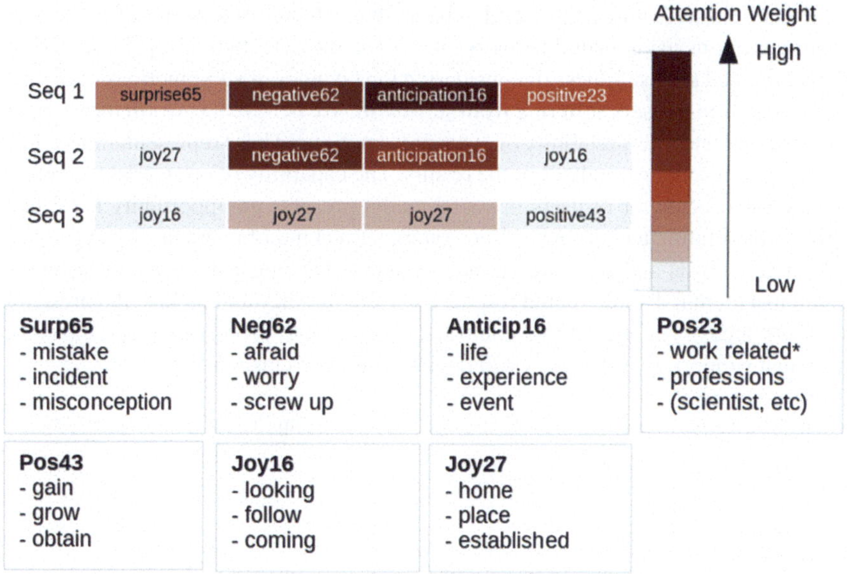

Fig. 16 Examples of weighted sequences of sub-emotions with different contexts. Each sequence corresponds to the label of the sub-emotion assigned to each word in a sequence of words. The lower part shows the topics related to each sub-emotion

that is related to life experiences and events. In the first sequence, the weight assigned is high because it is close to a context of worries, mistakes, and incidents. But if we analyze the second sequence, the weight is lower because is closer to a context of gain, growth, and home. Using an attention model allows capturing the importance of the sub-emotions in the post history using the context around it. These weights in the sub-emotions help the model to learn patterns related to people that commit self-harm.

8 Conclusion

In this work, we presented different representations based on fine-grained emotions, which we called sub-emotions. These sub-emotions allow capturing more specific topics and issues in posts shared by users that commit self-harm. On the one hand, our representations based on sub-emotions obtained better results than the proposed baselines, including some deep learning approaches and a representation based on broad emotions as features. On the other hand, the inclusion of dynamic analysis over the sub-emotions using neural networks improved the detection of self-harm. These models showed the usefulness of considering the changes of sub-emotions over time for the detection of users suffering from self-harm. We believe it is worth mentioning the simplicity and interpretability of our representations. These representations allow a more straightforward analysis of the results. The capability of our model to capture the emotional behavior of users in social media presents an opportunity for future wellness facilitating technologies. For example, this kind of technology can provide wide-area analysis and serve as warning systems. This analysis of the information related to a mental disorder could respect the users' privacy and include the presence in certain areas. The authorities could decide to create professional assistance or emotional support, that the users will decide whether to take or not.

Acknowledgements Ezra Aragón thanks for doctoral scholarship CONACyT-Mexico 654803.

References

1. Andover, M., & Morris, B. (2014). Expanding and clarifying the role of emotion regulation in nonsuicidal self-injury. *The Canadian Journal of Psychiatry.*
2. Aragón, M., López-Monroy, A., González-Gurrola, L., & Montes-y Gómez, M. (2019). Detecting depression in social media using fine-grained emotions. In *Proceedings of the 2019 Conference of the North American Chapter of the Association for Computational Linguistics: Human Language Technologies, Volume 1 (Long and Short Papers).*
3. Aragón, M., López-Monroy, A., González-Gurrola, L., & Montes-y Gómez, M. (2020). Attention to emotions: Detecting mental disorders in social media. In *International Conference on Text, Speech, and Dialogue.*

4. Aragón, M., López-Monroy, A., González-Gurrola, L., & Montes-y Gómez, M. (2021). Detecting mental disorders in social media through emotional patterns - the case of anorexia and depression. *IEEE Transactions on Affective Computing*.
5. Bahdanau, D., Cho, K., & Bengio, Y. (2015). Neural machine translation by jointly learning to align and translate. In *The International Conference on Learning Representations (ICLR)*.
6. Bahdanau, D., Cho, K., & Bengio, Y. (2015). Neural machine translation by jointly learning to align and translate. In *3rd International Conference on Learning Representations, Conference Track Proceedings*.
7. Bojanowski, P., Grave, E., Joulin, A., & Mikolov, T. (2016). Enriching word vectors with subword information. *Transactions of the Association for Computational Linguistics*.
8. Canales, L., & Martínez-Barco, P. (2014). Emotion detection from text: A survey. In *Processing in the 5th Information Systems Research Working Days (JISIC)*.
9. Coopersmith, G., Dredze, M., & Harman, C. (2014). Quantifying mental health signals in twitter. In *Workshop on Computational Linguistics and Clinical Psychology*.
10. Dyson, M., Hartling, L., Shulhan, J., Chisholm, A., Milne, A., Sundar, P., Scott, S., & Newton, A. (2016). A systematic review of social media use to discuss and view deliberate self-harm acts. *PLOS ONE*.
11. Hilton, C. (2016). Unveiling self-harm behaviour: What can social media site twitter tell us about self-harm? a qualitative exploration. *Journal of Clinical Nursing*.
12. Htait, A., Fournier, S., & Bellot, P. (2017). Lsis at semeval-2017 task 4: Using adapted sentiment similarity seed words for english and arabic tweet polarity classification. In *Proceedings of the 11th International Workshop on Semantic Evaluation (SemEval-2017)*.
13. Ji, S., Li, X., Huang, Z., & Cambria, E. (2020). Suicidal ideation and mental disorder detection with attentive relation networks. arXiv:2004.07601.
14. Kang, K., Yoon, C., & Kim, E. (2016). Identifying depressive users in twitter using multimodal analysis. In *2016 International Conference on Big Data and Smart Computing (BigComp)* (pp. 231–238). IEEE.
15. Kim, Y. (2014). Convolutional neural networks for sentence classification. In *Proceedings of the 2014 Conference on Empirical Methods in Natural Language Processing (EMNLP)*.
16. Laye-Gindhu, A., & Schonert-Reichl, K. A. (2005). Self-harm among community adolescents: Understanding the "whats" and "whys" of self-harm. *Journal of Youth and Adolescence*.
17. LeCun, Y., Bengio, Y., & Hinton, G. (2015). Deep learning. *Nature, 521*(7553).
18. Losada, D., Crestani, F., & Parapar, J. (2019). Overview of erisk 2019: Early risk prediction on the internet. In *Experimental IR Meets Multilinguality, Multimodality, and Interaction. 10th International Conference of the CLEF Association, CLEF 2019, Lugano, Switzerland*.
19. Losada, D., Crestani, F., & Parapar, J. (2020). Overview of eRisk 2020: Early Risk Prediction on the Internet. In *Experimental IR Meets Multilinguality, Multimodality, and Interaction Proceedings of the Eleventh International Conference of the CLEF Association (CLEF 2020)*.
20. Mohammad, S., & Turney, P. (2013). Crowdsourcing a word-emotion association lexicon. *Computational Intelligence*.
21. Preotiuc-Pietro, D., Eichstaedt, J., Park, G., Sap, M., Smith, L., Tobolsky, V., Schwartz, H., & Ungar, L. (2015). The role of personality, age and gender in tweeting about mental illnesses. In *Proceedings of the 2nd Workshop on Computational Linguistics and Clinical Psychology*.
22. Ragheb, W., Aze, J., Bringay, S., & Servajean, M. (2019). Attentive multi-stage learning for early risk detection of signs of anorexia and self-harm on social media. In *Proceedings of the 10th International Conference of the CLEF Association, CLEF 2019, Lugano, Switzerland*.
23. Thavikulwat, P. (2008). Affinity propagation: A clustering algorithm for computer-assisted business simulation and experimental exercises. *Developments in Business Simulation and Experiential Learning*.
24. Trifan, A., & Oliveira, J. (2019). Bioinfo@uavr at erisk 2019: Delving into social media texts for the early detection of mental and food disorders. In *Proceedings of the 10th International Conference of the CLEF Association, CLEF 2019, Lugano, Switzerland*.
25. Van Rijen, P., Teodoro, D., Naderi, N., Mottin, L., Knafou, J., Jeffryes, M., & Ruch, P. (2019). A data-driven approach for measuring the severity of the signs of depression using reddit posts.

In *Proceedings of the 10th International Conference of the CLEF Association, CLEF 2019, Lugano, Switzerland*.
26. Xuetong, C., Martin, D., Thomas, W., & Suzanne, E. (2018). What about mood swings? Identifying depression on twitter with temporal measures of emotions. In *Companion Proceedings of the The Web Conference 2018, International World Wide Web Conferences Steering Committee*.

On the Estimation of Depression Through Social Mining

Alina Trifan, Pedro Salgado, João Ribeiro, and José Luís Oliveira

Abstract This paper describes the work conducted by the Bioinformatics group of the Institute of Electronics and Engineering Informatics of University of Aveiro through several participations in the CLEF eRisk shared tasks related to the estimation of the level of depression. The eRisk initiative fosters Natural Language Processing research for the automatic detection of risk situations on the internet and provide a scientifically enriching infrastructure for evaluating and collaborating on social mining for mental health. Our participations in the eRisk tasks leveraged both standard machine learning algorithms and behavioral and linguistic patterns identified in the specialized literature. The results we present in this paper with respect to the estimation of a mental health condition advocate for a possible use of social monitoring as a digital complement to other standard public health surveillance and intervention practices.

1 Introduction

Social monitoring focuses on analyzing social media content in order to gather both generalized or more targeted knowledgeable insights that can be useful for addressing different societal issues. Examples of social monitoring cover a wide range of areas, including political sentiment analysis, financial marketing or public health. With

http://early.irlab.org/.

A. Trifan (✉) · P. Salgado · J. Ribeiro · J. L. Oliveira
DETI/IEETA, University of Aveiro, Aveiro, Portugal
e-mail: alina.trifan@ua.pt

P. Salgado
e-mail: psalgado@ua.pt

J. Ribeiro
e-mail: joaoantonioribeiro@ua.pt

J. L. Oliveira
e-mail: jlo@ua.pt

F. Crestani et al. (eds.), *Early Detection of Mental Health Disorders by Social Media Monitoring*, Studies in Computational Intelligence 1018,
https://doi.org/10.1007/978-3-031-04431-1_10

respect to generating health evidence from social media data, we find numerous studies on diverse topics. Most disease surveillance systems were developed for influenza before the COVID-19 virus. Eysenbach [16] presented one of the first studies which introduced the term infodemiology, where Internet data is used to derive health-related information.

In recent years many new studies explored the potential of utilizing social media and extracting behavioral traits, such as emotions and language patterns. There are different types of platforms that generate social data like blogs, microblogs, social networks, and media sharing platforms. Twitter,[1] Reddit[2] and Facebook[3] are all social media networks that have been used as data sources for conducting research in this area. The ultimate goal of social media mining for health is to complement traditional clinical information. Such approaches can provide new opportunities for early detection and intervention and they have the potential to reveal new insights on research of the causes and mechanisms of mental health [4]. Research initiatives such as CLEF eRisk [21] dynamize the scientific advances and societal impact that this research area can have. They foster collaborative work on the topic of mental health and social data, and push forward new discoveries and insights that can potentially benefit public health.

This paper describes the participation of the BioInfo@UAVR team in the CLEF eRisk 2019 and 2020 task of estimating the level of depression of social media users. We addressed the challenge of online risk detection from the perspective of quantifying the signs of depression trough social mining. As such, we combined standard machine learning algorithms with extended psycholinguistics and behavioral patterns derived from the literature. The rest of this paper is organized as follows: Sect. 2 overviews the current background in social data mining for mental health. The next section (Sect. 3) is dedicated to the methodologies we used in each of the two participations and the results obtained. We discuss the implication of our work in Sect. 4 and we draw our final remarks in Sect. 5.

2 Background

Depression is a mental disorder that can affect people of all ages and can range from a mild and transient negative mood state (dysphoria) to a debilitating set of symptoms that is associated with significant cognitive, emotional, behavioural, physiological and interpersonal impairment. The most common symptom is sadness or loss of interest/anhedonia. Additional symptoms can be changes in appetite/weight, disturbed sleep, psychomotor retardation or agitation, loss of energy or fatigue, worthlessness and impaired concentration/ability to make decisions. In most severe cases, it can lead to suicide ideation or even attempted suicide. Also, depression is characterized

[1] www.twitter.com.

[2] www.reddit.com.

[3] www.facebook.com.

by relapse and recurrence. Between 50% and 85% of depressed patients experience multiple subsequent episodes. The risk of future episodes also increases, and the time for an episode to recur decreases with each episode. Depression co-occurs with a number of psychiatric disorders and medical conditions. Particularly high rates of comorbidity have been noted between depression and anxiety (exceeds 50%), substance abuse, schizophrenia and eating disorders. Each year, approximately 800 000 people affected by depression die by suicide and the period of life with increased risk of a depressive episode occurs around mid to late adolescence and early adulthood. Also, females are consistently two times more likely than males to experience depression since adolescence. Approximately 25% of adults with unipolar mood disorders report an onset prior to young adulthood with 50% by age 30 years [18].

The relation between social media and well-being is well recognized, as users of social media networks often share very personal feelings and beliefs. The large volume of written data in the form of accessible common language available through social media attracted the attention of natural language processing researchers over the last years. Natural Language Processing (NLP) is a subfield of artificial intelligence situated in the intersection of linguistics and computer science, that targets the processing and analysis of natural language. It started by having a set of hand-coded rules, which are still useful today if we are working with specific use cases. Statistical NLP eventually came up and is currently the mainstream approach. It relies on large amounts of input data converted into a set of features that are fed to learning models. This strategy has the advantage of being adaptable and flexible. One can also use a combination of both strategies. For example, it is often the case that a rule-based system gathers the data that is then fed to a machine learning model.

Several mental illnesses have been explored during the years through social mining. Choudhury et al. studied emotion and behavior changes in new mothers, both in Twitter [7] and Facebook [8]. Similarly, Trifan et al. also conducted a preliminary study to identify mothers at risk of postpartum depression based on Reddit writings [28]. Depression affects more than 264 million people worldwide and is on the rise[14], one of the major causes leading to suicide. Luxton et al. [22] addresses this severe topic and shows how social media can influence suicidal behavior and evaluates the risk. Won et al. [30] showed that social media might have valuable information for forecasting and preventing suicide. Other studies, such as [6], used Twitter to show that machine learning classifiers can identify users at high risk of suicide. Nowadays, we face the Covid-19 crisis, and some research has already proven that social media to be useful in obtaining insights related to the virus [15]. Social monitoring can be active or passive. Active monitoring requires explicit participation from users, for example, a user inquiry, while passive monitoring makes use of data already published by a user.

On the previous edition of CLEF eRisk, several different approaches were taken by the participants. Uban et al. [29] presented three different models. One was a logistic regression model with the lexicon-based features as numerical vectors, the second was a Support Vector Machine (SVM) with RBF kernel, using the same features as the first one, and the last was a SVM with RBF kernel with Universal Sentence Encoder (USE) features. Maupome et al. [25] presented an approach in which the models with better performances were user-based (relate users to each other) instead of answer-based (relate a user to the text in the questionnaire), since they did not require annotated data (users with known BDIs). These models were a Latent Dirichlet Allocation (LDA) which is the most widely known topic modelling algorithm, a Contextualizer encoder that encoded each document in parallel using the angular similarity and a Stylometry method that focuses on the writing style of a document in order to characterize its author. Madani et al. [23] presented two Deep Learning models. One consisted in using a CNN with a ReLU activation function and the other was a combination of a Recurrent Neural Network (RNN) with Long Bi-Long Short Term Memory(BiLSTM) with one LSTM analysing from the beginning of the sentence to the end and the other analysing from the end to the beginning. Both models calculated for a question the frequency of each generated answer to choose the most recurrent answer. Martinez et al. [24] presented three models, all of them were based on Bidirectional Encoder Representations from Transformers (BERT). Two of these models used RoBERTa, which is a replication study of BERT, developed by Facebook AI. The other model is XLM- RoBERTa, also developed by Facebook AI, in an attempt to improve multilingual language models.

The eRisk task of estimating the level of depression is a living task, that has been evolving since its inception in 2019, both in terms of dataset enrichment, as well as the development of the solutions for tackling it. The initial results obtained by the teams participating in 2019 and 2020 might still be far from ideal, but they have an important role of building bricks that over time could enable the development of more mature solutions, to be potentially considered as complementary practices for standard clinical procedures. As such, the widespread use of social media, combined with the rapid development of computational infrastructures to support big data and the maturation of natural language processing and machine learning technologies, offer exciting possibilities for the improvement of both population-level and individual-level health [10].

3 Measuring Depression

This task was aimed at exploring the viability of automatically estimating the severity of multiple symptoms associated with depression [21]. Given the user's history of writings, participants had to work out a solution for predicting the user's response to each individual question included in Beck's Depression Inventory Questionnaire (BDI) [5]. The questionnaire assesses the presence of feelings like sadness, pessimism, loss of energy, hunger/loss of appetite, etc. For each individual question, a numeric value between 0 and 3 is considered a valid answer, with the exception of two questions, whose possible answers were: 0, 1a, 1b, 2a, 2b, 3a or 3b.

Our approaches for addressing the task of estimating the severity of depression at eRisk 2019 and 2020 are a combination of rule-based analysis and machine learning, more specifically analysis of psycholinguistic and behavioral patterns and supervised machine learning. Supervised learning refers to the machine learning methods that learn a function that maps the input/features to output/labels using the training set. The function's goal is to predict the correct label for the new input, the testing set. Before performing any type of analysis on any of the datasets, we conducted some text cleaning and pre-processing steps that are conceptually common to all the methods we will address.

3.1 Dataset Description

The training dataset was the dataset used in the test stage of the task's first edition, CLEF eRisk 2019 [20]. It contained 20 files, with one file per user provided. For each user, a file containing the history of writings on a social network was also provided. An annotation file, or ground truth file was also provided, containing the answers of all users to each of the questions in the questionnaire. The number of writings per user varied from 30 to 1511. The average number of writings of the dataset was 548, with a median of 328.5.

3.2 Metrics

The organizers of this task collected questionnaires filled by social media users together with their history of writings. For each user, the history of writings was extracted right after the user provided us the filled in questionnaire. The questionnaires filled by the users were considered the ground truth and were used to assess the quality of the responses provided by each participating team.

The evaluation metrics reflected the differences between the answers of the questionnaire provided by the task participants and the ones provided by the users that were part of the dataset. Moreover, in the psychological domain it is customary to associate depression levels with categories. Depression levels are defined as the sum of all answers of the 21 questions of the questionnaire. The following depression categories were used for further extension of the evaluation metrics:

- minimal depression—[0–9]
- mild depression—[10–18]
- moderate depression—[19–29]
- severe depression—[30–63]

The following metrics were considered for the evaluation of the results [21]:

- *Hit Rate (HR)*—the ratio of cases where the automatic questionnaire has exactly the same answer as the real questionnaire.
- *Average Hit Rate (AHR)*—HR averaged over all users.
- *Closeness Rate (CR)*—the absolute difference between the real and the participant provided answer.

- *Average Closeness Rate (ACR)*—CR averaged over all users.
- *Difference between overall depression levels (DODL).*
- *Average DODL (ADODL)*—DODL averaged over all users.
- *Depression Category Hit Rate (DCHR)*—the fraction of cases where the automated questionnaire led to a depression category that is equivalent to the depression category obtained from the real questionnaire.

3.3 Methods

Our initial approach for solving this task was a rule-based one and each rule was modelled with reference to several behavioral and psycholinguistics patterns that are known to be associated with the state of depression (Table 1). The reduced size of the dataset, in terms of users and the small number of writings per user, along with the lack of a training set or any ground truth for the 2019 eRisk edition, led to the choice of a rule-based approach rather than the use of standard machine learning algorithms.

Moreover, we explored the correlation between some of the questions by dividing the 21 questions into 6 groups. All questions belonging to a given group were scored

Table 1 Details of the textual features considered for each category score

Depression	Lexical category of a user's text—depressed users tend to have an overall more negative connotation of their texts [11, 26]. To this purpose we employed the TextBlob library [1] in order to calculate the average polarity of a user's writings
	Use of self-related words (e.g.: I, myself, mine)—depressed users tend to use them more often in their writings [9, 27]
	Use of absolutist words—Al-Mosaiwi et al. [3] recently showed that anxiety, depression, and suicidal ideation forums contained more absolutist words than control forums. The list of absolutist words used is presented next in Table 2
	Referrals to any of the anti-depressants listed by WebMD [2]
	Mentions of words related to mental disorders, (e.g.: depression, bipolar, schizophrenia, psychotic, ocd)
	Writings timestamps—depressed users tend to write more at late hours of the night
Guilt	Use of the words cry, guilt and their derivatives
Appetite	Use of the words hunger, appetite, eat, food and their derivatives
Anxiety	Use of the words sleep, anxious and their derivatives
	Writings timestamps
Fatigue	Use of the words irritated, fatigue, tired and their derivatives
Sleep	Same as for fatigue, along with the writing timestamps

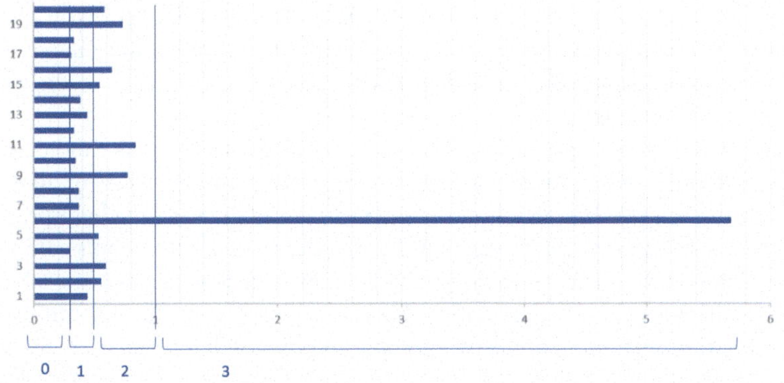

Fig. 1 Histogram of the depression scores calculated for each of the 20 users of the dataset. The vertical bold lines represent the threshold values for the normalization of the scores to the integer values defined as possible answers. In this example user 6 stands out as her text history led to a much higher depression score than the average. This is the case of what seems to be a support pal-this particular user employed extensive depression related vocabulary to provide support and comfort

with the same answer or numeric value. The 6 groups and the included categories (or question names) were:

1. Depression—suicidal thoughts, pessimism, past failure, self dislike, sadness, loss of pleasure, loss of interest and loss of sex
2. Guilt—guilty and punishment feelings, self criticalness, crying, worthlessness
3. Appetite—changes in appetite
4. Anxiety—agitation, indecisiveness, irritability
5. Fatigue—tiredness, loss of energy, concentration difficulty
6. Sleep—sleeping patterns

Table 1 overviews the textual and behavioral patterns modelled for each of the 6 groups. For each category, a score was calculated for each user as a normalized value of the number of occurrences of the features considered for each category with respect to the total number of occurrences of the same features over the dataset. These scores were then normalized to the interval [0, 3] based on predefined thresholds extracted from the histograms of occurrences. An example of such histogram and the threshold derived from it are shown in Fig. 1. In this example, a depression score lower than 0.3 would be converted to a 0, a score in the range of (0.3, 0.5) leads to a 1, a score equal or higher than 0.5 but lower than 1 represents a final score of 2 and anything over 1 means the final answer for the questions in the depression category will be 3.

For our second participation in the task, our approach built upon algorithms that we used in CLEF eRisk 2019 edition for solving not only this task, but also Task 1. This task considered the early detection of users of social media prone to self-harm themselves. As no training dataset was provided, we approached this task as a cross-validation task rather that an unsupervised classification. Self-harm ideation often relates to depression and poor mental health, therefore we were interested in understanding how a classifier trained on a depression corpus of social media writing would perform in the test stage.

The first step was to predict whether a user was depressed using the classifier previously trained of the Yates et al. dataset [31]. The dataset consists of all Reddit users who made a post between January and October 2016, matching high-precision patterns of self-reported diagnosis (e.g. "I was diagnosed with depression"). The depressed users were matched by control users, who have never posted in a subreddit related to mental health and never used a term related to it. In order to avoid a straight-forward separation of the two groups, all posts of diagnosed users related to depression or mental health were removed. For this part of our pipeline we followed a standard processing stream for text classification. We initially split the dataset into training and validation chunks, with a ratio of 2:1. We considered Bag of Words (BoW) and tf-idf based feature weighting with linear Support Vector Machine with Stochastic Gradient Descent.

Next, we conjugated the score of this classification with several psycholinguistics and behavioral patterns, as presented next. For each category, a score was calculated for each user as a normalized value of the number of occurrences of the features considered for each category with respect to the total number of occurrences of the same features over the dataset. These scores were then normalized to the interval [0, 3].

- Lexical category of a user's text—depressed users tend to have an overall more negative connotation of their texts [11, 26]. To this purpose we employed Empath,[4] an NLP framework for calculating the average polarity of a user's writings.
- Use of self-related words (e.g.: I, myself, mine)—depressed users tend to use them more often in their writings [9, 27].
- Use of absolutist words—Al-Mosaiwi et al. [3] recently showed that anxiety, depression, and suicidal ideation forums contained more absolutist words than control forums. The list of absolutist words used is presented next in Table 2.
- Mentions of words related to mental disorders, (e.g.: depression, bipolar, schizophrenia, psychotic, ocd).
- Use of the words cry, guilt and their derivatives.
- Use of the words sleep, anxious and their derivatives.

Table 2 Absolutist words validated by Al-Mosaiwi et al. [3]

Absolutely	All	Always	Complete	Completely
Constant	Constantly	Definitely	Entire	Ever
Every	Everyone	Everything	Full	Must
Never	Nothing	Total	Whole	

[4] https://github.com/Ejhfast/empath-client.

Table 3 Evaluation of BioInfo@UAVR's submission. The best results for each metric were added for comparison. It is important to note that no single team achieved the best results for all metrics

	AHR (%)	ACR (%)	ADODL (%)	DCHR (%)
BioInfo@UAVR	38.30	69.21	76.01	30.00
Best scores	38.30	69.41	83.15	35.71

- Use of the words irritated, fatigue, tired and their derivatives.

Compared to the approach that we took in our first participation in this task, we decided to remove some of the features that we used last year and we explored the use of Empath [17]. A statistical analysis of the training corpus revealed that the non-depressed users had relatively low depression scores, as it would be expected. As such, the users that our trained model would consider non-depressive were scored with low scores in all categories. Regarding the psycholinguistic features, our follow-up analysis of our eRisk2019 submission revealed that some of the features we included last year did not significantly contribute to the overall scores.

3.4 Results

Task participants had to provide a result file with one line per user in the test dataset. Each line contained the username and 21 values that corresponded to the answers of the 21 questions included in Beck's Depression Inventory. The results obtained by our team are presented in Table 3, along with the best results obtained in this task, for each of the metrics. The results of all participating teams can be found in [21]. While the general results obtained in this task have slightly improved since last year, they stand as proof of its difficulty. One important aspect to be mentioned is that our team obtained the best score for the AHR metric and second best score for ACR.

4 Discussion

Social media mining has the potential to reveal users' feelings, mood and detect underlying mental illnesses. This information can be an improvement and assistance to the medical system, if we can provide a link of this stream of information to clinical experts. In order to gain more confidence into these computational models, a classification that takes into account multiple feature extraction techniques seems to be a better alternative. Learning different ways of finding the best set of parameters for the models, through intensive validation, adds to the reliability of social mining as a possible extension of clinical monitoring.

While we recognize the potential that social mining has for signaling a user's mental health status and for the early detection of risk situation, we have come to understand that one possible limitation of our work is the lack of clinical knowledge. As researchers with computational backgrounds, who are often unfamiliar with existing practices in mental healthcare, we are in the frontline of developing new algorithms for social data. In order to better understand the tasks that we have in our hands and to improve the end solution we will focus on having the missing clinical perspective on our future participations.

Another important aspect that we identified as future working direction is the existance of other publicly available datasets that could enrich our methodology. As an example, The DAIC dataset was the result of an experiment led by DeVault et al. [13], which created a virtual interviewer called Ellie so that possibly depressed users could feel more comfortable talking with it. It was specifically designed to create interactional situations that assist the automatic assessment of distress indicators correlated with depression, anxiety or post-traumatic stress disorder. In order to simulate a human interviewer, Ellie was developed with the capability of audiovisual sensing and non-verbal behaviour understanding, natural language understanding and dia-logue management and non-verbal behaviour generation and realization. For Natural Language understanding, there were developed 4 statistically trained utterance classifiers to capture different aspects of user utterance meaning. For perception of non-verbal behaviour, a consultation with experts and trained clinicians helped to identify the right communicative behaviours to form a diagnosis. One important aspect to be mentioned is that the DAIC dataset provides the PHQ-8 questionnaire [19] results while CLEF eRisk dataset and evaluation methods require a BDI questionnaire prediction. However, since PHQ-8 and BDI questionnaires have high correlation, it is possible to convert one result into other [12].

5 Conclusions

We presented in this paper research on the topic of social mining, conducted in the context of the CLEF eRisk challenges. We participated in these tasks in two consecutive years and our approaches were built incrementally. While we recognize there is still room for improving the computational models that we present, we argue they are a significant contribution towards raising awareness on the capabilities of social mining for mental health. We are confident that future CLEF eRisk challenges will push this research topic forward, through shared tasks and collaborative research for online risk prediction.

The current pandemic came to enhance the importance of redesigning mental health interventions. The World Health organization reports the under-supply of mental health care, with depression leading to suicide being one of the major causes of death among young adults all around the world. Social media is a great part of our daily existence and can be used for monitoring personal well-being. More than just monitoring, as we live in the big data era we can explore all current technologies in connection with the large volume of social media data to work towards a more personalized and alternative mental healthcare approach. The already available scientific evidence previously introduced strongly suggests that a shift in mental health care provision towards online prevention and treatment in the near future is needed. Workshops such as eRisk appeal to an interdisciplinary audience sharing findings, models, and methods to increase access to and scalability of mental health care, by providing a closer union between clinical psychology and natural language processing. Moreover, they release extensive annotated corpora, that grow each year, containing public, anonymous texts of thousands of users, retrieved from social networks.

Acknowledgements This work was supported by the Integrated Programme of SR&TD SOCA (Ref. CENTRO-01-0145-FEDER-000010), co-funded by Centro 2020 program, Portugal 2020, European Union, through the European Regional Development Fund.

References

1. Textblob (2019).
2. WebMD (2019).
3. Al-Mosaiwi, M., & Johnstone, T. (2018). In an absolute state: Elevated use of absolutist words is a marker specific to anxiety, depression, and suicidal ideation. *Clinical Psychological Science*, 2167702617747074.
4. Arseniev-Koehler, A., Mozgai, S., & Scherer, S. (2018). What type of happiness are you looking for?-A closer look at detecting mental health from language. In *Proceedings of the Fifth Workshop on Computational Linguistics and Clinical Psychology: From Keyboard to Clinic* (pp. 1–12).
5. Beck, A. T., Ward, C. H., Mendelson, M., Mock, J., & Erbaugh, J. (1961). An inventory for measuring depression. *Archives of General Psychiatry, 4*(6), 561–571.
6. Braithwaite, S., Giraud-Carrier, C., West, J., Barnes, M., & Hanson, C. (2016). Validating machine learning algorithms for twitter data against established measures of suicidality. *JMIR Mental Health, 3*, e21.
7. Choudhury, M., Counts, S., & Horvitz, E. *Predicting postpartum changes in emotion and behavior via social media* (pp. 3267–3276).
8. Choudhury, M., Counts, S., Horvitz, E., & Hoff, A. *Characterizing and predicting postpartum depression from shared facebook data* (pp. 626–638).
9. Chung, C., & Pennebaker, J. W. (2007). The psychological functions of function words. *Social Communication, 1*, 343–359.
10. Conway, M., & O'Connor, D. (2016). Social media, big data, and mental health: Current advances and ethical implications. *Current Opinion in Psychology, 9*, 77–82.
11. De Choudhury, M., Gamon, M., Counts, S., & Horvitz, E. (2013). Predicting depression via social media. *ICWSM, 13*, 1–10.
12. Demiroglu, C., Beşirli, A., Ozkanca, Y., & Çelik, S. (2020). Depression-level assessment from multi-lingual conversational speech data using acoustic and text features. *EURASIP Journal on Audio, Speech, and Music Processing, 2020*(1), 1–17.
13. DeVault, D., Artstein, R., Benn, G., Dey, T., Fast, E., Gainer, A., Georgila, K., Gratch, J., Hartholt, A., Lhommet, M., et al. (2014). Simsensei kiosk: A virtual human interviewer for healthcare decision support. In *Proceedings of the 2014 international conference on Autonomous agents and multi-agent systems* (2014), pp. 1061–1068.

14. Disease, G., Murray, C., Chattopadhyay, A., Chin, K. L., Lorkowski, S., & Fareed, M. (2018). Global, regional, and national incidence, prevalence, and years lived with disability for 354 diseases and injuries for 195 countries and territories, 1990-2017: A systematic analysis for the global burden of disease study 2017. *The Lancet, 392*(11 2018), 10–16.
15. Drias, H., Drias, Y. (2020). *Mining twitter data on covid-19 for sentiment analysis and frequent patterns discovery.*
16. Eysenbach, G. (2006). Infodemiology: Tracking flu-related searches on the web for syndromic surveillance. In *AMIA ... Annual Symposium Proceedings/AMIA Symposium. AMIA Symposium* (Vol. 244(02 2006), pp. 244–248).
17. Fast, E., Chen, B., & Bernstein, M. S. (2016). Empath: Understanding topic signals in large-scale text. In *Proceedings of the 2016 CHI Conference on Human Factors in Computing Systems*, pp. 4647–4657. ACM.
18. Hofmann, S., & Reinecke, M. (2010). *Cognitive-Behavioral Therapy with Adults: A Guide to Empirically-Informed Assessment and Intervention.* Cambridge University Press.
19. Kroenke, K., Strine, T. W., Spitzer, R. L., Williams, J. B., Berry, J. T., & Mokdad, A. H. (2009). The PHQ-8 as a measure of current depression in the general population. *Journal of Affective Disorders, 114*(1–3), 163–173.
20. Losada, D. E., Crestani, F., & Parapar, J. (2019). Overview of eRisk 2019: Early risk prediction on the internet. In *Experimental IR Meets Multilinguality, Multimodality, and Interaction. 10th International Conference of the CLEF Association, CLEF 2019, Lugano, Switzerland, 2019.* Springer International Publishing.
21. Losada, D. E., Crestani, F., & Parapar, J. (2020). Overview of eRisk 2020: Early risk prediction on the internet. In T. T. S. V. H. J. C. L. C. E. A. N. L. C. N. F. E. A. Arampatzis, E. Kanoulas, (Eds.), *Experimental IR Meets Multilinguality, Multimodality, and Interaction Proceedings of the Eleventh International Conference of the CLEF Association (CLEF 2020).* Springer International Publishing.
22. Luxton, D., June, J., & Fairall, J. (2012). Social media and suicide: A public health perspective. *American Journal of Public Health 102 Supply, 2*(03 2012), S195–200.
23. Madani, A., Boumahdi,, F., Boukenaoui, A., Kritli, M. C., & Henabli, H. (2020). *Usdb at erisk 2020: Deep learning models to measure the severity of the signs of depression using reddit posts.*
24. Martınez-Castano, R., Htait, A., Azzopardi, L., & Moshfeghi, Y. *Early risk detection of self-harm and depression severity using bert-based transformers.*
25. Maupomé, D., Armstrong, M. D., Belbahar, R., Alezot, J., Balassiano, R., Queudot, M., Mosser, S., & Meurs, M.-J. *Early mental health risk assessment through writing styles, topics and neural models.*
26. Park, M., Cha, C., & Cha, M. (2012). Depressive moods of users portrayed in twitter. In *Proceedings of the ACM SIGKDD Workshop on Healthcare Informatics (HI-KDD)* (Vol. 2012, pp. 1–8). NY: ACM New York.
27. Rude, S., Gortner, E.-M., & Pennebaker, J. (2004). Language use of depressed and depression-vulnerable college students. *Cognition & Emotion, 18*(8), 1121–1133.
28. Trifan, A., Semeraro, D., Drake, J., Bukowski, R., & Oliveira, J. L. (2020). Social media mining for postpartum depression prediction. *Studies in Health Technology and Informatics, 270*(6 2020), 1391–1392.
29. Uban, A.-S., & Rosso, P. *Deep learning architectures and strategies for early detection of self-harm and depression level prediction.*
30. Won, H.-H., Myung, W., Song, G.-Y., Lee, W.-H., Kim, J.-W., Carroll, B., & Kim, D. K. (2013). Predicting national suicide numbers with social media data. *PloS One, 8*(04 2013), e61809.
31. Yates, A., Cohan, A., & Goharian, N. (2017). Depression and self-harm risk assessment in online forums. In *Proceedings of the 2017 Conference on Empirical Methods in Natural Language Processing* (pp. 2968–2978). Association for Computational Linguistics.

Automatically Estimating the Severity of Multiple Symptoms Associated with Depression

Diego Maupomé, Maxime D. Armstrong, Raouf Belbahar, Josselin Alezot, Rhon Balassiano, Fanny Rancourt, Marc Queudot, Sébastien Mosser, and Marie-Jean Meurs

Abstract This chapter describes the participation of the RELAI team in the eRisk 2020 second task. The 2020 edition of eRisk proposed two tasks: (T1) Early assessment of the risk of self-harm and (T2) Signs of depression in social media users. The second task focused on automatically filling a depression questionnaire given the user's writing history. The RELAI team addressed it using Latent Dirichlet Allocation (LDA), a topic modelling algorithm, and an approach based on writing styles. The proposed system based on LDA performed well according to all the evaluation metrics. According to the Average Difference between Overall Depression Levels (ADODL), it achieved the best performance among participants with a score of

D. Maupomé · M. D. Armstrong · R. Belbahar · J. Alezot · R. Balassiano · F. Rancourt · M. Queudot · M.-J. Meurs (✉)
Université du Québec à Montréal (UQAM), Montreal, QC, Canada
e-mail: meurs.marie-jean@uqam.ca

D. Maupomé
e-mail: maupome.diego@courrier.uqam.ca

M. D. Armstrong
e-mail: darmstrong.maxime@courrier.uqam.ca

R. Belbahar
e-mail: belbahar.raouf@courrier.uqam.ca

J. Alezot
e-mail: alezot.josselin_louis_auguste@courrier.uqam.ca

R. Balassiano
e-mail: balassiano.rhon@courrier.uqam.ca

F. Rancourt
e-mail: rancourt.fanny.2@courrier.uqam.ca

M. Queudot
e-mail: queudot.marc@courrier.uqam.ca

S. Mosser
Faculty of Engineering, Department of Computing and Software, McMaster University, Hamilton, ON, Canada
e-mail: mossers@mcmaster.ca

F. Crestani et al. (eds.), *Early Detection of Mental Health Disorders by Social Media Monitoring*, Studies in Computational Intelligence 1018,
https://doi.org/10.1007/978-3-031-04431-1_11

83.15%. Overall, the submitted systems achieved promising results and suggested that social media evidence could help early mental health risk assessment.

1 Introduction

The World Health Organization (WHO) estimates that depression affects more than 264 million people of all ages worldwide and that depressive disorders are a leading factor in morbidity and disability worldwide [31]. Depression and anxiety disorders cost the global economy US$1 trillion per year [33]. Furthermore, depression can conduct to self-harming or even to suicide. Worldwide, over 800 000 people die due to suicide every year, making it the second leading cause of death in 15–29 year-olds. There are indications that for each adult who died of suicide, there may have been more than 20 others attempting suicide [32]. Studies report that the choice of words that users can make or even topics of interest discussed on social media can tell about their psychological situation [22, 25, 26]. Therefore, mining textual content from social media could be a promising method for early detection of high-risk situations in order to provide support to those afflicted [4, 9, 10, 19].

The global goal of the eRisk challenges is the early detection of at-risk people from their textual production on social media, using Natural Language Processing (NLP) techniques. In 2020, one of the tasks put forth was measuring the severity of the signs of depression (T2) using textual data from related Reddit fora,[1] a follow-up of task 3 from the 2019 edition. T2 consists of automatically filling the BDI [2] for a set of users, based on a history of their postings on social media. In this work, we describe the participation of the RELAI team from Université du Québec à Montréal (UQAM) at the Conference and Labs of the Evaluation Forum (CLEF) 2020 eRisk tasks for early detection of depression [14, 16].

The chapter is organized as follows. Sections 2 and 3 presents the data and the metrics considered for our experiments. The following section discusses the research background they rely on. Section 5 describes the proposed approaches, presents the applied methodology, experimental setup and results obtained on T2. Sections 6 and 7 concludes this chapter with a discussion about the results, and suggests possible future improvements.

2 Task and Data

The second task of the eRisk 2020 lab was introduced in 2019 to explore much finer-grained prediction of the severity of depression symptoms [14]. For this purpose, each subject was asked to fill the Beck's Depression Inventory (BDI) questionnaire. This questionnaire was designed specifically for use in clinical settings to identify

[1] https://www.reddit.com.

depression and measure its depth. It allows assessing the presence of feelings like sadness, pessimism, loss of energy, etc. The BDI is composed of 21 questions with 4 possible answers (from 0 to 3), except for questions 16 and 18, where there are seven possible answers (0, 1a, 1b, 2a, 2b, 3a, 3b). The answers to each question represent an ordinal scale, each one associated with an integer value. The total of a subject's answers is considered their score. Additionally, these scores are associated with the following categories: minimal depression (depression levels 0–9), mild depression (10–18), moderate depression (19–29) and severe depression (30–63).

The participants' systems then had to estimate every user's answer to each question given users' writing history. To assess the correctness of the participants' responses, several metrics are used. Some are concerned with obtaining the exact answers, whereas others are concerned with the proximity in individual answers or overall BDI score. These metrics are described in detail in the following Section.

Table 1 Summary statistics of the training and test sets for T2 (Depression)

Total nb. users	Training	Test
	20	70
Nb. minimal depression users	4 (20%)	10 (14%)
Nb. mild depression users	4 (20%)	23 (33%)
Nb. moderate depression users	4 (20%)	18 (26%)
Nb. severe depression users	8 (40%)	19 (27%)
Total nb. writings	10941	35562
Nb. minimal depression writings	3338	5618
Nb. mild depression writings	2205	11858
Nb. moderate depression writings	3540	10476
Nb. severe depression writings	1858	7610

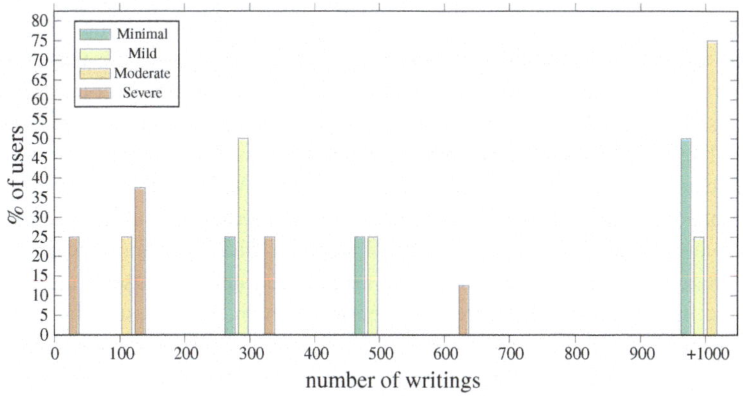

Fig. 1 Distribution of users from T2 (depression) by number of writings (bin size = 100)

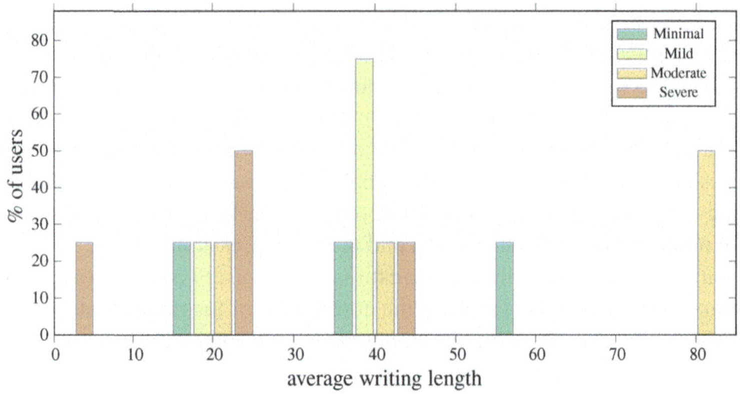

Fig. 2 Distribution of users from T2 by average length of writings (in words) (bin size = 20)

While participants in the previous iteration did not have training data at their disposal, 20 users were made available for eRisk 2020 participants, with 70 more used for evaluation. Their distributions according to the standard categorization used on BDI scores are shown in Table 1. The training and test sets differ in this respect, as well as in the verbosity of users. Interestingly enough, as shown in Figs. 1 and 2, the verbosity of users, both in terms of the number of writings and in the average length of writings, seems to oscillate, taking a sharp increase for subjects with moderate depression, followed by a sharp decrease for those with severe depression.

3 Evaluation Metrics

Four metrics evaluate the systems trying to address T2. The first one is the *Average Hit Rate* (AHR). For a given user, the hit rate is simply the number of matches between the system automatic answers of the questionnaire and the user answers, i.e., the rate of correct guesses over the total. The questionnaire is composed of 21 questions, the HR will return a decimal number between 0 (worst case) and 1 (perfect match). The AHR is then the mean hit rate across all users.

The second metric is the *Average Closeness Rate* (ACR). The closeness rate is a finer-grained measure of the disparity between the prediction and the ground truth for each answer, as defined by the ordinal scale on which the answers are placed. To calculate this, for each question, one takes the system and user's answers and computes the absolute differences (ad) between them. If the user chooses 1 for the first question and the system chooses 3 the absolute difference would be equal to 2. For questions 16 and 18, where there are seven possible answers, each pair $([1a, 1b], [2a, 2b], [3a, 3b])$ are considered to have the same value. As such, if a user answers 2a and the system predicts 2b the absolute difference is 0. In order to get an effectiveness score, the closeness rate for a question is simply: $\frac{mad-ad}{mad}$ where *mad* is the maximum absolute difference, and *ad* is the actual absolute difference. The closeness rate for a user is the mean closeness rate for each question. The ACR is then simply the mean closeness rate across users.

The third metric is the *Average Difference between Overall Depression Levels* (ADODL). As previously mentioned, the answers to each question in the BDI are tallied together to compute an overall depression level. The Difference between Overall Depression Levels (DODL) is simply the absolute difference between this total as per the ground truth and as per the system's predictions. This result is normalized: $DODL = \frac{63-ad}{63}$, 63 being the maximum possible depression level. If the user's depression level is of 30 and the predicted one is of 35, absolute overall difference is equal to 5 and the DODL is equal to $\frac{63-5}{63}$. As with the previous metrics, the ADODL is the mean DODL over all users.

The last metric is the *Depression Category Hit Rate* (DCHR). As previously mentioned, depression levels as measured by the BDI can be assigned to one of four categories. The DCHR for a system is the fraction of the cases where the system's score and user's score fall in the same category.

Since ADODL assesses the ability of a system to predict accurately the level of depression severity of an individual, our experiments are conducted to maximize it.

4 Related Work

In eRisk 2019, the highest AHR was achieved by a system called Sequential S3—*SS3* for Smoothness, Significance, and Sanction—trained using the dataset for the eRisk 2018 depression detection task [5]. Since the model was designed as a binary classifier [6], the authors had to make some modifications to return a depression level between 0 and 63 to be able to fill a BDI questionnaire.

To do so, after the SS3 classified a subject, they converted the obtained confidence vector into a single confidence value normalized between 0 and 1 and then divided the confidence value into four regions, one for each BDI depression category. Finally, the subject depression level was predicted by mapping the percentage of confidence value left inside the predicted region to its corresponding BDI depression level range (e.g. $(0.5, 0 : 75] \rightarrow [19, 29])$. To answer the 21 questions in the BDI, they decided for all users whose depression level was less or equal to 0 to answer all questions with 0. For the other users, they applied different methods. We describe below the methods used for the best runs. A question-centered variant was built, achieving the AHR mentioned above. The model filled the questionnaires with the expected number derived from the predicted depression level. However, the model answered this number only on questions for which a "textual hint" was found in the user's writings and answering using a uniform distribution. To achieve this, the model looked for the co-occurrence of the word "I" or "my" with at least one word matching a regular expression specially crafted for each question (e.g. Sad|unhappy for question 1) [5]. A variant of the previous system achieved the best ACR (distance-based variant).

Table 2 Summary of the best results obtained on eRisk 2019 T3

Run	AHR (%)	ACR (%)	ADODL (%)	DCHR (%)
CAMH GPT nearest unsupervised [1]	23.81	57.06	**81.03**	**45.00**
UNSLC [5]	**41.43**	69.13	78.02	40.00
UNSLE [5]	40.71	**71.27**	80.48	35.00

This time, without using a textual hint and uniform distribution, it uses a probability distribution depending on the value of the expected answer.

In terms of ADODL and DCHR, the best performances were reached with an unsupervised approach [1] using the distance between the answers and all the sentences of a user's writing history. To extract features, the participants used GPT-1 (Generative Pre-trained Transformer version 1) [10] language model trained on a corpus of books. They also fine-tuned the language model on the provided text from the 20 subjects in the eRisk dataset (3 epochs). To predict the BDI responses, they used the sentence-level feature vectors of each user's writings provided by GPT-1. Then, computed and picked the highest cosine similarity of each of the possible responses to all of this user's sentences. Table 2 reports the best results obtained by the participating teams of eRisk 2019. According to [13], these results show that it is possible to extract some depression signals from social media activity automatically. However, the performance is still modest and far from an effective depression screening tool.

In eRisk 2020, the approach achieving the highest AHR [28] was based on psycholinguistic features selected for each question, such as lexical categories, first-person pronouns, absolutist words and the Empathy framework [11]. The frequency of these features was compared among depressed and control users as separated by a CNN classifier [34] and normalized to the [0, 3] interval. A finer-grained approach by iLab [15] using pre-trained Transformers achieved the highest ACR. To this end, the labels for each user were spread to individual writings. To address the difficulty in handling long documents, the authors alternately tested truncating them and splitting them into smaller documents. The best ADODL was attained by the approach described in the present chapter. Finally, the highest DCHR was achieved by combining LIWC [27] features and logistic regression, or alternately, a support vector machine with a radial basis kernel [29].

5 Approaching the Task as One of Authorship Attribution

Authorship attribution is an essential topic in the field of Natural Language Processing (NLP). Authorship attribution is generally used to define an appropriate characterization of documents that captures authors' writing style. Thereby, given a set of documents written by a set of authors, the goal is to determine the author of a new unseen document.

Only 20 users filled the BDI. Treating each of these users as one observation to be mapped to the answers they gave to the questionnaire would lead to some examples far too limited to learn this mapping directly without extensive prior knowledge.

Instead, we approach the task as one of authorship attribution under two distinct hypotheses, leveraging unannotated data to train such models. Both methods rely on decision models taking two documents and calculating the probability that the same user wrote both documents. One method rests on the hypothesis that users writing similarly might present similar depression symptoms. The second method attempts to relate a user to the text contained in the BDI questionnaire. Under this hypothesis, the answers to the BDI being written from the user's perspective, a correct authorship decision model would assign a higher probability to the answer in a set that is truest to the user. These methods are referred to as **answer-based** and **user-based**, respectively.

The user-based method selects a set of documents for each user, v, for whom the BDI is known, denoted by P_v. Similar selection is performed for each test user u, denoting the set of documents by P_u. Given a decision model f, the *affinity* between users u and v as per f is defined as the average probability assigned by f to each pair of documents:

$$\alpha_f(u, v) = \frac{1}{|P_u||P_v|} \sum_{p \in P_u} \sum_{p' \in P_v} f(p, p') \tag{1}$$

For each question, the prediction for user u is computed as the highest-scoring answer among the set of known users, as weighted by their affinities to u.

In contrast, the answer-based approach attempts to match the user to the text contained in each answer. For a given question, the sentences accompanying each answer are paired with each document in P_u. The predicted answer is the one obtaining the highest average probability. We hypothesize that, given that the sentences associated with each answer are written from the user's perspective, a successful authorship attribution model would find the correct answer to be more plausible.

The decision models used for the methods previously described can be built in a variety of ways. As mentioned, given two documents, they must produce a probability that the same person wrote them. We distinguish two main categories of such models. The first one is representation models, which produce a vector representation of each document separately, and then pair them to a scalar by some standard operation such as cosine similarity or some distance function. These representations can be manually designed, as with stylistic measures, or learned in an unsupervised manner for a separate task, as with topic models. Additionally, these representations can be explicitly trained on the task at hand, predicting whether or not the same user wrote any two given documents.

The second category is models in which this prediction (the authorship decision task) is built into the model. We refer to these as authorship decision models. One key difference between these models and representation models trained on the task is that the mapping from vector representation to decision is also learned as part of the model. Another critical difference is that these models do not have to build a representation for each document separately but can compare documents as they are transformed.

One key advantage of this authorship framework is that decision models' training does not require the annotation provided for the training set; the models can be trained on unannotated data from the same domain. The dataset from the eRisk 2018 depression risk detection task could hence be used for the training of the authorship attribution models, using the 2020 training data for validation. These models include Latent Dirichlet Allocation (LDA) [3] and a Contextualizer [18] as well as a stylometry-based approach. As for validation, in the user-based approach, some users for whom the BDI is known were used as a knowledge base. Therefore, the set of users was split in half, using one half as a knowledge base and the other half for validation. On the contrary, the answer-based approach allows the validation of all 20 users.

5.1 Topic Models

It stands to reason that the topics discussed by users of social media could provide insight into their mental status. This line of inquiry has been studied extensively in the literature for a variety of disorders and behaviours [8, 23, 24]. Likewise, while the most widely known topic modeling algorithm is LDA [3], many variants exist, some more general [12, 36], some more specific to certain use-cases [21]. We opted to employ the standard LDA approach. Using topic modeling, the strategy is to create topic vectors for users and then measure the distance between these in the user-based approach or between these and the topic representation of answers for the answer-based approach.

This LDA model is trained on the eRisk 2018 depression risk detection dataset. Each user's posts are grouped into a single document. The pre-processing involves the removal of stop-words and short words (3 letters and fewer) and stemming. In addition to reducing the input space dimension, stemming does away with word inflections that are not relevant to the larger-grained strategy of LDA. Once stemmed, words appearing in fewer than 20 documents or over half of the documents are discarded.

The trained LDA model is then used to create vectors for the eRisk 2020 task 2 dataset documents. We find this approach to perform better on larger documents. Therefore, the posts gathered for each user are partitioned into temporally contiguous groups of roughly equal word count. Finally, the pairwise distance between such groups is measured using the cosine similarity between their topic model representations. This naturally falls in the unit interval, as the topic vectors are strictly positive.

LDA posits K topics from a corpus in its training process. As previous work [17, 23] demonstrated the capacity of different numbers of topics for the depression-

Table 3 Results for the **LDA answer-based approach** on T2 validation sets

Nb. of groups of documents per user	AHR (%)	ACR (%)	ADODL (%)	DCHR (%)
15	25.10	60.21	79.57	16.00
18	25.20	61.13	79.34	**37.00**
19	29.76	63.87	**80.41**	20.00
20	**32.86**	**64.27**	80.24	25.00
25	26.70	61.02	76.86	20.00

Table 4 Results for the **LDA user-based approach** on T2 validation sets

Nb. of groups of documents per user	AHR (%)	ACR (%)	ADODL (%)	DCHR (%)
10	32.67	66.57	78.44	**26.00**
15	32.67	66.57	**78.70**	20.00
18	33.52	**66.73**	78.41	22.00
19	33.52	66.44	78.12	24.00
20	**32.95**	66.51	77.68	20.00

related task, further investigation was made to optimize this parameter for our system. Validation results showed the best performances when using 30 topics for both approaches.

The different experiments show that the best ADODL is reached for the answer-based approach when combining each user's documents into 19 groups, as presented in Table 3.

As shown in Table 4, the ADODL attained by the user-based approach is approximately even when concatenating users' posts into 10–19 groups. We opt to use 19 groups at test time as we posit this will allow for finer-grained predictions.

5.2 *Contextualizer*

The Contextualizer [18] is a natural language encoding algorithm based on iteratively adjusting a context vector over a set number of steps. The context vector is computed at each step as a weighted sum of the word vectors in the sentence or document being encoded. These word vectors are supplemented by a sinusoidal position encoding [30]. The weighting is provided by a second-order attention mechanism matching the context vector's previous value to each word vector. The initial value of the context vector is set to a vector of ones. Thus, the context vector's final value should represent a relevant summary of the sentence in question.

We tested two different approaches for the authorship decision task, each one corresponding to one of the categories described in Sect. 5: encoding each document separately (parallel) or together (simultaneous). Both encoders were trained for this authorship task, ultimately using the depression questionnaire task as a final validation in both the user- and answer-based form. For the parallel encoder, the angular similarity between the document vectors is used. On the other hand, the simultaneous encoder outputs the probability of the author to be the same by design.

In order to prevent overfitting, we cease training of the authorship models by monitoring their accuracy on unseen pairs of documents, including unseen pairs of familiar documents, unseen documents by familiar users, as well as unseen users. After extensive testing, we select the parallel encoder for the user-based approach and the simultaneous one for answer-based prediction. Validation results are shown in Table 7.

5.3 Stylometry

While the previous approaches can arguably be catalogued as looking to the *content* of documents to characterize their author, one could instead focus on the *writing style* to make this characterization. To this end, several linguistic features served as document representations, such as length of words and sentences, word and character frequencies and word and sentence lengths. These features were primarily inspired by stylometric approaches to authorship attribution in instant messaging [7, 20] as well as legal proceedings and film reviews [35]. They are presented in Table 5. As with the LDA system, users' documents have been concatenated together to have the same number of documents per user while still accounting for all their production. Features are normalized considering these groups' length, whether this length pertains to words, characters or sentences. These features result in document representations of size 585. These vector representations are then compared using cosine similarity.

As previously mentioned, validation was performed with the subjects for whom the BDI was available. The parameters we were most concerned with tuning were the number of frequent words and characters to consider as well as the number of groups of documents to combine the users' documents into. As for the overall approach filling in the questionnaire, the user-based approach was expected to perform better than the answer-based one, as the answers are very brief and written in a neutral tone. Our results in terms of validation were consistent with this hypothesis, and only the user-based approach was used at test time. In terms of the number of groups, we obtain the best performance when set to 5.

Table 5 Linguistic features and their associated number of dimensions used for the stylometry-based authorship model. The frequencies of the most frequent tokens are computed and compared irrespective of what these tokens are or whether they are the same for any two users

Type	Feature
Syntactic	Frequency of select Parts of Speech (46)
Lexical	Frequency of most frequent word unigrams (100)
	Frequency of most frequent word bigrams (100)
	Frequency of most frequent character unigrams (100)
	Frequency of most frequent character bigrams (100)
	Frequency of most frequent character trigrams (100)
	Number of unique words (1)
	Number of alphanumeric characters (1)
	Number of digits (1)
	Number of non-ASCII characters (1)
	Punctuation ratio (1)
Morphological	Average length of words (1)
	Number of long words (1)
	Number of short words (1)
	Number of uppercase words (1)
	Number of uppercase characters (26)
Pragmatical	Average length of sentences (1)
	Number of hyperlinks (1)

Table 6 Validation results for the user-based stylometry system

Nb. of groups of documents per user	AHR (%)	ACR (%)	ADODL (%)	DCHR (%)
1	33.43	66.13	75.08	18.00
2	34.10	66.35	75.37	18.00
5	**35.24**	**69.40**	**77.05**	**18.00**
10	34.10	66.86	76.00	14.00

6 Results and Discussion

As shown in Table 7, no approach or authorship model proved to be convincingly superior on the validation sets. Therefore, models from all approaches were selected for prediction. The results achieved on the test set are shown in Table 8. As for the validation, the more severe metrics, the hit rates, were fairly low for all five models. On the contrary, by smoother metrics, ACR and ADODL, all models achieved results comparable to those seen in the validation. The user-based approach produced superior results across metrics and authorship models, consistent with validation. This is

Table 7 Results on the validation set for T2 (Depression)

Model	AHR (%)	ACR (%)	ADODL (%)	DCHR (%)
Stylometry (answer-based)	35.24	66.98	74.60	30.00
Stylometry (user-based)	35.24	**67.33**	76.73	18.00
LDA (answer-based)	29.76	63.87	80.40	20.00
LDA (user-based)	33.52	66.44	78.19	24.00
Context (answer-based, parallel)	18.57	55.40	75.40	40.00
Context (user-based, simultaneous)	**35.71**	67.14	**81.06**	30.00
Context (answer-based, parallel)	28.10	62.14	79.76	**45.00**
Context (user-based, simultaneous)	37.14	66.67	80.95	30.00

Table 8 Results on the test set for T2 (Depression)

Model	AHR (%)	ACR (%)	ADODL (%)	DCHR (%)
LDA (answer-based)	28.50	60.79	79.07	30.00
LDA (user-based)	36.39	68.32	**83.15**	34.29
Contextualizer (answer-based, simultaneous)	21.16	55.40	73.76	27.14
Contextualizer (user-based, parallel)	36.80	68.37	80.84	22.86
Stylometry (user-based)	37.28	68.37	80.70	20.00
BioInfo@UAVR [28]	**38.30**	69.21	76.01	30.00
iLab run 2 (split) [15]	37.07	**69.41**	81.70	27.14
iLab run 3 (truncated) [15]	35.99	69.14	82.93	34.29
prhlt_logreg_features [29]	34.01	67.07	80.05	**35.71**
prhlt_svm_features [29]	34.56	67.44	80.63	**35.71**

unsurprising for LDA, where considerable parts of users' activity will likely differ in subject matter from the BDI questionnaire. Also, given that the Contextualizer encoder matches documents individually to answers, there might be gains in performance to be obtained by considering the highest scoring document, rather than the average, for each answer. Nevertheless, although the user-based one outperformed the answer-based approach, it has the very appealing advantage of not requiring annotated data, i.e. users with known BDIs.

7 Conclusion

This chapter described the RELAI team's experiments from UQAM in the context of the eRisk 2020 second task. We approached the problem as one of authorship attribution by two different methods: **user-based** and **answer-based**. This approach affords the freedom to build decision models in a variety of ways. We relied again on

LDA and the Contextualizer as well as a stylometry-based approach, achieving the best result among participants for ADODL (83.15%) with the LDA model with the user-based approach. This metric is arguably the most relevant when it comes to an overall assessment of depression. Nonetheless, the ACR could be more interesting moving forward as it pertains to informing a clinician on the exact symptoms a patient is experiencing. Also, the LDA model shows a better balance between the different metrics. Almost all of the other approaches submitted achieved higher results than the average results for each metric. For example, the stylometric model user-based approach performed the second-best AHR.

We could also note some pertinent aspects. First, our systems are entirely independent of the domain; they make decisions only on extracted features from the provided texts without requiring heavy processes of feature engineering or domain-specific hand-crafted features. Also, the stark difference in the proportions in terms of the number of users and the number of writings between the training set and the test set for the two tasks could impact the performance of submitted models.

Overall, the test results show the promise of each approach. In future works, we will analyze in more detail the results obtained for each task. We plan to incorporate more carefully selected features into our decision models, which could better identify users at risk. Finally, given the unique nature of T2, we will explore different variations to improve predictions at a finer-grained level.

Reproducibility

The source code of the presented system is available under the GNU GPL v3 licence to ensure reproducibility. It can be found in the following repository:
https://gitlab.labikb.ca/ikb-lab/nlp/eRisk2020/erisk2020_task2

Acknowledgements This research was enabled in part by support provided by Calcul Québec (https://www.calculquebec.ca) and Compute Canada (https://www.computecanada.ca). MJM acknowledges the support of the Natural Sciences and Engineering Research Council of Canada (NSERC) [NSERC Grant number 06487-2017] and the support of the Government of Canada's New Frontiers in Research Fund (NFRF), [NFRFE-2018-00484].

References

1. Abed-Esfahani, P., Howard, D., Maslej, M., Patel, S., Mann, V., Goegan, S., & French, L. (2019). Transfer learning for depression: Early detection and severity prediction from social media postings. In *Working Notes of the Conference and Labs of the Evaluation Forum-CEUR Workshop Proceedings* (Vol. 2380).
2. Beck, A. T., Ward, C. H., Mendelson, M., Mock, J., & Erbaugh, J. (1961). An inventory for measuring depression. *Archives of General Psychiatry, 4*(6), 561–571.

3. Blei, D. M., Ng, A. Y., & Jordan, M. I. (2003). Latent dirichlet allocation. *Journal of Machine Learning Research, 3*, 993–1022.
4. Briand, A., Almeida, H., & Meurs, M.-J. (2018). Analysis of social media posts for early detection of mental health conditions. In *Canadian Conference on Artificial Intelligence* (pp. 133–143), Springer.
5. Burdisso, S. G., Errecalde, M., & Montes y Gómez, M. (2019). UNSL at eRisk 2019: A unified approach for anorexia, self-harm and depression detection in social media. In *Working Notes of the Conference and Labs of the Evaluation Forum-CEUR Workshop Proceedings* (Vol. 2380).
6. Burdisso, S. G., Errecalde, M., & y Gómez, M. M. (2019). A text classification framework for simple and effective early depression detection over social media streams. *Expert Systems with Applications, 133*, 182 – 197.
7. Cristani, M., Roffo, G., Segalin, C., Bazzani, L., Vinciarelli, A., & Murino, V. (2012). Conversationally-inspired stylometric features for authorship attribution in instant messaging. In *Proceedings of the 20th ACM International Conference on Multimedia* (pp. 1121–1124).
8. De Choudhury, M., & De, S. (2014). Mental health discourse on Reddit: Self-disclosure, social support, and anonymity. In *Eighth International AAAI Conference on Weblogs and Social Media* (Vol. 8, pp. 71–80).
9. De Choudhury, M., Gamon, M., Counts, S., & Horvitz, E. (2013). Predicting depression via social media. In *Seventh International AAAI Conference on Weblogs and Social Media* (Vol. 7, pp. 128–137).
10. Eichstaedt, J. C., Smith, R. J., Merchant, R. M., Ungar, L. H., Crutchley, P., Preoţiuc-Pietro, D., Asch, D. A., & Schwartz, H. A. (2018). Facebook language predicts depression in medical records. *Proceedings of the National Academy of Sciences, 115*(44), 11203–11208.
11. Fast, E., Chen, B., & Bernstein, M. S. (2016). Empath: Understanding topic signals in large-scale text. In *Proceedings of the 2016 CHI Conference on Human Factors in Computing Systems* (pp. 4647–4657).
12. Griffiths, T. L., Jordan, M. I., Tenenbaum, J. B., & Blei, D. M. (2004). Hierarchical topic models and the nested Chinese restaurant process. In *Advances in Neural Information Processing Systems* (pp. 17–24).
13. Losada, D. E., Crestani, F., & Parapar, J. (2019). Overview of eRisk 2019 early risk prediction on the internet. In *International Conference of the Cross-Language Evaluation Forum for European Languages* (pp. 340–357), Springer.
14. Losada, D. E., Crestani, F., & Parapar, J. (2020). Overview of eRisk 2020: Early risk prediction on the internet. In A. Arampatzis, E. Kanoulas, T. Tsikrika, S. Vrochidis, H. Joho, C. Lioma, C. Eickhoff, A. Névéol, L. Cappellato, & N. Ferro (Eds.), *Experimental IR Meets Multilinguality, Multimodality, and Interaction Proceedings of the Eleventh International Conference of the CLEF Association (CLEF 2020)*. Springer International Publishing.
15. Martínez-Castaño, R., Htait, A., Azzopardi, L., & Moshfeghi, Y. (2020). Early risk detection of self-harm and depression severity using BERT-based transformers: iLab at CLEF eRisk 2020. In *Working Notes of the Conference and Labs of the Evaluation Forum-CEUR Workshop Proceedings* (Vol. 2696).
16. Maupomé, D., Armstrong, M. D., Belbahar, R., Alezot, J., Balassiano, R., Queudot, M., Mosser, S., & Meurs, M.-J. (2020). Early mental health risk assessment through writing styles, topics and neural models. In *Working Notes of the Conference and Labs of the Evaluation Forum-CEUR Workshop Proceedings* (Vol. 2696).
17. Maupomé, D., & Meurs, M.-J. (2018). Using topic extraction on social media content for the early detection of depression. In *Working Notes of the Conference and Labs of the Evaluation Forum-CEUR Workshop Proceedings* (Vol. 2125).
18. Maupomé, D., & Meurs, M.-J. (2021). An iterative contextualization algorithm with second-order attention. arXiv:2103.02190.
19. Maupomé, D., Queudot, M., & Meurs, M.-J. (2019). Inter and intra document attention for depression risk assessment. In *Canadian Conference on Artificial Intelligence* (pp. 333–341), Springer.

20. Mudit Bhargava, P. M., & Asawa, K. (2013). Stylometric analysis for authorship attribution on Twitter. In *Big Data Analyctics: Second International Conference* (pp. 37–47).
21. Nguyen, V.-A., Ying, J. L., & Resnik, P. (2013). Lexical and hierarchical topic regression. In *Advances in Neural Information Processing Systems* (pp. 1106–1114).
22. Pennebaker, J. W., Mehl, M. R., & Niederhoffer, K. G. (2003). Psychological aspects of natural language use: Our words, our selves. *Annual Review of Psychology, 54*(1), 547–577.
23. Resnik, P., Armstrong, W., Claudino, L., Nguyen, T., Nguyen, V.-A., & Boyd-Graber, J. (2015). Beyond LDA: Exploring supervised topic modeling for depression-related language in Twitter. In *Proceedings of the 2nd Workshop on Computational Linguistics and Clinical Psychology: From Linguistic Signal to Clinical Reality* (pp. 99–107).
24. Resnik, P., Garron, A., & Resnik, R. (2013). Using topic modeling to improve prediction of neuroticism and depression in college students. In *Proceedings of the 2013 Conference on Empirical Methods in Natural Language Processing* (pp. 1348–1353).
25. Rude, S., Gortner, E.-M., & Pennebaker, J. (2004). Language use of depressed and depression-vulnerable college students. *Cognition & Emotion, 18*(8), 1121–1133.
26. Schwartz, H. A., Eichstaedt, J., Kern, M., Park, G., Sap, M., Stillwell, D., Kosinski, M., & Ungar, L. (2014). Towards assessing changes in degree of depression through facebook. In *Proceedings of the Workshop on Computational Linguistics and Clinical Psychology: From Linguistic Signal to Clinical Reality* (pp. 118–125).
27. Tausczik, Y. R., & Pennebaker, J. W. (2010). The psychological meaning of words: LIWC and computerized text analysis methods. *Journal of Language and Social Psychology, 29*(1), 24–54.
28. Trifan, A., Salgado, P., & Oliveira, L. (2020). BioInfo@ UAVR at eRisk 2020: On the use of psycholinguistics features and machine learning for the classification and quantification of mental diseases. In *Working Notes of the Conference and Labs of the Evaluation Forum-CEUR Workshop Proceedings* (Vol. 2696).
29. Uban, A.-S., & Rosso, P. (2020). Deep learning architectures and strategies for early detection of self-harm and depression level prediction. In *Working Notes of the Conference and Labs of the Evaluation Forum-CEUR Workshop Proceedings* (Vol. 2696).
30. Vaswani, A., Shazeer, N., Parmar, N., Uszkoreit, J., Jones, L., Gomez, A. N., Kaiser, Ł., & Polosukhin, I. (2017). Attention is all you need. In *Advances in Neural Information Processing Systems* (pp. 5998–6008).
31. World Health Organization. World Health Organization Fact Sheets - Depression. Retrieved April 14, 2021, from https://www.who.int/news-room/fact-sheets/detail/depression.
32. World Health Organization. (2014). *Preventing suicide: A global imperative*. World Health Organization.
33. World Health Organization. (2019). *The WHO special initiative for mental health (2019–2023): Universal health coverage for mental health*. Technical documents: World Health Organization.
34. Yates, A., Cohan, A., & Goharian, N. (2017). Depression and self-harm risk assessment in online forums. In *Proceedings of the 2017 Conference on Empirical Methods in Natural Language Processing* (pp. 2968–2978).
35. Sari, Y., Stevenson, M., & Vlachos, A. (2018). Topic or Style? Exploring the Most Useful Features for Authorship Attribution. In *Proceedings of the 27th International Conference on Computational Linguistics* (pp. 343–353).
36. Zhai, K., & Boyd-Graber, J. (2013). Online latent dirichlet allocation with infinite vocabulary. In *International Conference on Machine Learning* (pp. 561–569).

Beyond eRisk

Beyond Risk: Individual Mental Health Trajectories from Large-Scale Social Media Data

Johan Bollen, Marijn ten Thij, Lorenzo Lorenzo-Luaces, and Lauren A. Rutter

Abstract Depression and anxiety are now the 1st and 10th leading causes of disability worldwide. However, their variegated presentation and symptoms complicate efforts to develop a better understanding of the complex factors that shape the dynamics of their development within individuals. The development of personalized detection, diagnostics, and treatment options has been hindered by the lack of within-subject longitudinal observations at high temporal resolution and for large samples of individuals across the spectrum of internalizing disorders. Here, we discuss our efforts in the burgeoning field of precision mental health which leverages large-scale data of the behavioral, cognitive, emotional and social traces that billions of individuals leave behind when they interact with social media platforms. Our results point towards the possibility of modeling individualized mental health trajectories at population scale to identify high-precision targets for the detection, intervention, and mitigation of internalizing disorders.

1 Introduction

Internalizing disorders (IDs) like depression and anxiety account for a substantial proportion of morbidity associated with mental illness because of their high prevalence,

J. Bollen (✉)
Indiana University, Center for Social and Biomedical Complexity, Bloomington, IN, USA
e-mail: jbollen@indiana.edu

M. ten Thij
Department of Advanced Computing Sciences, Maastricht University, Maastricht, The Netherlands
e-mail: m.tenthij@maastrichtuniversity.nl

L. Lorenzo-Luaces · L. A. Rutter
Indiana University, Psychological and Brain Sciences, Bloomington, IN, USA
e-mail: lolorenz@indiana.edu

L. A. Rutter
e-mail: larutter@iu.edu

F. Crestani et al. (eds.), *Early Detection of Mental Health Disorders by Social Media Monitoring*, Studies in Computational Intelligence 1018,
https://doi.org/10.1007/978-3-031-04431-1_12

associated disability, and low rates of treatment utilization [42, 70, 96]. Major depression alone is experienced by at least 20% of US individuals at some point in their lives [44], with higher rates in prospective longitudinal studies [62]. Dimensional models of psychopathology like the Hierarchichal Taxonomy of Psychopathology (HiTOP) [54] highlight that depression and anxiety are part of a broader internalizing factor of psychopathology that underlies multiple disorders [3, 15, 16, 36, 57, 58, 60, 79].

However, in spite of their high and possibly rising prevalence [19, 52, 69] and being a leading cause of disability worldwide [25, 70, 98], these disorders often go unrecognized and undertreated, in part due to the heterogeneity of their presentation. Characterizing individual cognitive, linguistic, and social trajectories of IDs can yield a better understanding of the contributing mechanisms involved in their development, ultimately improving prevention, early detection, and more personalized treatments [63].

In the past two decades, social media platforms have attracted billions of individual users who, on a daily basis, share the most minute details of their behavioral, psychological, and social state. Social media posts are generally free-form, unstructured text-based messages, that may include images, in which the individual authors report on their activities, opinions, sentiment, preferences, and location, among other pertinent information.

Social media use has become a hallmark of modern life. Most (75%) of the United States (U.S.) population uses at least one social media platform [43]. Twitter, for example, is used daily by over a fifth of the United States population [87], with each user leaving behind detailed traces of their behavior, cognition, and social lives. This high level of social media use is not limited to adolescents and young adults. While most (90%) individuals 18–29 years old use social media daily, similarly high rates of use are found in 30–49 year olds (82%), and 50–64 year olds (69%). Even among adults over the age of 65, a substantial proportion (40%) still uses a social media platform daily.

There is an ongoing debate around whether social media negatively impacts mental health, especially among adolescents, women, and racial-ethnic minorities [37, 61, 67, 71]. Cross-sectional analyses largely support the idea that there is an association between perception of social media use and symptoms of IDs [76]. For example, Rutter et al. [82] reported that greater use of social media was associated with higher symptoms of depression and anxiety. Some longitudinal research also finds this association between social media use and IDs [80], but in other studies the direction of causality is unclear. Depression and anxiety may lead individuals to use social media, but increased social media use may lead to depression and anxiety [48].

Part of the reason why it is difficult to identify potentially-iatrogenic effects of social media is that researchers often employ rather crude measures of social media use and individuals' social networks, e.g. retrospective self-reports of time spent on social media, the number of social media platforms utilized [76], or one's number of close friends. Furthermore, not all social media use may equally affect mental health [85]. Internalizing symptoms may be associated with social media use that involves upward social comparison, (e.g., fear of missing out or FOMO), or negative interactions. For example, Bollen et al. [8, 9] established the existence of a "happiness paradox", a consequence of the "friendship paradox" prevalent in social networks whereby the majority of individuals have fewer friends than their friends do, on average [34, 40, 45, 50, 53]. The results suggest that most individuals will be led to negative social comparisons on social media which may act as a contributing mechanism to IDs. In other studies, however, social support and social connectedness has been associated with lower levels of depression and anxiety [24]. There are also connections between social comparison, social connectedness, and loneliness, and whereas social media may be a suitable outlet for some individuals who are lonely, for other lonely individuals, it may increase comparison and despair [48].

Researchers have increasingly leveraged social media to address these questions, and to model the dynamics of mental health trajectories [27]. The continuous use of social media represents a detailed longitudinal trail of the affective, cognitive, behavioral, and social states of individuals in the general population. In fact, Twitter alone has a user base of approximately 250 M. Assuming the latest estimate of the 12-month prevalence of *DSM-5* major depression [44], one could expect around 25 million depressed users. Previous research, including our own work, has shown that detailed indicators of mood [29, 31, 39, 83], emotions [14, 88], sleep/wake cycles [41], and social life [9, 47] can be extracted from social media content for millions of individuals.

Coppersmith et al. [26] and DeChoudhury [23] have pioneered methods establishing the feasibility of predicting the presence of internalizing disorders in online individuals from ensembles of indicators and risk factors observed in large-scale social media such as Twitter feeds. Eichstaedt [33] likewise demonstrated the ability to extract risk factors from social media to screen individuals for depression. Caution has been urged that such approaches, in particular those that rely on supervised learning to map risk factors to diagnostics, may confound sample selection criteria with genuine risk factors [22, 35]. The eRisk initiative [64] has extensively investigated opportunities for early risk detection of mental health disorders (depression, anorexia, and self-harm) from a variety of markers in social media streams, e.g. Reddit, including the construction of testbeds and challenges to develop capabilities to diachronically extract evidence of risk from social media streams. In spite of these successful efforts, and the ubiquity of social media use, the latter remains an untapped source of longitudinal data to model the dynamics of the individual development and trajectories of IDs.

Social media continues to represent a unique opportunity of publicly available real-time data to characterize the affective, cognitive, behavioral, and environmental risk factors of individual and longitudinal trajectories of mental illness at unprecedented resolution and large scale. Social media is ideally-suited for characterizing risk trajectories for mental illness because individual and social data can be collected on large samples and across multiple dimensions [46, 59, 102].

There is a great need to examine trajectories of psychopathology across the lifespan. Many of the data sets that can be used to characterize the developmental pathways of IDs are either data-rich but very small (e.g., developmental cohorts) or are large-scale, e.g., nationally representative, studies that are either cross-sectional or have a limited number of waves, e.g., the National Comorbidity Survey (NCS). Even studies designed for studying developmental processes like the National Longitudinal Study of Adolescent Health ("Add Health") have several limitations for modeling complex longitudinal processes. First, these studies are remarkably expensive. The sixth wave of Add Health *alone* may cost more than $6 million (NIH RFA-AG-21-008). While these datasets provide important information about the prevalence and risk factors for internalizing symptoms, they are not well-suited to characterize dynamic and temporal changes characteristic of IDs because they have few observations over time. In addition, the NIMH RDoC Initiative [28, 101], highlights the importance of measuring transdiagnostic processes across units of analysis that can complement self-reports and move beyond *DSM-5* categories. While social media analytics have been used to study depression, anxiety, and related disorders, few studies take IDs as a class, instead focusing on specific *DSM* disorders that are often heterogeneous and comorbid.

Throughout existing research efforts, individual social context emerges as an important, but difficult to operationalize, contributing factor in the development of IDs, in particular at high levels of temporal resolution and at scale. Social media however codifies the trajectories of interpersonal relationships and interactions at the scale of billions of individuals. As such, it provides a unique source of data to investigate the role of social network structure as a contributing and interacting mechanism of IDs. In previous research we retrieved the ego-centric social networks of large numbers of individuals from their social media interactions. From these data, we analyzed network structures to determine a range of indicators relevant to the mechanisms underlying the development of IDs: indicators of mood assortativity [8] (i.e., do users with similar indicators of ID preferentially associate on social media?) and social comparisons in online networks [9] (i.e., do negative social comparisons affect within-subject mental health?). Other researchers have investigated whether the directionality of information exchange via social networks traces patterns of support or "contagion" through transfer entropy of lexical indicators [66].

Beyond providing a detailed record of the cognitive, behavioral, and social traces left behind by billions of individuals in their online messages, social media can offer a degree of "ground truth" with respect to mental health diagnostics. Many individuals discuss their mental health on social media even to the point of reporting their diagnoses and treatments (e.g., medication, therapy) [46, 68, 74, 92] (see

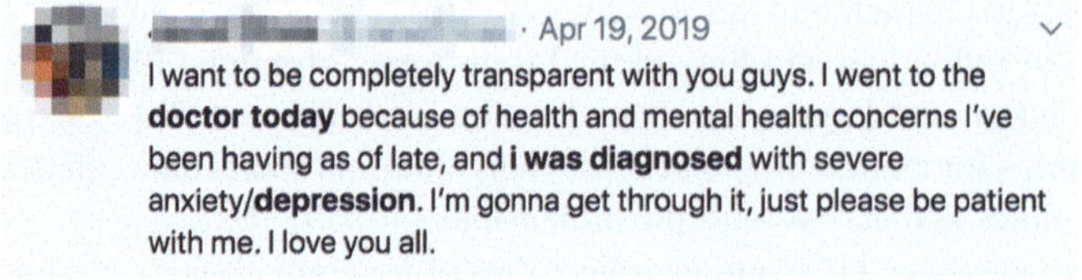

Fig. 1 Twitter users frequently report changes to their mental health. The individual's report may be publicly available for further analysis respecting Twitter's Terms of User, user privacy, and IRB regulations

Fig. 1 for an anonymous example). Data-driven approaches that leverage advances in machine learning (ML), artificial intelligence (AI), and natural language processing (NLP) techniques suggest that mental health diagnoses can predict online behavior. For example, depressed individuals more frequently use a variety of terms describing negative emotions [81, 89], first-person pronouns [7, 18, 86, 103], and symptoms of depression [1, 20]. These findings from social media data fit with basic research in IDs which finds increased self-referential processing [65], higher levels of negative affect, and more rigid and repetitive thinking in individuals with IDs.

Social media thus enables a variety of sampling strategies depending on the application. While social media data can be used for classification tasks, it may be even better-suited for complex modeling of social processes as well as modeling of dynamic inter-individual processes given its longitudinal and individual nature. Data can be collected to support analysis at the within-subject (individual timelines of social media data), between-cohort (stratified by demographics or diagnostics), and societal level (public health) through a number of sampling strategies each starting from sub-samples of populations established from medical records, social media feeds, and surveys:

Medical records sampling: Individuals are sampled from medical records, and social media data is retrieved pertaining to the respective individuals [33].

Survey sampling: Surveyed individuals complete mental health screenings and donate their social media data [22, 75].

Social media sampling: Individuals are sampled from (random) sets of social media users.

Diagnostic sampling: Individuals report clinical diagnostics in online statements [22, 26].

Some researchers have cautioned against the indiscriminate use of classifiers and machine learning in detection and diagnostics tasks from social media, in particular when samples can be biased by specific sample inclusion criteria that may be confounded with disorder features and characteristics [22, 32]. These findings suggest that, rather than focusing on cross-sectional classification, the field of data-driven mental health studies should focus on methods to develop a better understanding of the mechanics of the risk trajectories that give rise to the disorder.

Here we outline two of our own investigations that rely on social media data and a diagnostic sampling approach. They highlight many of the promises and challenges with respect to the development of applications of social media data to study the dynamics of the trajectories of mental health. First, we discuss an investigation of the association between specific changes in circadian sleep-wake rhythms, and a variety of other cognitive indicators, in individuals with depression. Second, we outline an effort to capture the cognitive risk factors of depression by examining the lexico-semantic structure of the online language of individuals with depression finding a higher prevalence of language segments that express the semantic structure of cognitive distortions.

2 Studying Behavioral Traces of Sleep and Emotions

The affective state of individuals with internalizing disorders can exhibit consistent and rapid changes which may be observed at the individual, longitudinal level by tracking the sentiment of tweet posted by individuals or groups of individuals over time. Similar changes can take place in an individual's activity level which may be observed from the number and frequency of tweets posted per time window. Note that such changes in activity levels may take place across multiple time spans, ranging from hours, days, and weeks, to months.

However, beyond specific transitions in time between different mental health states, other longitudinal and diachronic effects can shape the development of internalizing disorders, including the association between changes in circadian sleep-wake cycles and internalizing disorders [13, 55, 72, 77, 93], with evidence accumulating for the involvement of social media use [84]. Since many Twitter users tweet daily or more frequently, social media offers a unique opportunity to observe their circadian activity levels from the timing of their Twitter activity, i.e. the time at which a user posts a tweet or not. Hence, we investigated the degree to which social media activity data could be leveraged to study the association between circadian sleep-wake cycles and internalizing disorders.

2.1 *Sampling Approach*

We created two cohorts of individuals on Twitter: (1) a cohort of individuals who had been clinically diagnosed with depression (*D* cohort, N = 1,211) and (2) a random sample of individuals (*R* cohort, N = 8,791) with similar features as the individuals in the *D* cohort, but no indication of a clinical diagnosis of depression. We applied a sample inclusion criterion that in previous research was shown to provide the most accurate and reliable results [23, 26]. Specifically, we searched the Twitter API for cases where an individual had received a clinical diagnosis of depression and explicitly reported this on Twitter posting a variation of the statement `"I (was/have been) diagnos .+ depress*"` in their tweet. All such statements were manually vetted by a team of 3 experts; only cases that received unanimous approval were retained. This resulted in a sample of Twitter users who thus reported receiving a clinical diagnosis of depression (*D* cohort). Next we retrieved a random sample of individuals (*R* cohort) that had a similar distribution of account creation dates as the *D* cohort to account for community and platform changes over time.

Subsequently, we queried the Twitter API to retrieve the timelines of these individuals (3,200 most recent tweets before time of retrieval) thereby collecting a record of most, if not all, tweets they posted over time creating the *D* cohort (Fig. 2). These timelines served as the longitudinal records of the individuals' messages on Twitter. We note that because the Twitter API restricts timeline harvests to the 3,200 most

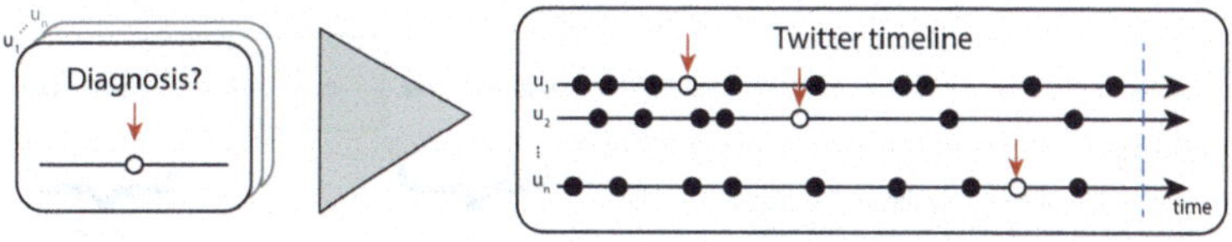

Fig. 2 Example of the diagnostic sampling approach. A cohort of individuals is constructed by searching for messages that report a clinical diagnosis of a chosen disorder (left). After ratifying these expressions, timelines of all individuals in the cohort retrieved through the Twitter API (right). A filled black dot represents a tweet and a white filled dot with a red arrow above represents a tweet that references a diagnosis. The blue dashed line represents the time of timeline retrieval

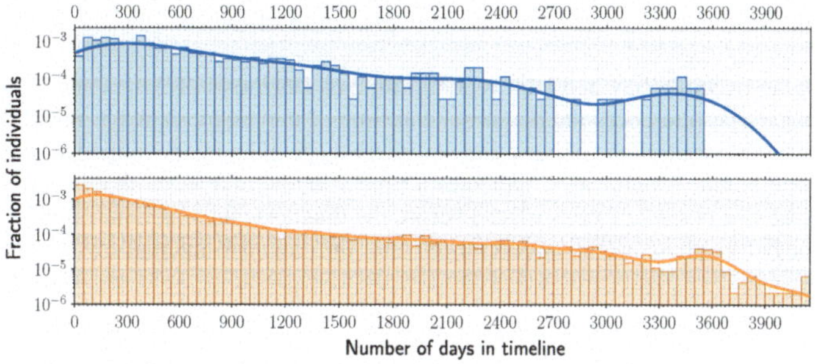

Fig. 3 Distribution of fraction of timelines with a given length in days shows that a wide range of timeline lengths can be harvested with the Twitter API restriction of returning only the 3,200 most recent tweets

recent tweets by the respective individual, the retrieved timelines can vary in length (time span), because some individuals can be more active than others and will thus reach this limit in a shorter amount of time. However, very few users are extremely active to the degree that their timeline lengths would be disproportionately affected. The distribution of the fraction of timelines of a given length in days is shown in Fig. 3, revealing a wide range of timeline lengths and no indications of discontinuities as a result of this criterion. Timeline length is furthermore unlikely a confounding factor in our analysis; we normalize our data for user activity levels and our random cohort was balanced to have a similar distribution of account creation dates to account for changes in user samples and platform effects over time (see ten Thij [90] and Bathina [4] for more details).

In addition to expressing a diagnosis, some individuals also mention a time when this diagnosis was given (see the examples in Figs. 1 and 4) or an interval in which they received the diagnosis (e.g., `"This year, I was diagnosed with depression"`). Based on these expressions, we are able to not only compare our *D* and *R* cohorts, but also compare the behavior of individuals before and after their diagnosis. Figure 4 shows how we assign tweets in the timeline to the before/after groups based on any expressed time of diagnosis (denoted by ToD, following the notation in [90]).

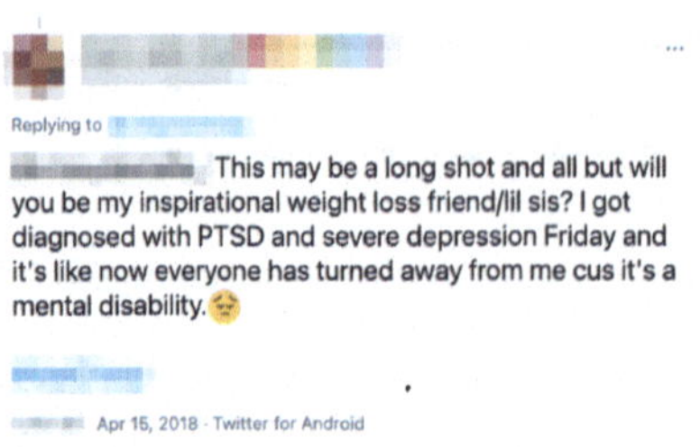

Example of a tweet that mentions a time of diagnosis.

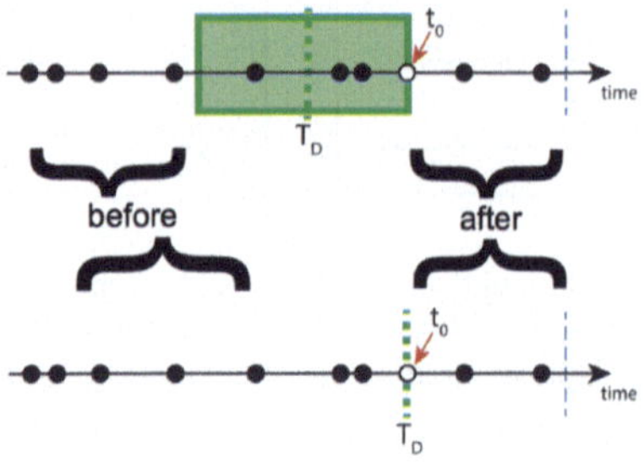

Definition of before and after diagnosis grouping of tweets

Fig. 4 Grouping tweets before and after reported time of Diagnosis (ToD). t_0 and T_D denote the time of the tweet that references the diagnosis and time of the diagnosis itself, respectively. ToD is determined by interpreting the point in time or interval specified by the individual in their tweet (e.g. "I was diagnosed 3 weeks ago" indicates a time window of 1 week that occurred 3 weeks before the tweet was posted). Tweets placed before the diagnosis interval (annotated in green) are assigned to the before phase and all tweets posted after the diagnosis interval are assign to the after phase

Many diagnosis tweets do not specify an exact date of diagnosis, e.g. "I was diagnosed July 10th", but rather specify an informal, approximate time range in which the diagnosis took place relative to the point in time at which the tweet was posted. For example, on July 24th, 2021 an individual may write "I was diagnosed with depression about 2 weeks ago". We therefore manually estimate an interval in which the diagnosis likely took place based on the magnitude and time unit stated. In this case, the magnitude is 2 weeks, and the unit of time is "a week", therefore the statement would be interpreted as referring to an interval of 1 week centered around the date that occurred 2 weeks before the tweet was posted, i.e. July 6th to July 13th. If an individual reported multiple diagnoses with a ToD designation, we determined the intersection of the extracted intervals as the most likely period of time in which the diagnosis took place (e.g., "I was diagnosed about a month ago" and "as I said, I was diagnosed 3 weeks ago"). Lacking an intersection, we assumed the ToD was uncertain or erroneous, and the individual was excluded from the ToD analysis. Finally, we assumed that "I was recently diagnosed" refers to the past 3 months. More details are provided in ten Thij [90]. This analysis may be automated in future work using NLP techniques to extract approximate and relative time references in natural language.

2.2 Behavioral Analysis

We sub-sampled the individuals in both cohorts by removing all individuals for which we could not determine timezone information, to avoid confounding time zone shifts with circadian patterns. We then characterized the sleep-wake cycles of the resulting *D* versus the *R* cohort, reasoning that individuals cannot tweet if they are asleep and that their first interactions of the day indicate when they are awake [90].

For all individuals, i.e. the *D* and *R* cohort combined, online activity showed a pronounced and consistent circadian pattern with the lowest level of activity from 2 AM to 7 AM, increasing rapidly after 7 AM to a plateau from 10 AM to 8 PM, and a peak in activity at 10 PM. The *D* cohort showed significant changes in their circadian activity levels vs the random sample of individuals. Indeed, individuals who were diagnosed with depression were significantly less active in the early morning, possibly indicating they wake up later, and relatively more active at night, indicating they fall asleep later or have disturbed sleep patterns versus a random sub-sample of Twitter users.

We performed a similar analysis with a sub-sample of individuals for which we have a ToD and timezone information (N = 93). For these individuals, we construct a circadian rhythm of their activity before their ToD and after their ToD. The resulting circadian rhythms, displayed in Fig. 5, showed a pronounced and consistent circadian pattern with the lowest level of activity from 2AM to 7AM, increasing rapidly after 7AM to a plateau from 10 AM to 8 PM, and a peak in activity in the evening hours (9 PM to 11 PM). Furthermore, there is a shift in the circadian rhythm between the tweets posted before and after the ToD, where the circadian rhythm after the ToD is more similar to the circadian rhythm of the *R* cohort, which points towards a possible treatment effect in these timelines.

We can not only record the time at which tweets are posted to assess individual activity levels, but we may also examine the content of these tweets at that time for established language markers related to internalizing disorders, such as a greater or less prevalence of personal pronouns, words with emotional loadings, "absolutist" terms, etc. This provides an opportunity to examine the lexical and semantic correlates of divergences of circadian cycles of individuals with depression versus those of a random sample. Two experts in cognitive-behavioral therapy (CBT) selected a

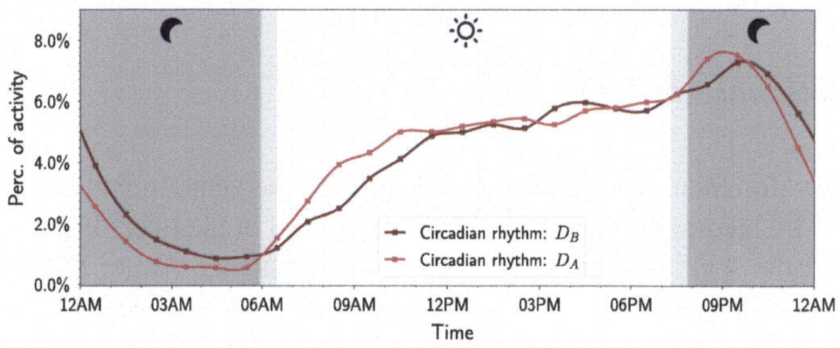

Fig. 5 Bootstrapped normalized activity levels for the *D* cohort using tweets before the time of diagnosis and tweets after the time of diagnosis. The markers display the median outcome of 10,000 runs, where we use the number of individuals in each cohort as the sample size per run. The solid lines display the cubic spline fit of these hourly values. The dark and light gray shaded areas indicate the day/night times during the cycle

Table 1 Overview of categories and corresponding tokens used for content analysis

Lexicon	Tokens					
Positive affect	Good	Happy	Hope	Like	Love	Thank	Thanks
	Well	Better	:)	:D			
Negative affect	Shit	Bad	Sad	Angry	Cry	Crying	Worse
	Worst	Horrible	Terrible	Frustrated	Annoyed	Overwhelmed	Stressed
	:(	:'(					
Personal pronouns	I	I	Me	My	Mine	Myself	
Rumination	Could	If	Know	Need	Only	Or	Want
	Will	Would					
Questioning	How	Think	What	When	Who	Why	Should
	Where						
Rigid thinking	All	Always	Because	Even	Ever	More	Much
	Never	No	Not	Really	Still		

sub-set of 76 tokens (listed in Table 1) that were deemed relevant markers of internalizing disorders from the 250 most used tokens in the Twitter feeds of our sample of individuals with depression (they were most frequent in each separate hour and occurred in each hour). The terms were organized in six different categories related to "self-reflection" and "rumination" (e.g., personal pronouns). A set of tokens related to "positive affect" were included as a control. We then analyzed the hourly circadian prevalence of the terms listed in Table 1 in the Twitter timelines of our cohort of individuals with depression [90].

Analyses of the content of the posts suggests greater levels of positive and negative emotionality when individuals are active, as well as a steady rise in rumination from midnight to dawn among individuals with depression [90].

2.3 Emotional Analysis

Based on the aforementioned results that show increased emotionality, we extended our analysis by incorporating the sentiment expressed in the tweet in the timelines. We assessed the sentiment in each tweet with the Valence Aware Dictionary and sEntiment Reasoner (VADER) [49], which scores texts on an affective scale ranging from -1 (negative) to $+1$ (postive), and recorded the number of daily tweets as an indicator of their activity levels, resulting in a time series that reveals sharp and distinct changes in affective as well as activity levels, possibly indicating changes from one mental health state to another. We provide an example of such changes in Fig. 6, based on the timeline gathered for the example diagnosis tweet in Fig. 4.

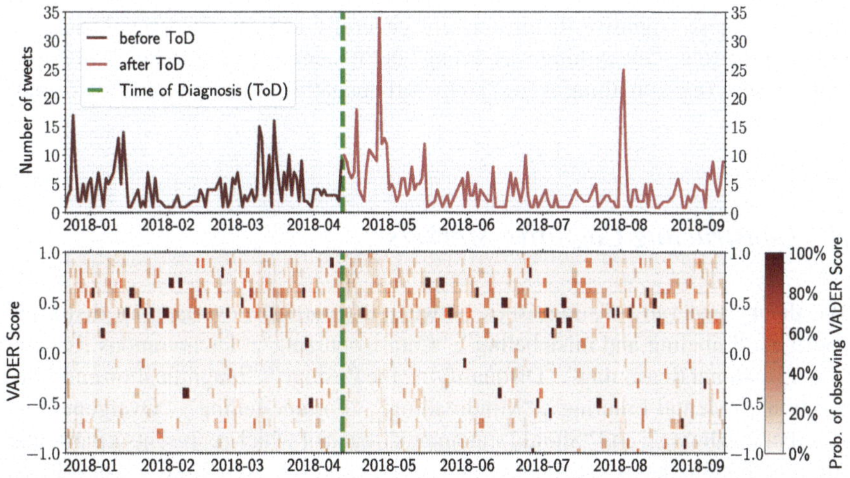

Fig. 6 Variations in emotional and sentiment levels of an individual over time. The top panel displays the activity level of the individual in number of tweets per day. The time of diagnosis is indicated by a dashed green line. The bottom panel displays the daily distribution of sentiment levels of the individual

Preliminary results indicate that the volume of tweets can be used as record of individual activity levels (shown in the top panel of Fig. 6 and evidenced by Ten Thij [90]), and that potentially meaningful changes in such activity levels can be related to the ToD. The bottom panel on the other hand shows the daily distributions of individual valence (measured by Tweet VADER ratings) as they change from the period *before* to the period *after* the Time of Diagnosis. Such analysis may reveal diachronic changes in activity levels and affectivity, in relation the point in time at which an individual was diagnosed with an ID. In this case, we see indications of greater variability of sentiment and potentially a skew towards lower valence after the ToD which may reveal pertinent changes in the individual's mental health status, possibly as a result of the ID or treatment effects.

3 Detecting Cognitive Markers of Mental Health Disorders

Beyond the presence of effects related to sleep-wake cycles, our team [4] investigated whether the language of depressed individuals on Twitter differs *semantically* from the language of a random sample of individuals on Twitter. In cognitive-behavioral therapy (CBT), a form of psychotherapy or "talk therapy," therapists work with their clients to identify malaptive patterns of thinking and behaviour. In practicing CBT, clients can begin to identify whether their thoughts contain cognitive distortions, i.e. patterns of thinking and experiencing the external world that are overly negative, untrue, and maladaptive, and that negatively affect their motivation, affect, and behaviour. These cognitive distortions are generally characterized by absolute or rigid thinking (e.g., "everything was wrong" or "it's unacceptable to fail"), distorted points of view (e.g., "nothing is fun"), or overly negative thinking (e.g., "my friends all hate me").

3.1 Constructing Cognitive Markers

CBT theory generally distinguishes between 12 partially overlapping distortion types, i.e. "Labeling and mislabeling", "Catastrophizing", "Dichotomous Reasoning", "Emotional Reasoning", "Disqualifying the Positive", "Magnification and Minimization", "Mental Filtering", "Mindreading", "Fortune-telling", "Overgeneralizing", "Personalizing", and "Should statements", each of which represents a particular pattern of thought that is maladaptive and overly rigid. This typology was developed by Beck (1964) [5] and has remained relatively stable since. The typology is intended as a means of organizing the general notion of cognitive distortions, not making theoretical claims with respect to their semantic properties nor their lexical structure. The process of identifying and mitigating cognitive distortions as part of CBT therapy remains an interactive conversational process engaged in by a trained CBT therapist and their clients.

The relationship between cognition and language is well-established, and is reflected in studies of the association between internalizing disorders and changes in language. However, the detection of cognitive distortions in individuals with depression has been poorly explored, particularly in the area of data-driven approaches which focus largely on the usefulness of any language features to predict risk factors and disorders.

Based on a theoretical and clinical understanding of cognitive distortions, and their important role in shaping the risk trajectories of individuals with depression (and consequently their language), our team of CBT experts employed an iterative and collaborative design process to construct an extensive lexicon of 241 n-grams that expressed the lexical and semantic core structure of a cognitive distortion. For each distortion type, e.g. "Fortune-telling", the panel proposed a set of n-grams of length 1 to 5, Cognitive Distortion Schemata (CDS), that captured the cognitive structure of that distortion in a stand-alone, context-free manner. For example, in the case of "fortune-telling", "I will fail" was one of the n-grams deemed to express a distortion of that type, regardless of its lexical context, i.e. it could be followed by a variety of terms such as "exam", "to succeed", "like always", etc without losing its distorted nature. Similarly, in the case of "Labeling and mislabeling", the trigram "I am a" was included to express the act of assigning a definite label to oneself, hence "I am" and "a" regardless of the actual label applied (e.g., "loser", "sad person", etc.) The list of 241 such n-grams was further vetted by a panel of 8 experts in CBT and revised based on their feedback.

Table 2 Examples of cognitive distortion schemata* for 12 commonly distinguished distortion types

Type	Definition
Catastrophizing:	Exaggerating the importance of negative events
will fail, will go wrong, will end, will be impossible, will not happen, will be terrible, ...	
Dichotomous Reasoning:	Thinking in terms of only two categories
always, perfect, the best, all, not a single, no one, nobody, nothing, never, the worst,...	
Disqualifying the Positive:	Unreasonably discounting positive experiences
great but, good but, OK but, not that great, not that good, it was not, not all that, fine but, ...	
Emotional Reasoning:	Thinking that something is true based on how one feels
but I feel, since I feel, because I feel, but it feels, since it feels, because it feels, still feels	
Fortune-telling:	Making predictions, usually negative ones, about the future
I will not, we will not, you will not, they will not, it will not, that will not, he will not, ...	
Labeling and mislabeling:	Labeling yourself or others
I am a, he is a, she is a, they are a, it is a, that is a, a burden, a complete, a loser, ...	
Magnification and Minimization:	Magnifying negative aspects or minimizing positive aspects
worst, best, not important, not count, not matter, no matter, the only thing, the one thing	
Mental Filtering:	Paying too much attention to negative details
I see only, all I see, all I can see, can only think, nothing good, nothing right, ...	
Mindreading:	Believing you know what others are thinking
everyone believes, everyone knows, everyone thinks, everyone will believe, ...	
Overgeneralizing:	Making sweeping negative conclusions
all of the time, all of them, all the time, always happens, always like, happens every time, ...	
Personalizing:	Believing others are behaving negatively because of oneself
all me, all my, because I, because my, because of my, because of me, I am responsible, ...	
Should statements:	Having a fixed idea on how you and/or others should behave
should, ought, must, have to, has to	

* n-grams of length 1 to 5

We show several examples of such CDS n-grams in Table 2 and a network visualizing the reciprocal Levenshtein similarities of its set of n-grams to highlight the degree of lexical overlap between the adopted n-grams in expressing a similar construct (Fig. 7).

3.2 Sampling Approach

We created two cohorts of individuals on Twitter: (1) a cohort of individuals who had been clinically diagnosed with depression (*D* cohort) and (2) a random sample of individuals (*R* cohort) on Twitter with similar features as the individuals in the *D* cohort but no indication of a clinical diagnosis of depression. To build the *D* cohort, we used the same diagnostic sampling approach as discussed in Sect. 2.1. We

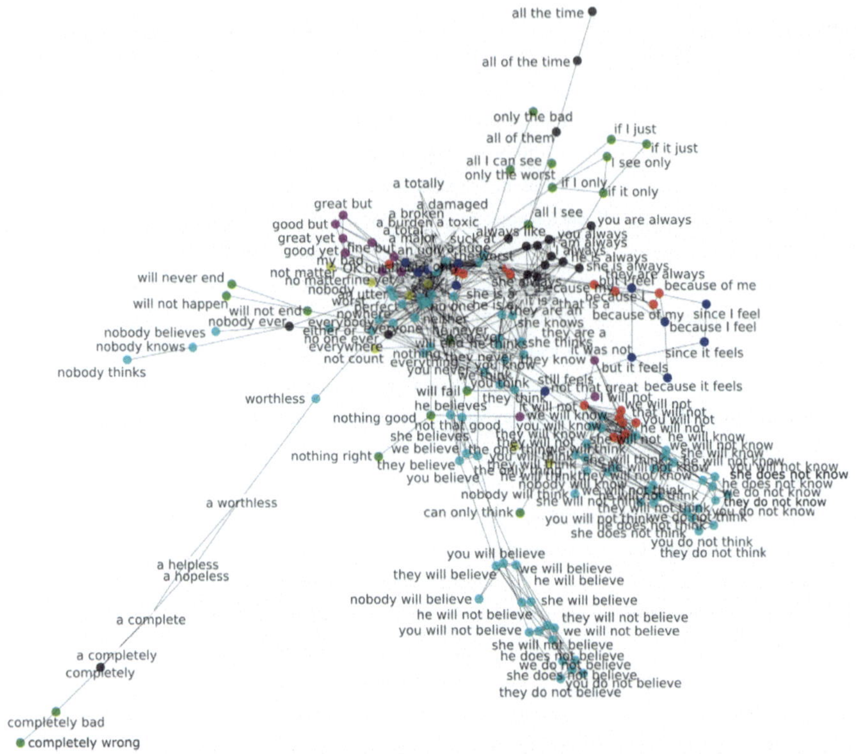

Fig. 7 Network visualizing the lexical overlap between the CDS n-grams from the Bathina (2021) lexicon [4] based on n-gram Levenshtein distances. Nodes are colored by cognitive distortion type. Edges are drawn only if the Levenshtein distance between the n-grams is less than 6. Node label positions are approximate with some labels removed to enhance readability

subsequently retrieved the timelines of all individuals in both cohorts, which served as the longitudinal records of the individuals' messages on Twitter (see Fig. 2).

3.3 *Lexical Analysis of Cognitive Distortion Markers*

We scanned each tweet for the occurrence (sub-string match) of each of the 241 CDS n-grams, thereby recording their prevalence (number of matches normalized by number of tweets) at the within-individual and between-cohort levels.

We found that Twitter users in the D cohort were more likely to use cognitively-distorted language at the within-subject level as well as the between-cohort level. In fact, across *all* 12 distortion types combined, they were more than 20% more likely to have a Tweet that contained a CD (prevalence ratio: 95% CI $=1.16 - 1.22$, Cohen's d $= 0.56$), see Fig. 8. The distortion types "personalizing" and "emotional

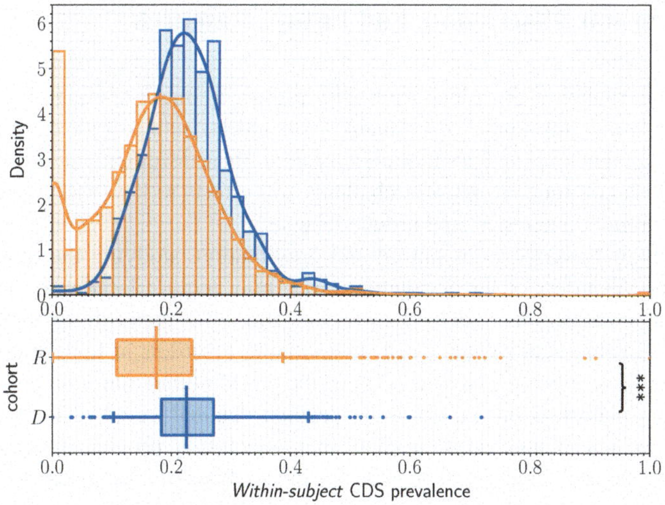

Fig. 8 Comparison of densities of cognitive distortion prevalence in the language of Twitter users (within-subject) with depression (N = 1,035) versus a random sample of Twitter users (N = 7,349) shows that the online language of individuals with depression contain higher levels of markers of cognitive distortions (241 CDS n-grams). Note the high number of Random Cohort individuals with zero CDS matches vs the D cohort

reasoning" occur approximately 2.3 times more frequently in the online language of the *D* cohort relative to the *R* cohort. Our findings indicated a significantly higher prevalence of most types of CDS in the *D* cohort, with medium to large effect sizes.

These results were *not* accounted for by the use of personal pronouns or by the emotional valence of the posted content, since an analysis without n-grams that contain personal pronouns produced identical results and our set of CDS n-grams was largely devoid of positive or negatively valenced words.

These results shed light onto how depression may affect public discourse on social media, and reveal the degree to which the distorted language styles used in depression are manifested in the colloquial language on social media platforms and potentially even in societal language over time [12]. Our results suggest a path for intervention strategies, including mobile and/or social media-based applications, that challenge particular expressions and types of depressogenic language. Future characterizations of the relations between depressogenic language and mood may aid in the development of automated interventions (e.g., "chatbots") or suggest promising targets for psychotherapy.

4 Conclusion, Discussion, and Future Research

Although internalizing disorders are highly prevalent, and a leading cause of disability worldwide, important gaps remain in the understanding of the dynamics, risk factors, and diagnostic markers that play a role in their development at the individual level. This continues to present challenges to efforts to lower their prevalence, improve treatment outcomes, and reduce relapse.

Due to their heterogeneous nature and presentation, studying the dynamics of internalizing disorders at the individual level, may require large-scale individual longitudinal observations. Such observations offer the opportunity to study the diachronic development dynamics of internalizing disorders at high temporal resolution at sufficient power. Nearly 1/7th of the world population now actively uses social media platforms on a *daily* basis, leaving detailed traces of their affective, cognitive, and social state on these platforms, which may provide a unique opportunity to enable such analysis. The need for the analysis of a multitude of traces of individual information ("big data") has driven the development of a myriad of tools across several fields within Computer Science, e.g., Natural Language Processing (NLP), Artificial Intelligence (AI) and Machine Learning (ML), to process the enormous quantities of categorical, nominal, and text data that comprise the longitudinal records of activity on social media for billions of individuals. Recently, the growing possibilities to cultivate and leverage this data has resulted in the development of the burgeoning fields of computational psychiatry and computational social science.

Significant challenges, however, remain. Much ongoing work is focused on feature selection and classification. Although these are important avenues to explore, our ability to detect and diagnose the presence of internalizing disorders in individuals, may be subject to a variety of biases, such as sample selection bias, overfitting, and ignoring the important complexities of the dynamics through which internalizing disorders develop within-subjects over time. The latter may in fact be a significant obstacle given extensive data showing the lack of reliable bio-markers or risk factors from which to predict the emergence of internalizing disorders and relapse within individuals. Importantly, DeChoudhury [22] and Ernala [35] caution extensively against purely data-driven approaches, showing that classifiers trained on data obtained from social media are subject to sample selection bias, an issue that may need to be addressed with carefully calibrated triangulation strategies whose effectiveness has been demonstrated in investigations that leverage a combination of survey and social media data for nowcasting [99].

Such a research program will, however, have to account for a number of significant challenges related to the acquisition of social media data, generally governed by platform-specific Terms of Service. In particular, ethics and user privacy and rights should be respected while acknowledging the role of social media platforms in shaping mental health. Recent results [17, 56, 73, 91] indicate that the use of social media platforms can have deleterious effects on mental health and social well-being. This association is likely complex, dependent on usage levels and modalities, demographically stratified, bidirectional, and subject to the specific characteristics of the platform in question. Significant non-stationarities of these effects can be expected given the outsized role of social media in both reporting on and shaping societal trends [2, 10, 11, 94, 100] which will affect samples and outcomes. Care should therefore be taken to disambiguate societal trends affecting language, e.g. large number of individuals reporting on elections [30] and other public events, from content that is indicative of individuals' psychological states [38]. In addition, much analysis will be retrospective, i.e. data is analyzed after it has been voluntarily made public by platform participants. This may attenuate issues of human subjects research (lack of interaction and the analysis of existing, public data), but complicates matters of consent. Individuals in social media can not anticipate their data being analyzed well after it has been made public, with possibly inadvertent implications for their social status and privacy. For example, an individual suffering from depression may not be aware that their public social media posts at that time may later be analyzed and used to make determinations about their mental health status. Careful consideration should thus be given to protecting user privacy and respecting prevailing norms of research ethics [6, 21, 22, 68, 78].

Most social media platforms offer a high degree of user anonymity, allowing users to voluntarily disclose demographic data and other pertinent personal data. This complicates efforts to establish balanced and equitable samples [51, 97] as well as the application of exclusion criteria to protect minors and other vulnerable populations. As a result, research based on social media data will need to carefully consider sample stratification on the basis of computationally determined demographics, e.g. through the use of classifiers that can estimate gender and age [4, 97], as well as platform effects, social factors, and inequities of access.

In light of these reflections, we envision a scientific program that seeks to unravel the individual complex dynamics and mechanics of the development of internalizing disorders [95], taking into account the full spectrum of affective, cognitive, behavioral, and social determinants that shape mental health. Machine learning and AI applications are crucial tools to support such a theory-driven research effort that aims to establish an understanding of the emergence of internalizing disorders from which advanced detection, diagnostics, and mitigation approaches can be established. Approaches that leverage social media itself as a platform for scalable, personalized prevention and intervention strategies may emerge that can benefit public health [63], and make treatment and support options available to millions of individuals that would otherwise be left under- or un-served by existing resources.

Acknowledgements Johan Bollen is grateful for support from the Urban Mental Health Institute of the University of Amsterdam, Wageningen University and Research, the NSF (NSF SMASBE #1636636), and the IU Vice Provost for COVID-19 Research.

References

1. Al-Mosaiwi, M., & Johnstone, T. (2018). In an absolute state: Elevated use of absolutist words is a marker specific to anxiety, depression, and suicidal ideation. *Clinical Psychological Science, 6*, 529–542.
2. Bahamonde, J., Bollen, J., Elejalde, E., Ferres, L., & Poblete, B. (2018). Power structure in chilean news media. *PLOS ONE, 13*(6), 1–18.
3. Barlow, D. H., DiNardo, P. A., Vermilyea, B. B., Vermilyea, J., & Blanchard, E. B. (1986). Co-morbidity and depression among the anxiety disorders: Issues in diagnosis and classification. *Journal of Nervous and Mental Disease*.
4. Bathina, K. C., Ten Thij, M., Lorenzo-Luaces, L., Rutter, L. A., & Bollen, J. (2021). Individuals with depression express more distorted thinking on social media. *Nature Human Behaviour,* 1–9.
5. Beck, A. T. (1964). Thinking and depression: II. Theory and therapy. *Archives of General Psychiatry, 10*(6), 561–571.
6. Benton, A., Coppersmith, G., & Dredze, M. (2017). Ethical research protocols for social media health research. In *Proceedings of the First ACL Workshop on Ethics in Natural Language Processing*, EthNLP, Association for Computational Linguistics (pp. 94–102).
7. Bernard, J. D., Baddeley, J. L., Rodriguez, B. F., & Burke, P. A. (2016). Depression, language, and affect: An examination of the influence of baseline depression and affect induction on language. *Journal of Language and Social Psychology, 35*(3), 317–326.
8. Bollen, J., Gonçalves, B., Ruan, G., & Mao, H. (2011). Happiness is assortative in online social networks. *Artificial life, 17*(3), 237–251.
9. Bollen, J., Gonçalves, B., van de Leemput, I., & Ruan, G. (2017). The happiness paradox: Your friends are happier than you. *EPJ Data Science, 6*(1), 4.
10. Bollen, J., Mao, H., & Pepe, A. (2011). Modeling public mood and emotion: Twitter sentiment and socio-economic phenomena. In *Fifth International AAAI Conference on Weblogs and Social Media* (Vol. 5, p. 1).
11. Bollen, J., Mao, H., & Zeng, X. (2011). Twitter mood predicts the stock market. *Journal of Computational Science, 2*(1), 1–8.
12. Bollen, J., ten Thij, M., Breithaupt, F., Barron, A. T. J., Rutter, L. A., Lorenzo-Luaces, L., & Scheffer, M. (2021). Historical language records reveal a surge of cognitive distortions in recent decades. *Proceedings of the National Academy of Sciences, 118*(30), e2102061118.
13. Borbély, A., & Wirz-Justice, A. (1982). Sleep, sleep deprivation and depression. *Human Neurobio1ogy, 1*, 205–210.
14. Brady, W. J., Wills, J. A., Jost, J. T., Tucker, J. A., & Van Bavel, J. J. (2017). Emotion shapes the diffusion of moralized content in social networks. *Proceedings of the National Academy of Sciences, 114*(28), 7313–7318.
15. Brown, T. A., & Barlow, D. H. (2009). A proposal for a dimensional classification system based on the shared features of the dsm-iv anxiety and mood disorders: Implications for assessment and treatment. *Psychological Assessment, 21*(3), 256.
16. Brown, T. A., Campbell, L. A., Lehman, C. L., Grisham, J. R., & Mancill, R. B. (2001). Current and lifetime comorbidity of the dsm-iv anxiety and mood disorders in a large clinical sample. *Journal of Abnormal Psychology, 110*(4), 585.
17. Burke, M., Marlow, C., & Lento, T. (2010). Social network activity and social well-being. In *Proceedings of the SIGCHI Conference on Human Factors in Computing Systems* (pp. 1909–1912), New York, NY, USA, 2010, CHI '10, ACM.
18. Cacheda, F., Fernandez, D., Novoa, F. J., & Carneiro, V. (2019). Early detection of depression: Social network analysis and random forest techniques. *Journal of Medical Internet Research, 21*, e12554.
19. Case, A., & Deaton, A. (2015). Rising morbidity and mortality in midlife among white non-hispanic Americans in the 21st century. *Proceedings of the National Academy of Sciences, 112*(49), 15078–15083.

20. Cavazos-Rehg, P. A., Krauss, M. J., Sowles, S., Connolly, S., Rosas, C., Bharadwaj, M., & Bierut, L. J. (2016). A content analysis of depression-related tweets. *Computers in Human Behavior, 54*, 351–357.
21. Chancellor, S., Birnbaum, M. L., Caine, E. D., Silenzio, V. M. B., & De Choudhury, M. (2019). A taxonomy of ethical tensions in inferring mental health states from social media. In *Proceedings of the Conference on Fairness, Accountability, and Transparency* (pp. 79–88), FAT, Association for Computing Machinery.
22. Chancellor, S., & Choudhury, M. D. (2020). Methods in predictive techniques for mental health status on social media: A critical review. *NPJ Digital Medicine, 3*, 43.
23. Choudhury, M. D., Gamon, M., Counts, S., & Horvitz, E. (2013). Predicting depression via social media. In *Proceedings of the Seventh International AAAI Conference on Weblogs and Social Media (ICWSM-13)* (pp. 128–137).
24. Coker, A. L., Smith, P. H., Thompson, M. P., McKeown, R. E., Bethea, L., & Davis, K. E. (2002). Social support protects against the negative effects of partner violence on mental health. *Journal of Women's Health & Gender-Based Medicine, 11*(5), 465–476.
25. Collishaw, S. (2015). Annual research review: Secular trends in child and adolescent mental health. *Journal of Child Psychology and Psychiatry, 56*(3), 370–393.
26. Coppersmith, G., Dredze, M., & Harman, C. (2014). Quantifying mental health signals in twitter. In *Proceedings of the Workshop on Computational Linguistics and Clinical Psychology: From Linguistic Signal to Clinical Reality* (pp. 51–60), CLPsych, ACM.
27. Correia, R. B., Wood, I. B., Bollen, J., & Rocha, L. M. (2020). Mining social media data for biomedical signals and health-related behavior. *Annual Review of Biomedical Data Science, 3*, 433–458.
28. Cuthbert, B. N., & Workgroup, N. R. (2014). The rdoc framework: Continuing commentary. *World Psychiatry, 13*(2), 196–197.
29. De Choudhury, M., Counts, S., & Gamon, M. (2012). Not all moods are created equal! exploring human emotional states in social media. In *Sixth International AAAI Conference on Weblogs and Social Media.*
30. DiGrazia, J., McKelvey, K., Bollen, J., & Rojas, F. (2013). More tweets, more votes: Social media as a quantitative indicator of political behavior. *PLOS ONE, 8*(11) , 1–5.
31. Doré, B., Ort, L., Braverman, O., & Ochsner, K. N. (2015). Sadness shifts to anxiety over time and distance from the national tragedy in newtown, connecticut. *Psychological Science, 26*(4), 363–373.
32. Dutta, S., Ma, J., & De Choudhury, M. (2018). Measuring the impact of anxiety on online social interactions. In *Twelfth International AAAI Conference on Web and Social Media.*
33. Eichstaedt, J. C., Smith, R. J., Merchant, R. M., Ungar, L. H., Crutchley, P., Preoţiuc-Pietro, D., Asch, D. A., & Schwartz, H. A. (2018). Facebook language predicts depression in medical records. *Proceedings of the National Academy of Sciences, 115*(44), 11203–11208.
34. Eom, Y.-H., & Jo, H.-H. (2014). Generalized friendship paradox in complex networks: The case of scientific collaboration. *Scientific Reports, 4.*
35. Ernala, S. K., Birnbaum, M. L., Candan, K. A., Rizvi, A. F., Sterling, W. A., Kane, J. M., & Choudhury, M. D. (2019). Methodological gaps in predicting mental health states from social media: Triangulating diagnostic signals. In *Proceedings of the 2019 CHI Conference on Human Factors in Computing Systems* (pp. 1–16), no. 134 in CHI, ACM.
36. Erwin, B. A., Heimberg, R. G., Juster, H., & Mindlin, M. (2002). Comorbid anxiety and mood disorders among persons with social anxiety disorder. *Behaviour Research and Therapy, 40*(1), 19–35.
37. Escobar-Viera, C. G., Whitfield, D. L., Wessel, C. B., Shensa, A., Sidani, J. E., Brown, A. L., Chandler, C. J., Hoffman, B. L., Marshal, M. P., & Primack, B. A. (2018). For better or for worse? A systematic review of the evidence on social media use and depression among lesbian, gay, and bisexual minorities. *JMIR Mental Health, 5*(3), e10496.
38. Fan, R., Varol, O., Varamesh, A., Barron, A., van de Leemput, I. A., Scheffer, M., & Bollen, J. (2019). The minute-scale dynamics of online emotions reveal the effects of affect labeling. *Nature Human Behaviour, 3*(1), 92–100.

39. Fardouly, J., Diedrichs, P. C., Vartanian, L. R., & Halliwell, E. (2015). Social comparisons on social media: The impact of facebook on young women's body image concerns and mood. *Body Image, 13*, 38–45.
40. Feld, S. L. (1991). Why your friends have more friends than you do. *American Journal of Sociology, 96*, 1464–1477.
41. Golder, S. A., & Macy, M. W. (2011). Diurnal and seasonal mood vary with work, sleep, and daylength across diverse cultures. *Science, 333*(6051), 1878–1881.
42. Greenberg, P. E., Fournier, A.-A., Sisitsky, T., Pike, C. T., & Kessler, R. C. (2015). The economic burden of adults with major depressive disorder in the United States (2005 and 2010). *The Journal of Clinical Psychiatry, 76*(2), 155–162.
43. Greenwood, S., Perrin, A., & Duggan, M. (2016). Social media update 2016. *Pew Research Center, 11*, 2.
44. Hasin, D. S., Sarvet, A. L., Meyers, J. L., Saha, T. D., Ruan, W. J., Stohl, M., & Grant, B. F. (2018). Epidemiology of adult DSM-5 major depressive disorder and its specifiers in the united states. *JAMA Psychiatry, 75*(4), 336–346.
45. Hodas, N. O., Kooti, F., & Lerman, K. (2013). Friendship paradox redux: Your friends are more interesting than you. In *Proceedings of the Seventh International AAAI Conference on Weblogs and Social Media*, AAAI Press.
46. Hswen, Y., Naslund, J. A., Brownstein, J. S., & Hawkins, J. B. (2018). Online communication about depression and anxiety among twitter users with schizophrenia: Preliminary findings to inform a digital phenotype using social media. *Psychiatric Quarterly, 89*(3), 569–580.
47. Huberman, B. A., Romero, D. M., & Wu, F. (2008). Social networks that matter: Twitter under the microscope. arXiv:0812.1045.
48. Hunt, M. G., Marx, R., Lipson, C., & Young, J. (2018). No more fomo: Limiting social media decreases loneliness and depression. *Journal of Social and Clinical Psychology, 37*(10), 751–768.
49. Hutto, C. J., & Gilbert, E. (2014). Vader: A parsimonious rule-based model for sentiment analysis of social media text. In *Eighth International AAAI Conference on Weblogs and Social Media*.
50. Jo, H.-H., & Eom, Y.-H. (2014). Generalized friendship paradox in networks with tunable degree-attribute correlation. *Physical Review E, 90*, 022809.
51. Kalimeri, K., Beiro, M. G., Bonanomi, A., Rosina, A., & Cattuto, C. (2020). Traditional versus facebook-based surveys: Evaluation of biases in self-reported demographic and psychometric information. *Demographic Research, 42*, 133–148.
52. Keyes, K. M., Gary, D., O'Malley, P. M., Hamilton, A., & Schulenberg, J. (2019). Recent increases in depressive symptoms among us adolescents: trends from 1991 to 2018. *Social Psychiatry and Psychiatric Epidemiology, 54*, 987–996.
53. Kooti, F., Hodas, N. O., & Lerman, K. (2014). Network weirdness: Exploring the origins of network paradoxes. In *Proceedings of the Eighth International AAAI Conference on Weblogs and Social Media*, AAAI Press.
54. Kotov, R., Krueger, R. F., Watson, D., Achenbach, T. M., Althoff, R. R., Bagby, R. M., Brown, T. A., Carpenter, W. T., Caspi, A., Clark, L. A., et al. (2017). The hierarchical taxonomy of psychopathology (hitop): A dimensional alternative to traditional nosologies. *Journal of Abnormal Psychology, 126*(4), 454.
55. Krause, A. J., Simon, E. B., Mander, B. A., Greer, S. M., Saletin, J. M., Goldstein-Piekarski, A. N., & Walker, M. P. (2017). The sleep-deprived human brain. *Nature Reviews Neuroscience, 18*, 404–418.
56. Kross, E., Verduyn, P., Demiralp, E., Park, J., Lee, D. S., Lin, N., Shablack, H., Jonides, J., & Ybarra, O. (2013). Facebook use predicts declines in subjective well-being in young adults. *PLoS ONE, 8*(8), e69841.
57. Krueger, R. F., & Finger, M. S. (2001). Using item response theory to understand comorbidity among anxiety and unipolar mood disorders. *Psychological Assessment, 13*(1), 140.
58. Krueger, R. F., Kotov, R., Watson, D., Forbes, M. K., Eaton, N. R., Ruggero, C. J., Simms, L. J., Widiger, T. A., Achenbach, T. M., Bach, B., et al. (2018). Progress in achieving quantitative classification of psychopathology. *World Psychiatry, 17*(3), 282–293.

59. Lachmar, E. M., Wittenborn, A. K., Bogen, K. W., & McCauley, H. L. (2017). # mydepressionlookslike: Examining public discourse about depression on twitter. *JMIR Mental Health, 4*(4), e43.
60. Lai, H. M. X., Cleary, M., Sitharthan, T., & Hunt, G. E. (2015). Prevalence of comorbid substance use, anxiety and mood disorders in epidemiological surveys, 1990–2014: A systematic review and meta-analysis. *Drug and Alcohol Dependence, 154*, 1–13.
61. Lin, L. Y., Sidani, J. E., Shensa, A., Radovic, A., Miller, E., Colditz, J. B., Hoffman, B. L., Giles, L. M., & Primack, B. A. (2016). Association between social media use and depression among us young adults. *Depression and Anxiety, 33*(4), 323–331.
62. Lorenzo-Luaces, L. (2015). Heterogeneity in the prognosis of major depression: From the common cold to a highly debilitating and recurrent illness. *Epidemiology and Psychiatric Sciences.*
63. Lorenzo-Luaces, L., Peipert, A., Romero, R. D. J., Rutter, L. A., & Rodriguez-Quintana, N. (2020). Personalized medicine and cognitive behavioral therapies for depression: Small effects, big problems, and bigger data. *International Journal of Cognitive Therapy*, 1–27.
64. Losada, D. E., Crestani, F., & Parapar, J. (2020). eRisk 2020: Self-harm and depression challenges. In *Advances in Information Retrieval: 42nd European Conference on IR Research, ECIR* (pp. 557–63), Lisbon, Portugal. Retrieved April 14–17, 2020.
65. Lou, Y., Lei, Y., Mei, Y., Paavo, L. H., & Li, H. (2019). Review of abnormal self-knowledge in major depressive disorder. *Frontiers in Psychiatry, 10*, 130.
66. Mao, X., & Shang, P. (2017). Transfer entropy between multivariate time series. *Communications in Nonlinear Science and Numerical Simulation, 47*, 338–347.
67. McCrae, N., Gettings, S., & Purssell, E. (2017). Social media and depressive symptoms in childhood and adolescence: A systematic review. *Adolescent Research Review, 2*(4), 315–330.
68. Mikal, J., Hurst, S., & Conway, M. (2016). Ethical issues in using twitter for population-level depression monitoring: A qualitative study. *BMC Medical Ethics, 17*(1), 22.
69. Mojtabai, R., Olfson, M., & Han, B. (2016). National trends in the prevalence and treatment of depression in adolescents and young adults. *Pediatrics, 138*(6), e20161878.
70. Murray, C. J., Vos, T., Lozano, R., Naghavi, M., Flaxman, A. D., Michaud, C., Ezzati, M., Shibuya, K., Salomon, J. A., Abdalla, S., et al. (2012). Disability-adjusted life years (dalys) for 291 diseases and injuries in 21 regions, 1990–2010: A systematic analysis for the global burden of disease study 2010. *The Lancet, 380*(9859), 2197–2223.
71. Nesi, J., & Prinstein, M. J. (2015). Using social media for social comparison and feedback-seeking: Gender and popularity moderate associations with depressive symptoms. *Journal of Abnormal Child Psychology, 43*(8), 1427–1438.
72. Nutt, D., Wilson, S., & Paterson, L. (2008). Sleep disorders as core symptoms of depression. *Dialogues in Clinical Neuroscience, 10*, 329–336.
73. Orben, A., & Przybylski, A. (2019). The association between adolescent well-being and digital technology use. *Nature Human Behaviour, 3*, 173–182.
74. Pavelko, R. L., & Myrick, J. G. (2015). That's so OCD: The effects of disease trivialization via social media on user perceptions and impression formation. *Computers in Human Behavior, 49*, 251–258.
75. Primack, B. A., Bisbey, M. A., Shensa, A., Bowman, N. D., Karim, S. A., Knight, J. M., & Sidani, J. E. (2018). The association between valence of social media experiences and depressive symptoms. *Depression and Anxiety, 5*, 784–794.
76. Primack, B. A., Shensa, A., Escobar-Viera, C. G., Barrett, E. L., Sidani, J. E., Colditz, J. B., & James, A. E. (2017). Use of multiple social media platforms and symptoms of depression and anxiety: A nationally-representative study among us young adults. *Computers in Human Behavior, 69*, 1–9.
77. Ranum, B. M., Wichstrøm, L., Pallesen, S., Falch-Madsen, J., Halse, M., & Steinsbekk, S. (2019). Association between objectively measured sleep duration and symptoms of psychiatric disorders in middle childhood. *JAMA Network Open, 2*(12), e1918281.
78. Reece, A. G., Reagan, A. J., Lix, K. L. M., Dodds, P. S., Danforth, C. M., & Langer, E. J. (2017). Forecasting the onset and course of mental illness with Twitter data. *Scientific Reports, 7*(1), 13006.

79. Regier, D. A., Rae, D. S., Narrow, W. E., Kaelber, C. T., & Schatzberg, A. F. (1998). Prevalence of anxiety disorders and their comorbidity with mood and addictive disorders. *The British Journal of Psychiatry, 173*(S34), 24–28.
80. Riehm, K. E., Feder, K. A., Tormohlen, K. N., Crum, R. M., Young, A. S., Green, K. M., Pacek, L. R., La Flair, L. N., & Mojtabai, R. (2019). Associations between time spent using social media and internalizing and externalizing problems among us youth. *JAMA Psychiatry, 76*(12), 1266–1273.
81. Rude, S., Gortner, E.-M., & Pennebaker, J. (2004). Language use of depressed and depression-vulnerable college students. *Cognition & Emotion, 18*(8), 1121–1133.
82. Rutter, L. A., Thompson, H., Riley, T. R., De Jesús-Romero, R., & Lorenzo-Luaces, L. (2021). Social media use, physical activity, and internalizing symptoms in adolescence: A cross-sectional analysis. *Journal of Medical Internet Research Pre-prints.*
83. Saha, K., Chan, L., De Barbaro, K., Abowd, G. D., & De Choudhury, M. (2017). Inferring mood instability on social media by leveraging ecological momentary assessments. *Proceedings of the ACM on Interactive, Mobile, Wearable and Ubiquitous Technologies, 1*(3), 1–27.
84. Scott, H., Biello, S. M., & Woods, H. C. (2019). Social media use and adolescent sleep patterns: cross-sectional findings from the UK millennium cohort study. *BMJ Open, 9*, 9.
85. Seabrook, E. M., Kern, M. L., & Rickard, N. S. (2016). Social networking sites, depression, and anxiety: A systematic review. *JMIR Mental Health, 3*(4), e50.
86. Smirnova, D., Cumming, P., Sloeva, E., Kuvshinova, N., Romanov, D., & Nosachev, G. (2018). Language patterns discriminate mild depression from normal sadness and euthymic state. *Frontiers in Psychiatry, 9*, 105.
87. Smith, A., & Brenner, J. (2012). Twitter use 2012. *Pew Internet & American Life Project, 4.*
88. Stieglitz, S., & Dang-Xuan, L. (2013). Emotions and information diffusion in social media-sentiment of microblogs and sharing behavior. *Journal of management information systems, 29*(4), 217–248.
89. Tackman, A. M., Sbarra, D. A., Carey, A. L., Donnellan, M. B., Horn, A. B., Holtzman, N. S., Edwards, T. S., Pennebaker, J. W., & Mehl, M. R. (2019). Depression, negative emotionality, and self-referential language: A multi-lab, multi-measure, and multi-language-task research synthesis. *Journal of Personality and Social Psychology, 116*, 817–834.
90. Ten Thij, M., Bathina, K., Rutter, L. A., Lorenzo-Luaces, L., van de Leemput, I. A., Scheffer, M., & Bollen, J. (2020). Depression alters the circadian pattern of online activity. *Scientific Reports, 10*(1), 1–10.
91. Tromholt, M., Lundby, M., Andsbjerg, K., & Wiking, M. (2015). The facebook experiment: Does social media affect the quality of our lives? Technical Report, The Happiness Institute.
92. Tsugawa, S., Kikuchi, Y., Kishino, F., Nakajima, K., Itoh, Y., & Ohsaki, H. (2015). Recognizing depression from twitter activity. In *Proceedings of the 33rd Annual ACM Conference on Human Factors in Computing Systems* (pp. 3187–3196).
93. Tsuno, N., Besset, A., & Ritchie, K. (2005). Sleep and Depression. *Journal of Clinical Psychiatry, 66*, 1254–1269.
94. Valdez, D., Ten Thij, M., Bathina, K., Rutter, L. A., & Bollen, J. (2020). Social media insights into us mental health during the covid-19 pandemic: Longitudinal analysis of twitter data. *Journal of Medical Internet Research, 22*(12), e21418.
95. van de Leemput, I. A., Wichers, M., Cramer, A. O. J., Borsboom, D., Tuerlinckx, F., Kuppens, P., van Nes, E. H., Viechtbauer, W., Giltay, E. J., Aggen, S. H., Derom, C., Jacobs, N., Kendler, K. S., van der Maas, H. L. J., Neale, M. C., Peeters, F., Thiery, E., Zachar, P., & Scheffer, M. (2014). Critical slowing down as early warning for the onset and termination of depression. *PNAS, 111*, 87–92.
96. Wang, P. S., Lane, M., Olfson, M., Pincus, H. A., Wells, K. B., & Kessler, R. C. (2005). Twelve-month use of mental health services in the united states: Results from the national comorbidity survey replication. *Archives of General Psychiatry, 62*(6), 629–640.
97. Wang, Z., Hale, S. A., Adelani, D., Grabowicz, P. A., Hartmann, T., Flöck, F., & Jurgens, D. (2019). Demographic Inference and Representative Population Estimates from Multilingual Social Media Data. In *Proceedings of the 2019 World Wide Web Conference* (pp. 2056—2067), WWW, ACM.

98. Whiteford, H. A., Degenhardt, L., Rehm, J., Baxter, A. J., Ferrari, A. J., Erskine, H. E., Charlson, F. J., Norman, R. E., Flaxman, A. D., Johns, N., et al. (2013). Global burden of disease attributable to mental and substance use disorders: Findings from the global burden of disease study 2010. *The lancet, 382*(9904), 1575–1586.
99. Wojcik, S., Bijral, A. S., Johnston, R., Ferres, J. M. L., King, G., Kennedy, R., Vespignani, A., & Lazer, D. (2021). Survey data and human computation for improved flu tracking. *Nature Communications, 21*, 194.
100. Wood, I. B., Varela, P. L., Bollen, J., Rocha, L. M., & Gonçalves-Sá, J. (2017). Human sexual cycles are driven by culture and match collective moods. *Scientific Reports* 7(1), 1–11.
101. Woody, M. L., & Gibb, B. E. (2015). Integrating nimh research domain criteria (rdoc) into depression research. *Current Opinion in Psychology, 4*, 6–12.
102. Yang, X., McEwen, R., Ong, L. R., & Zihayat, M. (2020). A big data analytics framework for detecting user-level depression from social networks. *International Journal of Information Management, 54*, 102141.
103. Zimmermann, J., Brockmeyer, T., Hunn, M., Schauenburg, H., & Wolf, M. (2017). First-person pronoun use in spoken language as a predictor of future depressive symptoms: Preliminary evidence from a clinical sample of depressed patients. *Clinical Psychology & Psychotherapy, 24*(2), 384–391.

Explainability of Depression Detection on Social Media: From Deep Learning Models to Psychological Interpretations and Multimodality

Ana-Sabina Uban, Berta Chulvi, and Paolo Rosso

Abstract Mental disorders are an important public health issue. Computational methods have the potential to aid with the detection of risky behaviors online, through extracting information from social media in order to detect users at risk of developing mental disorders. In this domain, understanding the behavior of the computational models used is crucial. Exploring the explainability of neural network models for mental disorder detection can make their decisions more reliable and easier to trust, and can help identify specific patterns in the data which are indicative of mental disorders. We present our attempts at predicting mental disorders in social media. We focus on depression detection and build models to detect users suffering from depression in multiple social media datasets, and additionally include experiments attempting to detect post-traumatic stress disorder (PTSD) users from similar social media data. We use approaches that combine deep learning with linguistic features including the emotions expressed and stylometry features. We continue with an in-depth analysis of the results and findings through different explainability techniques used to interpret the deep learning model's behavior, including feature analysis, hidden layer analysis and ablation studies. We include psychological interpretations for all our findings. We additionally collect a new multimodal dataset: *multiRedditDep*, consisting of social media data including texts and images posted by depressed users, and present our attempts at automatically discovering signs of depression in a multimodal setting. We include an in-depth analysis of the content of images posted by

A.-S. Uban (✉) · B. Chulvi · P. Rosso
PRHLT Research Center, Universitat Politècnica de València, València, Spain
e-mail: auban@fmi.unibuc.ro

B. Chulvi
e-mail: berta.chulvi@upv.es

P. Rosso
e-mail: prosso@dsic.upv.es

A.-S. Uban
Human Language Technologies Research Center, University of Bucharest, Bucharest, Romania

B. Chulvi
Social Psychology Department, Universitat de València, València, Spain

F. Crestani et al. (eds.), *Early Detection of Mental Health Disorders by Social Media Monitoring*, Studies in Computational Intelligence 1018,
https://doi.org/10.1007/978-3-031-04431-1_13

depressed users based on a semantic taxonomy of objects depicted in the images. We finalize by proposing directions for the future including approaches for depression detection based on conversational data.

1 Introduction

Mental health disorders are an important and pervasive public health issue. Depression in particular affects approximately 300 million people worldwide [79], and is a major factor leading to suicide, constituting the 3rd leading cause of death for individuals between 10 and 24 years old. Moreover, most of research in Public Health domain shows that depression is underdiagnosed and undertreated [2, 63], with more than half of the people suffering from depression not receiving any treatment [79]. For example, Williams et al. [78] show that the percentage of people suffering from depression who are not diagnosed in a given community is close to the percentage of people who are diagnosed. In the 2015 Washington Heights Community Survey [78], using a depression diagnostic test instrument, they found that 8% of the population had symptoms and a diagnosis of depression, while 7.6% had symptoms of depression but had not been diagnosed. People affected by mental disorders are often reluctant to approach a specialized clinician to seek help with treating the disorder [18] or do not have access to health insurance [78]. However, more and more frequently people turn to social media to discuss their issues and to seek emotional support. This opens up an important opportunity for automatic processing of social media data in order to identify changes in mental health status that may otherwise go undetected before they develop more serious health consequences. Recently, the COVID-19 pandemic is expected to exacerbate this problem, affecting mental health as well as physical health [32], through generating feelings of anxiety, depression and even trauma [33, 52, 62, 66, 67, 80].

The way mental disorders are manifested and can be recognized is primarily through everyday communication. It has been shown in previous computational studies that individuals suffering from mental disorders manifest changes in their language and their behavior, for example, greater negative emotions and high self-attentional focus [14, 27, 69].

Thus, there is a need for automation in detecting signs of mental disorders, motivated not only by the intractability of manually analyzing the high quantity of data produced daily on social media platforms, but also by the potential of artificial intelligence to exploit large quantities of data in order to uncover implicit markers of mental disorder risk, that can sometimes be difficult to notice even by the affected person. According to [27], automatic social media-based screening of depression reported so far in literature may reach prediction performance somewhere between unaided clinician assessment (diagnosis without the use of any screening questionnaire) and screening surveys. Data from social media, as a very rich and relatively easy to obtain type of data, as well as continuously growing source of real-time information, can thus be leveraged to gain many valuable insights into an individual's mental state and its evolution. Computational models capable of accurately predicting the development of mental disorders could then be integrated into applications with major social impact such as tools to alert users that they are at risk of developing a disorder or conversational bots. For clinicians, the computational analysis of mental health as seen in social media data could provide data for a deeper understanding of the mental disorders, and possibly lead to the development of improved instruments for diagnosis.

In practice, models based on neural networks are vastly successful for most NLP applications. Nevertheless, neural networks are notoriously difficult to interpret. Recently, there is increasing interest in the field of explainability methods in machine learning as well as in NLP [22], which aim for providing interpretations of the decisions of neural networks. If any system for mental disorder detection is to be developed as a tool to assist social media users, it is essential that its decision-making process is understandable in the name of transparency. Especially in the medical domain, using black-box systems can be dangerous for patients and is not a realistic solution [28, 85]. Recently, the need of explanatory systems is required by regulations like the General Data Protection Regulation (GDPR[1]) adopted by the European Union. Additionally, the behavior of powerful classifiers modelling complex patterns in the data has the potential to help uncover new manifestations of the disease, and thus assist clinicians in the diagnosis process.

Acknowledging the important social impact of modeling mental disorders with computational methods, and taking into account the knowledge provided by psychology in this area, we present several contributions to the automatic analysis of depression in social media, aiming to answer the following research questions:

RQ1. *To what extent can the analysis of deep learning models be used to interpret the signs of depression in social media data?*

RQ2. *Can computational models be used to describe the way individuals think, perceive, and remember information, from a psychological perspective, as a way to assist clinicians to improve the diagnosis of depression?*

RQ3. *What can multimodal data posted on social media, including text and images, reveal about patterns specific to users with depression?*

In this study, we bring several contributions to the research into the automatic detection of depression, at different levels.

We design models to automatically predict depression from social media data and study their performance; to this effect we explore the use of deep learning for detecting depression from text data, and compare various architectures, including hierarchical attention networks and transformers. We model our text data using a multi-aspect representation, through using features that reflect various complementary levels of the language, including content, style and emotions. Our choice of model architecture and features is motivated on one hand by its prediction power (through the capacity to model complex patterns in linguistic data at different levels), and on the other hand by its high interpretability (through the use of various features and through the hierarchical attention mechanisms). We attempt to interpret

[1] https://eur-lex.europa.eu/eli/reg/2016/679/oj.

the decisions of the developed classifiers, as well as perform feature analysis, in order to obtain a deeper understanding of mental disorder signs.

We finally move beyond the linguistic dimension and approach the problem of depression detection from a multimodal perspective: we introduce a new multimodal dataset of social media users suffering from depression, analyze patterns found in the data, as well as attempt to automatically detect users suffering from depression based on the texts and images they post online.

The chapter is structured as follows: Sect. 2 contains a summary of the existing literature on the computational analysis of depression and mental disorders more generally. In Sect. 3 we present the different social media datasets used in our experiments. In Sect. 4 we describe the models we used for the different experiments we performed, including deep learning models and features, and our solution for the temporal modelling of emotions. In Sect. 5 we attempt to explain the models' predictions through different techniques including feature analysis, hidden layer analysis and ablation experiments, and we include a discussion of our results and their relevance in the wider context of mental health research. In Sect. 6 we introduce the problem of multimodal mental disorder detection and present some preliminary results related to an enriched dataset for multimodal depression detection. Finally, in Sect. 7 we suggest directions for future development.

2 Previous Work

There is an extensive body of research related to automatic risk detection for mental disorders from social media data [8, 27]. The majority of research has focused on the study of depression [1, 15, 19, 83], but other mental illnesses have also been studied, including generalized anxiety disorder [65], schizophrenia [39], post-traumatic stress disorder [11, 12], risks of suicide [44], anorexia [37] and self-harm [37, 81]. Different social media platforms have been considered, such as Twitter [9], Facebook [14], or Reddit [36]. Research works related to depression have considered monitoring already diagnosed patients [83] as well as the detection of users showing signs of depression.

The vast majority of studies provide either quantitative analyses, or predictors built using simple machine learning models [14, 15]. Few studies have made use of more complex deep learning methods such as different types of convolutional (CNN) or recurrent neural networks (RNN) [59, 64, 75] or word embeddings [45, 70]. At the level of features, most previous works have used traditional bag of word n-grams [11], while some have also applied more domain-specific representations, such as hand-crafted lexicons [69], Linguistic Inquiry and Word Count (LIWC) [48] features [14], or latent semantic analysis (LSA) [56, 69].

Among the features used for mental disorder detection in previous literature, LIWC categories, emotions and personal pronouns usage have consistently been shown to be relevant for this task [10, 14, 15, 19, 27, 56, 58, 70]. Most studies using complex linguistic features such as emotion expression or psycholinguistic categories based on the LIWC lexicon are either simple quantitative analyses or use classical classifiers such as support vector machines or logistic regression [14, 15, 56]. To our knowledge, we are the first to use a deep neural architecture including multiple different types of linguistic features in order to model mental disorder manifestations in social media data. Recently, more studies have started employing deep learning for mental disorder detection, generally using word sequences as features [59, 64, 75]. Among these, few studies use hierarchical attention networks, showing their usefulness for this task. In [68], the authors use a hierarchical attention network for the prediction of several mental disorders from a dataset of psychiatric notes, with good results. One study on anorexia detection [41] uses a hierarchical attention network similar to ours (although using only word embedding features) obtaining the best results in the eRisk shared task on anorexia detection [37].

In the field of mental disorder detection, there are not many studies attempting to explain the behavior of models. We note one such example [3], where the authors analyze attention weights of a neural network trained for automatic anorexia detection. Nevertheless, recent studies have shown the limitations of using attention analysis for interpretability [61, 77].

Our choice of models is thus motivated not only by their modelling power and proven success in this area, but also by their higher interpretability through the use of attention, through the hierarchical structure and through the inclusion of multiple types of linguistic features.

There are few studies which jointly include in their models different aspects of the language for assessing risk of mental disorders [55, 64, 65]. In a previous study [73] on the early detection of self-harm tendencies, we propose using a hierarchical neural network composed of long short-term memory (LSTM) and CNN layers, trained on social media texts represented using content features, as well as emotion and style features. Few studies consider several disorders at the same time [82].

Quantitative analyses in existing research on mental disorders have found that people suffering from depression manifest changes in their language, such as a greater usage of negative emotions and high self-attentional focus [14], or increased first-person pronoun usage [70]. Other computational studies have used topic modeling or word usage analyses to discover increased prevalence of certain topics among depressed users, such as discussing medications or bodily issues such as lack of sleep, or expressing hopelessness or sadness [60, 69]. Nevertheless, correlation studies are limited in discovering more complex connections between features of the text and mental disorder risk.

Moreover, most computational studies model mental disorder symptoms as static phenomena, whereas the evolution of mental disorder markers, as well as their prevalence in texts posted by a user, is an important indicator of mental disorder risk. We mention one previous study [53] in which the authors attempt to classify time series representing the mood of social media users in order to predict occurrence of anorexia. The CLEF eRisk Lab [36–38] focuses on early detection of mental disorders, and in the associated shared task the participating systems are required to process a stream of social media posts ordered chronologically, and are evaluated taking into account the delay with which they manage to identify users who have been diagnosed with a disorder. However, annotations are provided at user-level and are static (do not identify the moment of the onset of the disorder), and few submissions attempt to model the input data as a reflection of a dynamical process.

From a practical perspective, models based on neural networks are vastly successful for most NLP applications, even though they have been only briefly explored in existing computational studies on mental disorders. Nevertheless, neural networks are notoriously difficult to interpret. Recently, there is increasing interest in the field of explainability in machine learning research, including NLP [22], which aims for providing interpretations of the decisions of neural networks. For a mental disorder detection tool whose aim is to assist social media users, it is essential that its behavior is understandable. Moreover, explaining the behavior of powerful classifiers modeling complex patterns in the data has the potential to help uncover signs of the disease that are difficult to observe otherwise, and thus assist clinicians in the diagnosis process.

In the field of mental disorder detection, there are not many studies attempting to explain the behavior of classifiers. We note one such example [3], where the authors analyze attention weights of a neural network to show that attention at the user level correlates with the importance of individual texts for classification performance in automatic anorexia detection.

Finally, research on mental disorders from a computational perspective has been generally disconnected from mental health research in psychology, with virtually no computational studies providing in-depth interpretations of their findings from a psychological perspective.

Much less is known about the use of other kinds of information in automatic mental disorder detection, such as the images and audio data shared online, with only a few studies taking a multimodal approach. Of these, most use video and image data collected from interviews of the person being assessed [57], which is more costly to collect, and assumes a prior suspicion of mental health problems, excluding the possibility of early detection. Few exceptions have considered multi-modal data shared online by the user, such as [65] who proposed a multimodal depressive dictionary learning model to detect depressed users on Twitter, by considering users' avatars in their home pages. In a notable study, [54] attempt to detect suicidal ideation using texts and images posted by users on social media, and show that image data can help improve prediction performance.

3 Datasets

In order to perform our different experiments based on textual social media data, we rely on different datasets that are publicly available and annotated with labels indicating whether the user suffers from depression. We use two different Twitter datasets annotated for depression: the first is a dataset introduced as part of the CLPsych workshop [12] and shared task, and the second was introduced in [64]. The CLPsych dataset also contains labels corresponding to users suffering from PTSD, so for a comparison with the results obtained on depression labels, we also include this PTSD dataset in our experiments. Finally, we perform the same experiments on the Reddit dataset annotated for depression proposed as part of the eRisk shared task, and compare results across the different datasets. All datasets follow a similar annotation methodology based on self-stated diagnoses, as described in [11].

CLPsych Twitter dataset on depression and PTSD. CLPsych (Computational Linguistics and Clinical Psychology) is a workshop and shared task organized each year around a different topic concerning computational approaches for mental health. In 2015 [12], the shared task challenged participants to detect Twitter users suffering from depression and PTSD. Labelling of the data was done semi-automatically, through an initial selection based on self-stated diagnoses, followed by human curation. For each user, their most recent public tweets were included in the dataset.

Twitter dataset on depression. To complement the CLPsych dataset, we include a second Twitter dataset labelled for depression. This dataset was collected and introduced in [64], following a similar methodology, based on self-stated diagnoses. Tweets published within a month of the diagnosis statement were included for each positive user. This short time frame is an exception compared to the other datasets considered. Control users were selected among Twitter users never having posted any tweet containing the character string "depress".

eRisk Reddit dataset on depression. In our experiments we also use the datasets introduced as part of the eRisk shared task annotated for depression [36]. The data is collected from Reddit posts and comments selected from specific relevant subreddits. Users suffering from a depression are annotated by automatically detecting self-stated diagnoses, followed by a manual curation step (not involving clinical experts). The control cases are selected from participants in the same subreddits (having similar interests), thus making sure the gap between control cases and diagnosed users is not trivially detectable. Moreover, a long history of posts are collected for the users included in the dataset, up to years prior to the diagnosis.

In all the datasets, the posts containing the mention of a diagnosis were excluded. Table 1 contains statistics describing all datasets considered.

Table 1 Datasets statistics

Dataset	Users	Positive%	Posts	Words
CLPsych PTSD	1078	72.6%	2,541,214	~19 M
CLPsych depression	822	64.1%	1,919,353	~26 M
Twitter depression [64]	519	50.2%	52,080	~500 K
eRisk depression	1304	16.4%	811,586	25 M

4 Models

In this section we present the various models used for our experiments in detection of depression, as well as methods used as part of the effort to provide interpretability of depression detection on social media.

We start by presenting the various linguistic features used. We then describe the deep learning architectures used for our classification experiments. In previous literature on automatic prediction of mental disorders, when neural networks are employed their architectures are relatively simple [6, 65]. We propose exploring more sophisticated deep architectures, including RNNs and CNNs, as well as hierarchical attention networks and transformers. Each of the architectures used are briefly described below, starting with the main deep learning model used, and continuing with various baseline models.

4.1 Features

As previous studies have shown, mental disorders are manifested in language at different levels: topics discussed, emotions conveyed, as well as the author's style. In psychology, the notion of "cognitive style" has been used to explain that it is possible to identify some dimensions in a person's reasoning style that reflects how this individual organizes and structures information. Some research [84] has pointed out that thinking styles are associated with emotions and also that thinking styles had predictive power for emotions beyond age.

At a computational level, we aim to build multi-dimensional representations of the texts in our datasets to account for the different levels of the language where markers of depression can manifest. We extract various features from the texts, which will be used as input to our subsequent text classification models, as well as in our other analyses in the following sections.

Content features. We include a general representation of text content by transforming each text into word sequences. The obtained sequences will constitute the main input of the recurrent and convolutional layers of our neural networks. Preprocessing of texts includes lowercasing and tokenizing, and removing punctuation and numbers. Stopwords are not excluded. The most frequent 20,000 words in all datasets were selected to form a common vocabulary. When passed as input to the neural networks, words within a sequence were encoded as embeddings of dimension 300. In order to initialize the weights of the embedding layers, we started from pre-trained GloVe [49] embeddings.

Style features. We aim at representing the stylistic level of texts through including stopwords and pronoun features. The usage pattern of stopwords is known to be reflective of an author's style, at an unconscious level [30]. In the study of mental disorders, the increased use of pronouns, especially first person pronouns, has been shown to correlate with mental disorder risk [69]. We include two separate stylistic features: firstly, we extract from each text a numerical vector representing stopword frequencies as bag-of-words, normalized by text lengths. We complement these with other stylistic features extracted from the LIWC lexicon, including syntactic features such as usage of pronouns or other parts of speech, as described below.

LIWC features. The LIWC lexicon [48] has been widely used in computational linguistics as well as in some clinical studies for analysing how suffering from mental disorders manifests in an author's writings. LIWC is a lexicon mapping words of the English vocabulary to lexico-syntactic features of different kinds, with high quality associations curated by experts in psycholinguistics having the potential to capture different levels of language: including style (through syntactic categories such as "pronoun", "verb", "future", "past" etc.), emotions (through affect categories such as "sad", "anxiety", "affect", "positive emotion", "negative emotion" etc.) and topics (through content-oriented categories such as words referring to cognitive or analytical processes (e.g. "cogmech", "analytical", "because", "effect"), or to topics such as "money", "health" or "religion"). We use LIWC 2007 [47] and include all 64 categories in the lexicon in our classification experiments, which we represent as a numerical vector for each input example by computing for each category the ratio of words in a text that are related to the category, according to the lexicon (obtaining one vector for each input text, with elements of each vector representing the ratio corresponding to one category in the lexicon).

Emotions and sentiment. We dedicate a few features to representing emotional content in our texts, since the emotional state of a user is known to be highly correlated with their mental health. Several of the LIWC categories aim to capture sentiment polarity and emotion content, from more general ones, such as *negative emotion*, *positive emotion*, *affective processes*, to more specific emotions, such as *sadness* and *anxiety*. We additionally include a second lexicon, the NRC emotion lexicon [40], which is dedicated exclusively to emotion representation, containing eight categories corresponding to a more fine-grained selection of emotions, based on Plutchik's [50] eight basic emotions: *anger*, *anticipation*, *disgust*, *fear*, *joy*, *sadness*, *surprise*, *trust*, along with two additional categories corresponding to *negative* and *positive* sentiment, respectively. We represent NRC features similarly to LIWC features, as numerical vectors of ratios for each text, and include all NRC features in the classification experiments.

4.2 Hierarchical Attention Networks

Hierarchical attention networks for text classification were introduced in [81] where they were used for review classification, by representing a text as a hierarchical structure. We propose that social media data in our setup are very well suited to such a hierarchical representation; in our case the hierarchy consists of user post histories, which are composed of social media posts, composed of word sequences. Especially since the evolution of the mental state of a user is in itself a relevant indicator for the development of a disorder [41, 53], user-level representations are expected to be natural and useful for modeling this problem. This structure will also allow us to include hierarchical attention mechanisms, to weigh separately words within a post and posts within a user's history, which is useful especially since the evolution of the mental state of a user can be in itself a relevant indicator for the development of a disorder [41, 53].

The hierarchical network is composed of two components: a *post-level encoder*, which produces a representation of a post, and a *user-level encoder*, which generates a representation of a user's post history.

Post-level encoder. For encoding the word sequence at post-level, we experiment with two different neural architectures: LSTM with attention, and CNN.

We denote the layer encoding the word sequences (LSTM/CNN) as $\overrightarrow{f}$, the input word sequence as $w_{it}, t \in [1, T], i \in [1, C]$, where T is the number of words in a post, C is the number of a user's posts in an input chunk, and H is the dimensionality of the post-level encoder (number LSTM units or CNN feature maps). The embedding matrix is denoted as W_e, E is the dimensionality of the embedding space, and V is the size of the vocabulary.

In the LSTM setup, the post-level attention weights α_{it} are applied to the resulted hidden layer, obtaining the final representation (s_i) of the input word sequence:

$$\begin{aligned} x_{it} &= W_e w_{it}, t \in [1, T], i \in [1, C], w_{it} \in \mathbb{N}^V, W_e \in \mathbb{R}^{E\times V}, x_{it} \in \mathbb{R}^E \\ \overrightarrow{h}_{it} &= \overrightarrow{f}(x_{it}), \overrightarrow{h}_{it} \in \mathbb{R}^{T\times H} \\ v_{it} &= tanh(W_w h_{it} + b_w), W_w \in \mathbb{R}^{H\times 1}, b_w \in \mathbb{R}^H, v_{it} \in \mathbb{R}^T \\ \alpha_{it} &= \frac{exp(v_{it}^T v_w)}{\sum_t exp(v_{it}^T v_w)}, v_w \in \mathbb{R}^H, \alpha_{it} \in \mathbb{R}^{T\times H} \\ s_i &= \sum_t \alpha_{it} h_{it}, s_i \in \mathbb{R}^H \end{aligned} \tag{1}$$

The bag-of-stopwords feature f_{it} and the lexicon features l_{it} for each post are passed to dense layers (with parameters W_f, b_f and W_l, b_l respectively, where F denotes the number of stopwords considered, L denotes the number of lexicon features considered, and D denotes the number of units in the dense layers used to encode the bag-of-stopwords and lexicon features), and concatenated to the word sequence representations to obtain the post encoding p_i:

$$\begin{aligned} hf_{it} &= W_f f_i + b_f, hf_{it} \in \mathbb{R}^D, f_i \in \mathbb{R}^F, W_f \in \mathbb{R}^{F\times D}, b_f \in \mathbb{R}^D \\ hl_{it} &= W_l l_i + b_l, hl_{it} \in \mathbb{R}^D, l_i \in \mathbb{R}^L, W_l \in \mathbb{R}^{L\times D}, b_l \in \mathbb{R}^D \\ p_i &= s_i \oplus hf_{it} \oplus hl_{it}, p_i \in \mathbb{R}^{H+2D} \end{aligned} \tag{2}$$

For the CNN post-level encoder, the pooling layer output is used to encode the word sequences, and further concatenated with the other features' representations, to obtain the post-level encoding.

User-level encoder. Each of the posts in the input datapoint is encoded with the post-level encoder, and then they are stacked to form the bi-dimensional representation s_i, which is then concatenated with encodings of the other features, and passed to the user-level encoder, modeled as an LSTM with attention. User-level attention

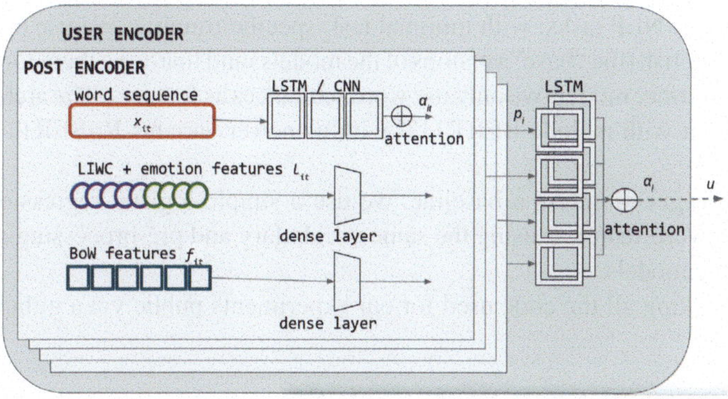

Fig. 1 Hierarchical attention network architecture

weights are denoted by α_i and the final user representation is u, where U is the number of LSTM units in the user-level encoder. The output of the user encoder is connected to the final output layer which generates the prediction.

$$\begin{aligned} h_i &= \overrightarrow{LSTM}(p_i), h_i \in \mathbb{R}^{C \times U} \\ v_i &= tanh(W_p h_i + b_p), W_p \in \mathbb{R}^{U \times 1}, b_p \in \mathbb{R}^U, v_i \in \mathbb{R}^L \\ \alpha_i &= \frac{exp(v_i^T v_p)}{\sum_i exp(v_i^T v_p)}, v_p \in \mathbb{R}^U, \alpha_i \in \mathbb{R}^{C \times U} \\ u &= \sum_i \alpha_i h_i, i \in [1, C], u \in \mathbb{R}^U \end{aligned} \tag{3}$$

A depiction of the hierarchical architecture is shown in Fig. 1.

In all architectures we use batch normalization and L_2 regularization. Binary cross-entropy is used as a loss function. For training our models we use the Adam optimizer. Other hyperparameters are chosen through hyperparameter tuning on the validation set.

4.3 Baseline Classifiers

BiLSTM with attention. We use a traditional bidirectional LSTM network. Word sequences (truncated/padded at 512 words), with words encoded as embeddings, are passed as input to the BiLSTM layer, which is then fed to an attention layer. The bag-of-stopwords features are passed through a dense layer; and the remaining extracted features (including pronouns, emotions and LIWC categories usage) are concatenated into one vector. The output of the BiLSTM is concatenated along with the other features and the final representation passed through an output layer that generates the final prediction.

Transformers. We experiment with state-of-the-art language models based on transformer architectures, which have been shown to obtain high performances on a wide range of NLP tasks, with minimal task-specific training. We use pre-trained models for English (the "base" versions of the models) and fine-tune them for our task. For the transformer models we only use word sequences as features. The architectures we experiment with include BERT [17] with its newer variants RoBERTa [35] and AlBERT [31].

Logistic regression. As a baseline, we use a simple logistic regression model with bag-of-word features, using the same vocabulary and pre-processing as for the deep learning models.

We are making all the code used for our experiments public via a github repository.[2]

4.4 Classification Results

We start by performing classification experiments on the datasets described above. We model the problem as a binary classification task, training a deep learning model separately for each of the disorders and datasets considered.

We follow the typical machine learning workflow, and split each of the datasets into training, validation and test subsets. For the datasets released as part of a shared task, we maintain the original train/test split provided by the shared task organizers, to ensure consistency and comparability with previous results, even though the test sets are sometimes larger than the training sets. For the [64] Twitter dataset, we use a random 70/30 split for generating the training and test set. We make sure to split train and test sets at the user level: no texts in the training set have common authors with texts in the test set. In this way we ensure models are not learning any user-specific artifacts, and instead are modeling markers of the disorders themselves.

We show results for the classification experiments on all datasets and using the different classifiers in Table 2. We include results of experiments on the different depression datasets, as well as results for the PTSD dataset. We use F1-score and area under the ROC curve (AUC) as our metrics.

We find that our proposed HAN model with LSTM-based user encoder and post encoder and linguistic features generally outperforms the baseline models considered, and we focus on this model in our following analyses related to explainability.

5 Explainability of Depression Detection

In order to explore more in depth the problem of depression detection from social media data, we attempt to explain predictions of the models previously discussed and interpret our findings.

---

[2] https://github.com/ananana/mental-disorders/.

Table 2 F1 and AUC scores for all datasets and models

Model	PTSD CLPsych		Depr. CLPsych		Depr. Shen et al.		Depr. eRisk	
	F1	AUC	F1	AUC	F1	AUC	F1	AUC
BiLSTM seq	0.55	0.78	0.56	0.72	0.75	0.83	0.40	0.82
LSTM hierarch (HAN)	0.57	**0.70**	0.53	**0.73**	0.77	0.81	0.45	**0.83**
CNN + LSTM hierarch	0.61	0.77	0.56	0.72	0.88	**0.94**	0.35	0.80
RoBERTa	0.40	0.57	0.54	0.65	0.84	0.84	0.45	0.71
AlBERT	0.36	0.53	0.41	0.59	0.84	0.85	0.20	0.61
LogReg	0.49	0.69	0.55	0.72	0.71	0.81	0.36	0.76

We intend to explore the explainability of depression prediction models from different perspectives. In the following subsections we present different analyses meant to uncover insights into how the model arrives at its predictions [71, 72]. We first provide several feature-focused analyses of misclassifications, using the lexicon-based features (emotions and LIWC categories) in order to identify particular interpretable patterns among users which the model cannot classify correctly. We then look at the abstract internal representations of the data in the layers of the network. Finally, we perform some ablation studies in order to understand the contribution of each linguistic feature in predicting users with depression.

5.1 Error Analysis

We continue by analysing the behavior of the deep learning model (HAN), as a way to gain trust in the model, and also as a way to uncover patterns in the data that the trained model is able to capture.

In the case of models for detecting mental disorders, classification errors can have serious negative impacts on the users' well-being, if such as system would be deployed into a tool for assisting social media users. False negative predictions in particular can lead to missing cases of people with high risk of suffering from mental health disorders, and, left undetected, the disorders might further develop. We attempt to understand what causes misclassifications by comparing correctly versus incorrectly classified examples in terms of different features, including words, NRC emotions and LIWC categories. We thus compare the different types of misclassified and correctly classified examples, across the four groups: true positives (TP), false positives (FP), true negatives (TN) and false negatives (FN).

Vocabulary analysis. In Table 3 we show the vocabulary words which are most distinctive for misclassifications for each disorder, separately for FP and FN cases. We select these words by applying the chi^2 test to extract the most discriminative

Table 3 Top words (χ^2 test) that discriminate between incorrect and correct predictions

Experiment	False negatives	False positives
PTSD (CLPsych)	mpoints, earning, reward, thank, following, you, plz, ff, ptsd, cptsd	I, besties, gameinsights, ipadgames, thatsheartgiveaway, vietnam, coins, collected
Depression (CLPsych)	earning, mpoints, video, rewards, patientchat, thank, besties, you, gameinsight, ipadgames	dundee, I, my, me, lol, the, vitamin, win, of, fuck, mobile, syria, love
Depression (Shen et al.)	I, rt, to, you, the, and, my, is, of, me	rt, prayer, bestmusicvideo, iheartawards, zain, pillowtalk, location, hiphopnews, ghetsis, via
Depression (eRisk)	clemson, game, lemieux, team, uio, play, song, pka, you, season	I, my, her, she, me, is, was, the, are, trump, of

features between FN and FP cases on one hand, and FP and TP cases on the other hand, and report the words with the highest scores. In some cases, these keywords can shed some light on what characterizes the sub-clusters of FN users identified with the user embedding representations. For depression, the FN group (both for the CLPsych and the eRisk datasets) appear to be distinguished by discussing topics related to games. Another interesting finding is the occurrence of "Vietnam" for FP in PTSD: the model learns to excessively associate PTSD sufferers with the topic of Vietnam, possibly showing a topic bias in the dataset.

Feature biases. In order to understand the effect of lexicon features on the model's prediction, we measure for each of the lexicon categories their comparative prevalence in misclassified and correctly classified examples, separately for the control cases and users suffering from a disorder. We identify four categories of features, based on their prevalence in FP, FN, TP and TN examples comparatively. We compare the prevalence of each feature in each of the four groups using the same measures used for feature extraction in the classification experiments: for each lexicon feature, we compare average usage of words pertaining to that category across users in that group, normalized by text length.

Feature bias type 1 (FN<TP; FP>TN): features which occur to a lower degree in misclassified positive examples than in correctly classified positive examples; while for control examples they occur more in incorrectly classified ones than in correctly classified ones. The model likely relies too much on the connection between their high prevalence and high risk scores.

Feature bias type 2 (FN<TP; FP<TN): generally under-represented features in misclassified examples—if they are not well represented, the model tends to make mistakes.

Feature bias type 3 (FN>TP; FP>TN): features which are generally over-represented in misclassified examples—when they are highly prevalent, the model is less accurate.
Feature bias type 4 (FN>TP; FP<TN): features which are over-represented in FN cases and under-represented in FP cases. The model likely relies too much on their low prevalence to emit high risk scores.

For each dataset, we identify misclassifications grouped into the two categories (FP and FN), and find those features for which there is a statistically significant difference of the average value between the misclassified group and the correctly classified group, using Student's T-test. We do this separately for emotions (see Fig. 2) and for LIWC features (shown in Table 4), for a more strict selection we choose only categories with p-values below 10^{-6}.

Cognitive style is a concept used in cognitive psychology to describe the way individuals think, perceive, and remember information [25]. Research in psychology suggests that some cognitive styles are more prevalent in some patients suffering from depression. In our error analysis we find that some errors have a relation with the under-representation of these cognitive styles. Some of the features that are relevant to explain the misclassifications of the model (see Table 4) are related to cognitive styles.

For instance, for depression we find that in the case of FN, features as *cogmech*, that refers to cognitive processes (causation, discrepancy, tentative, certainty, etc.), occurs to a lower degree in FP examples. We can conclude that the model is confused

Table 4 LIWC features with highest differences for misclassified groups ($p < 10^{-6}$)

Experiment	Feat. bias 1	Feat. bias 2	Feat. bias 3	Feat. bias 4
PTSD (CLPsych)	money, number, article work, achieve, preps	–	–	cogmech, fear, assent, pronoun, bio, I, leisure, swear, affect, feel
Depression (CLPsych)	hear, conj, ipron, present, article, auxverb, certain, negative, verb,	–	–	–
Depression (Shen et al.)	–	–	–	ppron, adverb, bio, funct, verb past, funct, article, health, present
Depression (eRisk)	ppron, quant, auxverb, verb, present, you, pronoun, excl, I, conj, adverb, future, cogmech, funct	–	ipron	–

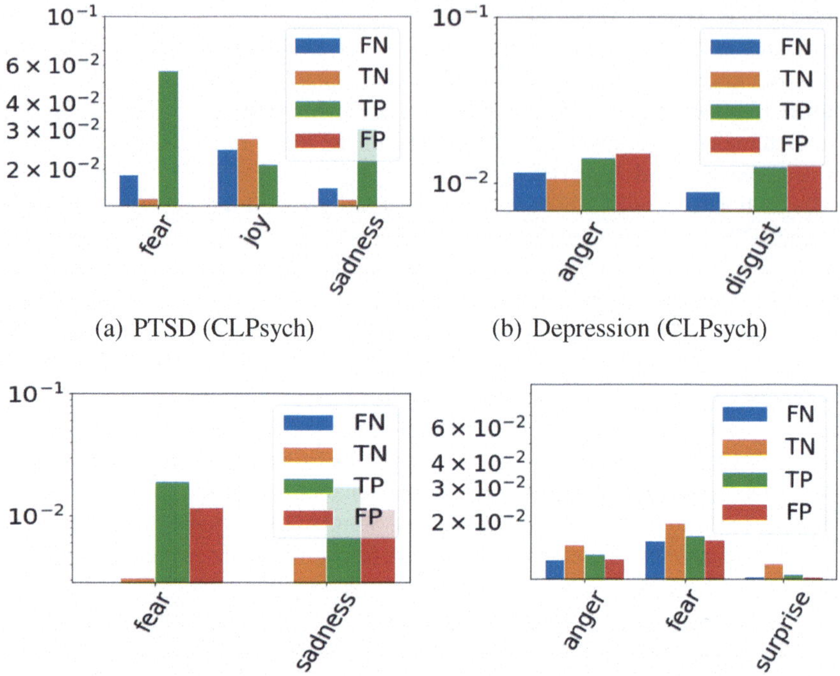

(a) PTSD (CLPsych) (b) Depression (CLPsych)

(c) Depression (Shen et al.) (d) Depression (eRisk)

Fig. 2 Mean values for emotions that are significantly different for misclassif. ($p<0.05$)

when the depressed users do not express themselves in the typical pattern that refers some way of reasoning about causes, consequences, etc.

There is an interesting result related to the use of the *future* feature of LIWC. We found that in depression (eRisk corpus), if this feature that speaks about *future* occurs to a lower degree, the model tends to make more mistakes in the classification of positive examples. We can infer that the model is able to detect the mental health disorders when people speak about what life is preparing for them, but has more difficulties when users that suffer from these mental health disorders do not speak about plans and focus more on the moment.

Considering the analysis of emotions (see Fig. 2) we found also that the unclear expression of some emotions leads the model to make mistakes and that these emotions are just the ones that are relevant for each mental health disorder. For instance, we see that the model makes more mistakes when people that suffer from depression do not express anger and fear.

5.2 Hidden Layer Analysis

We continue with an experiment that goes deeper into analysing the internal representations of the network. We can regard the final layer of the trained network as the most compressed representation of the input examples, which is, in terms of our trained model, the optimal representation for distinguishing between the control cases and those suffering from a mental disorder. Thus, the final layer (the output of the 32-dimensional user-level LSTM) can be interpreted as a 32-dimensional embedding for the input points, corresponding to the users to be classified.

We analyze the output of the *user embedding* layer by reducing it to 2 dimensions using principal component analysis (PCA) and visualizing it in 2D space with a kernel density estimate (KDE) plot to show the distribution of scores across the 2 dimensions, separately for each dataset (Fig. 3). We make sure to train the PCA model on a balanced set of positive and control users, then we extract 2D representations for all users in the test set. By looking at these representations, we can gain insight into the separability of the classes, from the perspective of the trained model, and better understand where it encounters difficulties in separating between the datapoints belonging to different classes.

We notice that, in accordance with the classification performance reported previously, the highest separation in user embedding space seems to be achieved for the Twitter (Shen et al.) dataset, while depressed users in the other datasets (CLPsych and eRisk) show higher overlap with control cases. Moreover, we notice an interesting pattern of multiple clusters of positive users, while control cases' representations seem to be more compact.

5.3 Ablation Experiments

In order to understand the relative importance of the features used to represent the text data, corresponding to the different levels of the language, we train and evaluate our classifier separately excluding each of the features, through ablation experiments. Through these experiments, we can gain insight into the relative importance of each feature for predicting mental disorders, and further, into the levels of the language (topics, style, emotions, etc.) where mental disorder symptoms are manifested.

Results of the ablation studies are shown in Table 5, with performance measured in terms of F1-score and AUC. We find that, for most datasets, using all features leads to the best prediction performance, suggesting that each of the features we include has a relevant contribution to detecting signs of mental disorders, including the lexicon features and the bag-of-stopwords feature, which are rarely used in deep learning models for mental disorder detection in previous research. We find that word sequences have the biggest impact on performance.

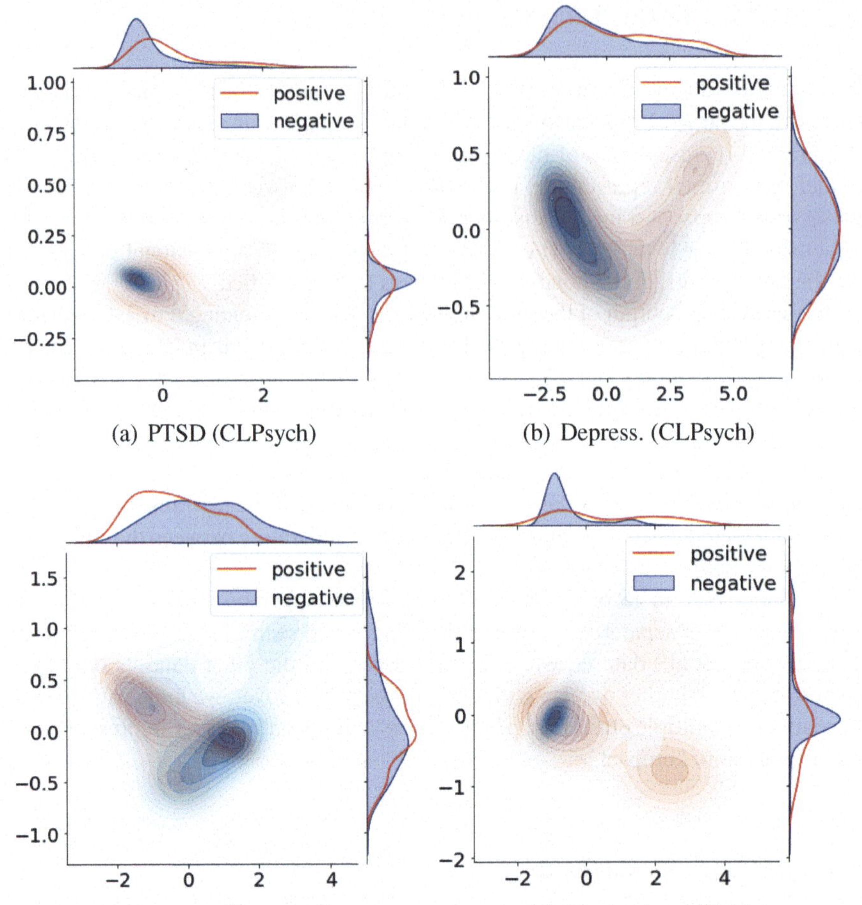

(a) PTSD (CLPsych) (b) Depress. (CLPsych)

(c) Depress. (Shen et al.) (d) Depression (eRisk)

Fig. 3 User embeddings for classification of users with a disorder versus control cases

Table 5 F1 and AUC scores for ablation experiments, using the HAN model

Model	PTSD CLPsych		Depr. CLPsych		Depr. eRisk	
	F1	AUC	F1	AUC	F1	AUC
All-word seq	0.50	0.53	0.51	0.68	0.34	0.79
All-stopwords	0.57	0.71	0.53	0.69	0.50	0.81
All-lexicon feat	0.60	**0.72**	0.50	0.65	0.43	**0.84**
All features	0.57	0.70	0.53	**0.73**	0.45	0.83

6 Multimodal Depression Detection

Multimodality has rarely been explored in mental health analysis from social media, compared to text-based methods. However, text on social media is only a small part of the means of expression employed by users. It can be easily assumed that, for example, the images that the users share can be relevant for containing some signals related to their mental health, especially at the implicit level. Considering that in order to achieve early risk detection (detecting a mental health problem even before a user is aware of it) needs to be heavily based on implicit markers, analysing additional media such as images can be very valuable for capturing signals of a developing mental disorder, and even for uncovering specific interests and behaviors of users online as their mental health deteriorates, which are possibly unknown to clinicians.

We introduce *multiRedditDep*, a new multimodal dataset of social media users suffering from depression. For this purpose, we mine the Reddit platform, and to our knowledge we are the first to build a multimodal dataset for mental disorders sourced from Reddit.

As opposed to Twitter, messages on Reddit tend to be longer, which can constitute an advantage when training a model to detect depression based on the texts posted.

Moreover, previous datasets on mental disorders collected from social media rely on profile or avatar images [26, 34]. In our dataset, we collect instead images *posted* by the users. We claim this brings a separate challenge: the problem of depression detection then does not consist of detecting depression from an image depicting the user themselves, but rather needs to be based on the topics and content which the user is interested in and posts online. This is, in our opinion, a more difficult problem, especially due to the diversity of image content posted online and the difficulty to interpret the message intended by the user when posting an image. Moreover, analysing the images allows a comparison of the content of the image and the content of the text associated with the image. The relationship between these can be an independent indicator of the intentions and state of mind of the user (for example a message where the text and the image associated to it are contradictory could indicate sarcasm).

6.1 *multiRedditDep Dataset Collection*

We introduce a new multimodal social media dataset for depression detection: *multiRedditDep*.

We collect data from Reddit and annotate it semi-automatically, following the approach of previous studies introducing social media datasets annotated for depression [12, 36, 64]. Specifically, we label users based on self-stated diagnoses, including expressions such as "I was diagnosed with depression" and "I have been diagnosed with depression". We select the Reddit users where we find these phrases: they will constitute the positive group. Additionally, we select control users by selecting

Table 6 Multimodal *multiRedditDep* dataset statistics

	Images	Unique users
Depressed	48,121	1,419
Control	72,855	2,344

random users who have posted at least once on the */r/depression* forum, but that have not mentioned any diagnosis of depression in the recorded history of their activity. We choose to select users active in the depression forum rather than randomly selecting users active on any subreddit, since this makes the problem of distinguishing between the two groups less trivial, and encourages any trained model to learn more implicit markers of depression.

We then perform a post-processing step where we eliminate from the collected users the ones with suspicious authenticity, according to a manual inspection: we remove bots and a few users with very many posts, such that they could not be written by a single person (for example some official accounts of politicians). After building the two groups of users, we collect images posted by these users on any subreddit, as well as the titles associated with them.

The statistics of the obtained dataset are shown in Table 6.

6.2 *Classification Experiments*

We exploit this dataset to train multimodal classifiers for early depression prediction. Including visual information could help improve the detection performance; moreover, using explainability techniques on the trained multimodal models could uncover additional insights on the manifestations of depression in social media.

We experiment with simple feed-forward neural network architectures and different features, including visual and text features, and compare the performance of the classifier in the different settings. We measure accuracy and area under the ROC curve (AUC).

6.2.1 Feature Extraction

ImageNet image labels. In order to extract image features, we rely on the pretrained VGG-16 model in order to label images with labels in the ImageNet taxonomy [16], and use it in order to extract textual information regarding the contents of the image. For each image, the model provides 5 tags which refer to the objects present in the image. The most frequent tag for all images regardless of label is "web_site", which, after some manual inspection, we assume to be referring to screenshots. Since this

Table 7 Classification results on the multiRedditDep multimodal dataset

Model	Accuracy	AUC
Text only (word2vec embeddings)	62.73	65.29
Images only (word2vec embeddings)	61.88	61.63
Text and images (word2vec embeddings)	65.40	68.69
Text only (BERT+word2vec embeddings)	66.24	69.20
Text and images (BERT+word2vec embeddings)	**66.39**	**69.37**

is not an informative enough description of the contents of the image, we treat these images separately.

Text extraction from images. The previous step reveals a majority of images in our dataset are screenshots. In order to obtain some more semantic information about the content of these images, we set aside all images with this tag. Upon some manual inspection, we observe that the screenshots tagged with "web_site" are usually images of the user's screen containing some text posted on a social media platform. We then decide to treat these images separately, and extract the text in the screenshots using the OCR engine Tesseract.[3]

Word embeddings. After having transformed image data into a textual format through generating tags or extracting the text present in the image, we encode the textual information from the image and from the image's title using semantic representations. The first type of representations used are word embeddings, and we experiment with Word2Vec and FastText. We encode both the image title and the image tags using averages of word embedding vectors for each word in the title or tag set respectively.

Transformer-based sentence embeddings. We also experiment with more sophisticated representations based on pre-trained transformers. We use BERT [17] based sentence embeddings to represent the titles of the posts as one of the features. In the case of the set of image tags, we do not use this representation, since they are isolated words (as opposed to full sentences) which would not benefit from being encoded with contextual embeddings.

We split the dataset into train/validation/test subsets, using 70% of the data for training, 10% for validation, and 20% for test. We report the results on the test set in Table 7.

6.2.2 Classification Results

We notice that the best performing models use both textual and image features: the models based solely on textual features do not perform as well as the models which also include image features, showing that images contribute with additional relevant information for helping distinguished between depressed and control users, espe-

[3] https://github.com/tesseract-ocr/tesseract.

cially in the case of the models using only word2vec features. The BERT based models outperform the word embedding models, which is not surprising, given the superior capacity of the transformer models. We also notice that using only image features cannot outperform the models using only textual features, suggesting stronger image features (beyond word2vec embeddings based on image tags) could be promising for improving results in the future.

6.3 *Image Analyses and Psychological Interpretations*

We continue by performing some statistics on the extracted features, in order to better understand the type of content that depressed users post in comparison with the control group.

We first try to assess the similarity between the images posted and the texts associated to them. To this end, we compute the average word embedding similarity (based on the cosine distance) between the tags extracted from the images, and their titles, on average for all 5 tags, and separately for each tag. The distributions of the obtained similarities are shown in Figs. 4 and 5. We notice a low average similarity score of around or below 0.1 in both cases, and do not notice a notable difference between the distributions for each tag. This could mean that, in general, the text associated with the images does not match their content directly, nor in a metaphoric or ironic sense.

We further take a deeper look at the image labels in order to understand the differences in content posted by depressed users as compared to control cases. We extract the image labels which show significant differences between the depressed and con-

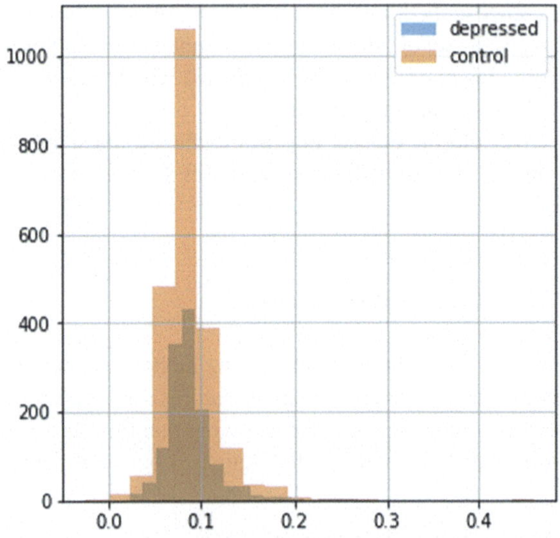

Fig. 4 Image label—image title similarities, on average for all tags

Fig. 5 Image label—image title similarities, for each of the extracted tags

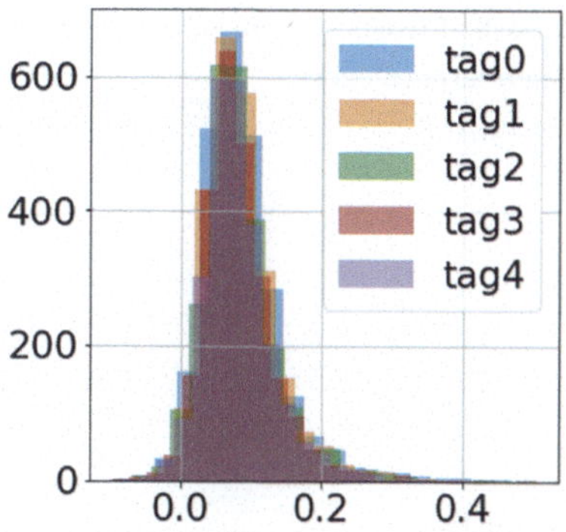

trol group as such: for each label type, we compute the proportion of images which are classified by the VGG feature extractor as pertaining to that label (considering only the first label, with the highest probability). We exclude labels which, after a manual inspection, we consider to correspond to screenshots (including 'web_site', 'menu', 'book_jacket', 'envelope', 'comic_book', 'crossword_puzzle', 'monitor', 'screen'). We then compare the distribution of obtained label proportions for each user between the depressed and the control group, and test its significance using the Mann-Whitney U test (p-value < 0.05). We find that 222 labels show significant differences between the two groups.

Given the high number of possible labels output by VGG (1,000 labels), and the fine granularity of these labels, we attempt to perform a more high-level analysis in order to obtain more interpretable insights into the differences between the image content posted by the two groups of users.

To this effect, we attempt to build a taxonomy of semantic groups in which the objects depicted in the images can be categorized. We do this in a semi-automatic fashion: we first automatically group the 1,000 labels based on their semantic content. We use pretrained word2vec embeddings to obtain semantic representations for all the labels in the embedding vector space. In the case of multi-word labels, we obtain a unique representation by averaging the vectors corresponding to each word in the label. We then apply the k-means algorithm in order to automatically cluster the obtained vectors into 20 clusters. We further manually curate the obtained categories, re-assigning some of the labels to different groups, and introducing new groups where necessary, and manually assigning each cluster a name describing its semantic content. We end up with 23 categories of labels which we use for further analysis. We finally group the obtained categories into the following higher-level categories as seen in Table 8.

We then measure the differences in image content between depressed and control users by comparing the average percent of images pertaining to each category at the user level (considering only the first image label), using the Mann-Whitney U Test. The differences between the average percent of images pertaining to that category posted by a user for the two groups (depressed and control) are shown in Table 9.

Table 8 Taxonomy of image object categories

High-level category	Category
ANIMALS	Dogs Cats
	Other domestic animals
	Mammal wild animals
	Aquatic animals
	Insects and reptiles
	Wild birds
	Rodents
VEGETAL	Plants
PEOPLE	Clothes
	Parts of human body
ACTIONS AND MOVEMENT	Sports
	Vehicles
	Shopping
	Leisure
THINGS	Food
	Domestic objects
	Work objects
	Health objects
	Weapons
	Technology
	Musical instruments
SCENERY	Landscapes and buildings

Images of animals. A first result is that the group of users suffering from depression post more images of animals than the control group, but especially more images of pets. There is good amount of research about animal-assisted therapy in the healing of psychological and emotional problems [20]. Our result is consistent with research that focuses on the relation between pets and depression as a way to fight social isolation. It is a controversial issue if pets help depression patients to heal or are a sign of depression. Some studies have, respectively, found that pet owners have similar [7] or higher [46] levels of depressive symptoms compared with non-owners. Recently Mueller et al. [43] focused on human-animal interaction module of a Health and Retirement study [76] and describe the characteristics of pet ownership in a population of older adults and examine the relation between pet ownership and multiple mental and physical health indicators such as health status, depression, and physical activity. Their results show that pet ownership was significantly associated with a higher likelihood of having had depression. However, pet ownership was not associated with having experienced depression within the last week, and they conclude that findings from this study could indicate a relationship between pet ownership and

Table 9 Average percent of images pertaining to each category for users in the depressed and control group, and p-value corresponding to significance of difference in the distributions at user level

	p-value	Depressed avg. usage	Control avg. usage
ANIMALS	2e-12	16.92	13.51
Dogs	4e-13	6.70	4.45
Cats	2e-6	1.83	1.32
Other domestic animals	0.48	0.17	0.19
Mammal wild animals	0.01	1.55	1.42
Aquatic animals	0.002	1.59	1.60
Insects and reptiles	0.0001	4.03	3.52
Wild birds	0.02	4.48	0.50
Rodents	4e-6	0.56	0.42
VEGETAL	0.12	0.07	0.06
Plants	0.12	0.07	0.06
PEOPLE	0.22	14.95	15.71
Clothes	0.28	14.04	14.95
Body parts	0.01	0.91	0.76
ACTIONS AND MOVEMENT	0.07	11.97	14.64
Sports	0.17	2.89	3.79
Vehicles	0.33	3.38	4.03
Shopping	0.02	1.84	1.74
Leisure	0.31	3.85	5.07
THINGS	0.36	48.45	48.53
Food	0.0009	5.06	4.20
Domestic objects	0.12	18.46	18.04
Work objects	0.47	13.51	14.39
Health objects	0.009	2.31	2.38
Weapons	0.49	0.83	1.26
Technology	0.01	7.23	6.83
Musical instruments	0.03	1.02	1.39
SCENERY	0.01	7.61	7.52
Landscapes and buildings	0.01	7.61	7.52

depression, but it is impossible to determine the directionality of that relationship. What is most intriguing about our results is that the differences are clearly significant between the two groups in all animal sub-categories, including wild animals, indicating a general attraction to the animal world that is greater among users suffering from depression than in the control group. Only in the category "other domestic animals" there are no statistically significant differences between the two groups of users.

Moscovici when elaborating his Theory of Social Representation [74] always points out the symbolic and general value of the distinction between nature and society [42] in terms that society is a human creation, and this is what we call culture. Following this hypothesis of the opposition of nature and culture in the way humans explain the world, some empirical research [51] has operationalised the nature dimension by referring it to animals and showing that they play an important role in terms of social classification. However, how the opposition “nature versus culture” works in relation to mental disorders such as depression has not been explored. More research is needed to understand these results.

Images of things. We do not find a significant difference in the category “things” as a whole but we find a clear one in the sub-categories “food” and “health-related objects”. Similarly, but less significantly, we find differences in “musical instruments” and “technology objects”. People suffering depression post more images about “food” and “technology objects” than the control group and less images of “health objects” and “musical instruments” than the control group.

To interpret the results about the “food” category we can refer to [4], a recent study of images that users post in Instagram with the hashtag *#depression*. They found that food images attract more positive social support, in terms of a greater number of positive comments, than other content categories. Their results could give an explanation for the difference that we found in our data, because it is well established that people, in general [23] and especially the ones that are suffering some kind of social stigma [24] or mental disorder [5], need to manage their everyday self-presentation in order to achieve social support. In consequence, posting food images is a good strategy in terms of getting a positive feedback. We also think that this explanation could be applied to the differences that we observe in landscape categories but we do not know any previous research related to it.

Images of health objects are a small quantity but present a clear significant difference between the two groups of users. There is no prior research that helps us to interpret this result. We know from the results of the Pew Research Center’s Internet and American Life Project [21] that 80% of internet users have looked online for information about a specific disease or treatment. Images of health objects could be related with a search for causes of health events which may vary if the user is suffering from depression. The authors have found some results that indicate a different pattern in the search for causal explanations in correlation with the expression of emotions in depressed people and control cases [71].

Images of technology objects are mostly related to computer devices and we could assume that this has some relation with a greater use of internet by depressed people. The findings regarding the impact of the use of internet on well-being are mixed and studies are often criticized due to small samples and lack of consistency in measurement. Cotten et al. [13] examined this issue among older adults, using data from the Health and Retirement Survey [76]. The study estimates the relationship between the use of internet and depression and the results indicate a positive contribution of the use of internet to mental well-being of retired people. However, in a meta-analysis of 40 studies that examines the relationship between various internet uses and measures of psychological well-being, including depression, loneliness, self-esteem, and life satisfaction, Huang [29] found a small detrimental effect of the use of internet on psychological well-being.

7 Conclusions and Future Directions

Mental disorders are an important and sensitive issue of public health. Using sophisticated computational solutions which leverage large amounts of data to assist with early detection of mental health issues can be very valuable, but such systems must be developed with corresponding attention to the complexity of the signs of mental health disorders, and to the impact they can have on the life of individuals. This is why a deep understanding of how mental disorders develop is necessary, from the early stages, accounting for explicit and implicit signs of the disorder, for their evolution and interactions over time.

We have presented a study on the automatic detection of mental disorders based on linguistic markers extracted from social media, targeting depression. We showed that deep learning models can be useful for successfully detecting social media users who risk developing a mental disorder, where the texts they post online are represented with linguistic features at different levels, including the content of the message, but also the user's writing style and the emotions conveyed. We provided interpretations of the model's decisions through various techniques (**RQ1**).

Moreover, we interpreted our findings through in-depth qualitative analyses grounded in well-established theories in psychology (**RQ2**). We suggest that linking computational findings to theoretical grounding provided by research in psychology is essential for more refined computational and linguistic models of mental health, and that such approaches have high potential for improving the performance of automatic tools for monitoring mental health, as well for aiding clinicians to better understand mental disorders.

We have also introduced a new multimodal dataset on depression based on social media data, including texts and images posted by depressed users, and have shown that a classifier can leverage the additional information in order to distinguish depressed users from the control group **(RQ3)**.

An interesting direction for the future would be the integration of a depression detection model into conversational agent tools: in this way, the benefit of the automatic depression detection model could have a more direct implication on the user, for example by providing a kind of "assisted therapy", or by detecting users who show a risk of developing a serious disorder in order to refer them to a human therapist.

We believe our models and findings can be very valuable to people suffering from depression, but any deployment of a tool for mental disorder detection should take into account potential ethical concerns. If such tools are used by third parties (such as employers seeking to filter candidates based on their mental health profile), this could compromise the privacy of the individuals. We suggest that the development of an ethical standard is necessary, such that launching such tools could be accompanied by an ethical statement to constrain their users.

Acknowledgements The authors thank the EU-FEDER Comunitat Valenciana 2014–2020 grant IDIFEDER/2018/025. The work of Paolo Rosso was in the framework of the research project PROMETEO/2019/121 (DeepPattern) by the Generalitat Valenciana.

References

1. Abd Yusof, N. F., Lin, C., & Guerin, F. (2017). Analysing the causes of depressed mood from depression vulnerable individuals. In *Proceedings of the International Workshop on Digital Disease Detection using Social Media 2017 (DDDSM-2017)* (pp. 9–17).
2. Allan, C. E., Valkanova, V., & Ebmeier, K. P. (2014). Depression in older people is underdiagnosed. *The Practitioner, 258*(1771), 19–22, 2–3.
3. Amini, H., & Kosseim, L. (2020). Towards explainability in using deep learning for the detection of anorexia in social media. In *International Conference on Applications of Natural Language to Information Systems* (pp. 225–235). Springer.
4. Andalibi, N., Öztürk, P., & Forte, A. (2017). Sensitive self-disclosures, responses, and social support on instagram: The case of #depression. In *Proceedings of the 2017 ACM Conference on Computer Supported Cooperative Work and Social Computing*.
5. Bell, C. M., R. J. A. O. J. C. Y. K. A. A. L. J. P. K. (2017). The role of perceived burden and social support in suicide and depression. *Suicide and Life-Threatening Behavior, 48*(1), 87–94.
6. Benton, A., Mitchell, M., & Hovy, D. (2017). Multi-task learning for mental health using social media text. arXiv:1712.03538.
7. Branson, S., Boss, L., Cron, S., & Turner, D. (2017). Depression, loneliness, and pet attachment in homebound older adult cat and dog owners. *Journal of Mind and Medical Sciences, 4*, 38–48.
8. Calvo, R. A., Milne, D. N., Hussain, M. S., & Christensen, H. (2017). Natural language processing in mental health applications using non-clinical texts. *Natural Language Engineering, 23*(5), 649–685.
9. Chen, X., Sykora, M. D., Jackson, T. W., & Elayan, S. (2018). What about mood swings: Identifying depression on twitter with temporal measures of emotions. In *Companion Proceedings of the the Web Conference* (pp. 1653–1660).
10. Conway, M., & O'Connor, D. (2016). Social media, big data, and mental health: Current advances and ethical implications. *Current Opinion in Psychology, 9*, 77–82.
11. Coppersmith, G., Dredze, M., & Harman, C. (2014). Quantifying mental health signals in twitter. In *Proceedings of the Workshop on Computational Linguistics and Clinical Psychology: From Linguistic Signal to Clinical Reality* (pp. 51–60).
12. Coppersmith, G., Dredze, M., Harman, C., Hollingshead, K., & Mitchell, M. (2015). Clpsych 2015 shared task: Depression and ptsd on twitter. In *Proceedings of the 2nd Workshop on Computational Linguistics and Clinical Psychology: From Linguistic Signal to Clinical Reality* (pp. 31–39).
13. Cotten, S. R., Ford, G., Ford, S., & Hale, T. M. (2012). Internet use and depression among older adults. *Computers in Human Behavior, 28*(2), 496–499.
14. De Choudhury, M., Counts, S., Horvitz, E. J., & Hoff, A. (2014). Characterizing and predicting postpartum depression from shared facebook data. In *Proceedings of the 17th ACM Conference on Computer Supported Cooperative Work & Social Computing* (pp. 626–638).
15. De Choudhury, M., Gamon, M., Counts, S., & Horvitz, E. (2013). Predicting depression via social media. In *Seventh International AAAI Conference on Weblogs and Social Media*.
16. Deng, J., Dong, W., Socher, R., Li, L.-J., Li, K., & Fei-Fei, L. (2009). Imagenet: A large-scale hierarchical image database. In *2009 IEEE Conference on Computer Vision and Pattern Recognition* (pp. 248–255). IEEE.
17. Devlin, J., Chang, M.-W., Lee, K., & Toutanova, K. (2019). Bert: Pre-training of deep bidirectional transformers for language understanding. In *NAACL-HLT (1)*.

18. Edwards, S., Tinning, L., Brown, J. S. L., Boardman, J., & Weinman, J. (2007). Reluctance to seek help and the perception of anxiety and depression in the united kingdom. *Journal of Nervous & Mental Disease, 195*(3), 258–261.
19. Eichstaedt, J. C., Smith, R. J., Merchant, R. M., Ungar, L. H., Crutchley, P., Preoţiuc-Pietro, D., Asch, D. A., & Schwartz, H. A. (2018). Facebook language predicts depression in medical records. *Proceedings of the National Academy of Sciences, 115*(44), 11203–11208.
20. Fine, A. H. (Ed.). (2015). *Handbook on animal-assisted therapy* (4th ed.). San Diego: Academic.
21. Fox, S. (2011). *The social life of health information.*
22. Gilpin, L. H., Bau, D., Yuan, B. Z., Bajwa, A., Specter, M., & Kagal, L. (2018). Explaining explanations: An overview of interpretability of machine learning. In *2018 IEEE 5th International Conference on Data Science and Advanced Analytics (DSAA)* (pp. 80–89). IEEE.
23. Goffman, E. (1959). *The presentation of self in everyday life.*
24. Goffman, E. (1963). *Stigma. Notes on the managament of spoiled identity.*
25. Grigorenko, E. L., & Sternberg, R. J. (1995). Thinking styles. In *International Handbook of Personality and Intelligence* (pp. 205–229). Springer.
26. Guntuku, S. C., Preotiuc-Pietro, D., Eichstaedt, J. C., & Ungar, L. H. (2019). What twitter profile and posted images reveal about depression and anxiety. In *Proceedings of the International AAAI Conference on Web and Social Media* (Vol. 13, pp. 236–246).
27. Guntuku, S. C., Yaden, D. B., Kern, M. L., Ungar, L. H., & Eichstaedt, J. C. (2017). Detecting depression and mental illness on social media: An integrative review. *Current Opinion in Behavioral Sciences, 18*, 43–49.
28. Holzinger, A., Biemann, C., Pattichis, C. S., & Kell, D. B. (2017). What do we need to build explainable ai systems for the medical domain? arXiv:1712.09923.
29. Huang, C. (2010). Internet use and psychological well-being: A meta-analysis. *Cyberpsychology, Behavior, and Social Networking, 13*(3), 241–249.
30. Koppel, M., Schler, J., & Argamon, S. (2009). Computational methods in authorship attribution. *Journal of the American Society for Information Science and Technology, 60*(1), 9–26.
31. Lan, Z., Chen, M., Goodman, S., Gimpel, K., Sharma, P., & Soricut, R. (2019). Albert: A lite bert for self-supervised learning of language representations. arXiv:1909.11942.
32. Lee, S. A., Mathis, A. A., Jobe, M. C., & Pappalardo, E. A. (2020). Clinically significant fear and anxiety of covid-19: A psychometric examination of the coronavirus anxiety scale. *Psychiatry Research*, 113112.
33. Lima, C. K. T., de Medeiros Carvalho, P. M., Lima, I. d. A. S., de Oliveira Nunes, J. V. A., Saraiva, J. S., de Souza, R. I., da Silva, C. G. L., & Neto, M. L. R. (2020). The emotional impact of coronavirus 2019-ncov (new coronavirus disease). *Psychiatry Research*, 112915.
34. Liu, L., Preotiuc-Pietro, D., Samani, Z. R., Moghaddam, M. E., & Ungar, L. (2016). Analyzing personality through social media profile picture choice. In *Tenth International AAAI Conference on Web and Social Media.*
35. Liu, Y., Ott, M., Goyal, N., Du, J., Joshi, M., Chen, D., Levy, O., Lewis, M., Zettlemoyer, L., & Stoyanov, V. (2019). Roberta: A robustly optimized bert pretraining approach. arXiv:1907.11692.
36. Losada, D. E., Crestani, F., & Parapar, J. (2018). Overview of erisk: Early risk prediction on the internet. In *International Conference of the Cross-Language Evaluation Forum for European Languages* (pp. 343–361). Springer.
37. Losada, D. E., Crestani, F., & Parapar, J. (2019). Overview of erisk 2019 early risk prediction on the internet. In *International Conference of the Cross-Language Evaluation Forum for European Languages* (pp. 340–357). Springer.
38. Losada, D. E., Crestani, F., & Parapar, J. (2020). Overview of erisk at CLEF 2020: Early risk prediction on the internet (extended overview).
39. Mitchell, M., Hollingshead, K., & Coppersmith, G. (2015). Quantifying the language of schizophrenia in social media. In *Proceedings of the 2nd workshop on Computational Linguistics and Clinical Psychology: From Linguistic Signal to Clinical Reality* (pp. 11–20).

40. Mohammad, S. M., & Turney, P. D. (2013). Nrc emotion lexicon. National Research Council, Canada 2.
41. Mohammadi, E., Amini, H., & Kosseim, L. (2019). Quick and (maybe not so) easy detection of anorexia in social media posts. In Cappellato, L., Ferro, N., Losada, D., & Müller, H. (Eds.) CLEF 2019 Labs and Workshops, Notebook Papers. CEUR Workshop Proceedings. CEUR-WS.org (Vol. 2380).
42. Moscovici, S. (1976). *Society against nature. The Emergence of Human Societies.*
43. Mueller, M. K., Gee, N. R., & Bures, R. M. (2018). Human-animal interaction as a social determinant of health: Descriptive findings from the health and retirement study. *BMC Public Health, 18*, 305.
44. O'dea, B., Wan, S., Batterham, P. J., Calear, A. L., Paris, C., & Christensen, H. (2015). Detecting suicidality on twitter. *Internet Interventions, 2*(2), 183–188.
45. Orabi, A. H., Buddhitha, P., Orabi, M. H., & Inkpen, D. (2018). Deep learning for depression detection of twitter users. In *Proceedings of the Fifth Workshop on Computational Linguistics and Clinical Psychology: From Keyboard to Clinic* (pp. 88–97).
46. Parslow, R.A., J. A. C. H. R. B., & Jacomb, P. (2005). Pet ownership and health in older adults. *Gerontology, 51*, 40–47.
47. Pennebaker, J. W., Boyd, R. L., Jordan, K., & Blackburn, K. (2015). The development and psychometric properties of liwc2015. Technical Report.
48. Pennebaker, J. W., Francis, M. E., & Booth, R. J. (2001). Linguistic inquiry and word count: Liwc 2001. *Mahway: Lawrence Erlbaum Associates, 71*(2001), 2001.
49. Pennington, J., Socher, R., & Manning, C. D. (2014). Glove: Global vectors for word representation. In *Proceedings of the 2014 Conference on Empirical Methods in Natural Language Processing (EMNLP)* (pp. 1532–1543).
50. Plutchik, R. (1980). A general psychoevolutionary theory of emotion. In *Theories of emotion* (pp. 3–33). Elsevier.
51. Pérez, J. A., Moscovici, S., & Chulvi, B. (2002). Natura y cultura como principio de clasificación social. anclaje de representaciones sociales sobre minorías étnicas. *Revista de Psicología Social, 17*(1), 51–67.
52. Qiu, J., Shen, B., Zhao, M., Wang, Z., Xie, B., & Xu, Y. (2020). A nationwide survey of psychological distress among chinese people in the covid-19 epidemic: Implications and policy recommendations. *General Psychiatry, 33*, 2.
53. Ragheb, W., Azé, J., Bringay, S., & Servajean, M. (2019). Attentive multi-stage learning for early risk detection of signs of anorexia and self-harm on social media. In *CLEF (Working Notes)*.
54. Ramírez-Cifuentes, D., Freire, A., Baeza-Yates, R., Puntí, J., Medina-Bravo, P., Velazquez, D. A., Gonfaus, J. M., & Gonzàlez, J. (2020). Detection of suicidal ideation on social media: Multimodal, relational, and behavioral analysis. *Journal of Medical Internet Research, 22*(7), e17758.
55. Reece, A. G., Reagan, A. J., Lix, K. L., Dodds, P. S., Danforth, C. M., & Langer, E. J. (2017). Forecasting the onset and course of mental illness with twitter data. *Scientific Reports, 7*(1), 1–11.
56. Resnik, P., Garron, A., & Resnik, R. Using topic modeling to improve prediction of neuroticism and depression in college students. In *Proceedings of the 2013 Conference on Empirical Methods in Natural Language Processing* (pp. 1348–1353).
57. Ringeval, F., Schuller, B., Valstar, M., Gratch, J., Cowie, R., Scherer, S., Mozgai, S., Cummins, N., Schmitt, M., & Pantic, M. (2017). Avec 2017: Real-life depression, and affect recognition workshop and challenge. In *Proceedings of the 7th Annual Workshop on Audio/Visual Emotion Challenge* (pp. 3–9).
58. Ríssola, E. A., Aliannejadi, M., & Crestani, F. (2020). Beyond modelling: Understanding mental disorders in online social media. *Advances in Information Retrieval, 12035*, 296.
59. Sadeque, F., Xu, D., & Bethard, S. (2017). Uarizona at the clef erisk 2017 pilot task: linear and recurrent models for early depression detection. In *CEUR Workshop Proceedings* (Vol. 1866). NIH Public Access.

60. Schwartz, H. A., Eichstaedt, J., Kern, M., Park, G., Sap, M., Stillwell, D., Kosinski, M., & Ungar, L. (2014). Towards assessing changes in degree of depression through facebook. In *Proceedings of the Workshop on Computational Linguistics and Clinical Psychology: From Linguistic Signal to Clinical Reality* (pp. 118–125).
61. Serrano, S., & Smith, N. A. (2019). Is attention interpretable? In *Proceedings of the 57th Annual Meeting of the Association for Computational Linguistics* (pp. 2931–2951).
62. Shah, K., Kamrai, D., Mekala, H., Mann, B., Desai, K., & Patel, R. S. (2020). Focus on mental health during the coronavirus (covid-19) pandemic: Applying learnings from the past outbreaks. *Cureus, 12*, 3.
63. Sheehan, D. V. (2004). Depression: Underdiagnosed, undertreated, underappreciated. *Managed care (Langhorne, Pa.), 13*(6 Suppl Depression), 6–8.
64. Shen, G., Jia, J., Nie, L., Feng, F., Zhang, C., Hu, T., Chua, T.-S., & Zhu, W. (2017). Depression detection via harvesting social media: A multimodal dictionary learning solution. In *IJCAI* (pp. 3838–3844).
65. Shen, J. H., & Rudzicz, F. (2017). Detecting anxiety through reddit. In *Proceedings of the Fourth Workshop on Computational Linguistics and Clinical Psychology-From Linguistic Signal to Clinical Reality* (pp. 58–65).
66. Shigemura, J., Ursano, R. J., Morganstein, J. C., Kurosawa, M., & Benedek, D. M. (2020). Public responses to the novel 2019 coronavirus (2019-ncov) in Japan: Mental health consequences and target populations. *Psychiatry and Clinical Neurosciences, 74*(4), 281.
67. Torales, J., O'Higgins, M., Castaldelli-Maia, J. M., & Ventriglio, A. (2020). The outbreak of covid-19 coronavirus and its impact on global mental health. *International Journal of Social Psychiatry*, 0020764020915212.
68. Tran, T., & Kavuluru, R. (2017). Predicting mental conditions based on "history of present illness" in psychiatric notes with deep neural networks. *Journal of biomedical informatics, 75*, S138–S148.
69. Trotzek, M., Koitka, S., & Friedrich, C. M. (2017). Linguistic metadata augmented classifiers at the clef 2017 task for early detection of depression. In *CLEF (Working Notes)*.
70. Trotzek, M., Koitka, S., & Friedrich, C. M. (2018). Word embeddings and linguistic metadata at the clef 2018 tasks for early detection of depression and anorexia. In Cappellato, L., Ferro, N., Nie, J., & Soulier, L. (Eds.) CLEF 2018 Labs and Workshops, Notebook Papers. CEUR Workshop Proceedings. CEUR-WS.org (Vol. 2125).
71. Uban, A.-S., Chulvi, B., & Rosso, P. (2021). An emotion and cognitive based analysis of mental health disorders from social media data. *Future Generation Computer Systems, 124*, 480–494.
72. Uban, A. S., Chulvi, B., & Rosso, P. (2021). On the explainability of automatic predictions of mental disorders from social media data. In *International Conference on Applications of Natural Language to Information Systems* (Vol. 12801). Springer.
73. Uban, A. S., & Rosso, P. (2020). Deep learning architectures and strategies for early detection of self-harm and depression level prediction. In Cappellato, L., Eickhoff, C., Ferro, N., & Névéol, A. (Eds.) CLEF 2020 Labs and Workshops, Notebook Papers. CEUR Workshop Proceedings. CEUR-WS.org (Vol. 2696).
74. Wagner, W. (2020). Social representation theory: An historical outline.
75. Wang, Y.-T., Huang, H.-H., & Chen, H.-H. (2018). A neural network approach to early risk detection of depression and anorexia on social media text. In Cappellato, L., Ferro, N., Nie, J., & Soulier, L. (Eds.) CLEF 2018 Labs and Workshops, Notebook Papers. CEUR Workshop Proceedings. CEUR-WS.org (Vol. 2125).
76. Weir, P. (2012). *The health and retirement study.*
77. Wiegreffe, S., & Pinter, Y. (2019). Attention is not not explanation. In *Proceedings of the 2019 Conference on Empirical Methods in Natural Language Processing and the 9th International Joint Conference on Natural Language Processing (EMNLP-IJCNLP)* (pp. 11–20).
78. Williams, S. Z., Chung, G. S., & Muennig, P. A. (2017). Undiagnosed depression: A community diagnosis. *SSM - Population Health, 3*, 633–638.
79. World Health Organization. (2012). W. Depression: A global crisis. World Mental Health Day, October 10 2012. World Federation for Mental Health, Occoquan, VA, USA.

80. Xiang, Y.-T., Yang, Y., Li, W., Zhang, L., Zhang, Q., Cheung, T., & Ng, C. H. (2020). Timely mental health care for the 2019 novel coronavirus outbreak is urgently needed. *The Lancet Psychiatry, 7*(3), 228–229.
81. Yang, Z., Yang, D., Dyer, C., He, X., Smola, A., & Hovy, E. (2016). Hierarchical attention networks for document classification. In *Proceedings of the 2016 Conference of the North American Chapter of the Association for Computational Linguistics: Human Language Technologies* (pp. 1480–1489).
82. Yates, A., Cohan, A., & Goharian, N. (2017). Depression and self-harm risk assessment in online forums. In *Proceedings of the 2017 Conference on Empirical Methods in Natural Language Processing* (pp. 2968–2978).
83. Yazdavar, A. H., Al-Olimat, H. S., Ebrahimi, M., Bajaj, G., Banerjee, T., Thirunarayan, K., Pathak, J., & Sheth, A. (2017). Semi-supervised approach to monitoring clinical depressive symptoms in social media. In *Proceedings of the 2017 IEEE/ACM International Conference on Advances in Social Networks Analysis and Mining 2017* (pp. 1191–1198).
84. Zhang, L.-F. (2008). Thinking styles and emotions. *The Journal of Psychology, 142*(5), 497–516.
85. Zucco, C., Liang, H., Di Fatta, G., & Cannataro, M. (2018). Explainable sentiment analysis with applications in medicine. In *2018 IEEE International Conference on Bioinformatics and Biomedicine (BIBM)* (pp. 1740–1747). IEEE.

The Future

The Future of eRisk

Javier Parapar, Patricia Martin-Rodilla, David E. Losada, and Fabio Crestani

Abstract eRisk constitutes now a reference forum in the study and detection of risk on the Internet. The five previous editions have shown how the Internet may be used to address personal risks. We have contributed to creating tools and datasets, identifying and improving risk detection and estimation techniques, and applying and defining evaluation metrics for them. However, it would be a mistake to continue our efforts without reflecting on the lessons learned from each of the challenges and editions, integrating them into future design decisions. This chapter captures this process of reflection and decision-making about eRisk in the future, detailing the strategic lines defined and their practical implications in future editions of eRisk.

1 eRisk so Far

As the previous chapters of this volume shown, researchers and practitioners may use early risk detection technologies in different areas, especially those related to mental health and safety. eRisk, as a reference forum in these technologies, has allowed us to define an interdisciplinary area with a joint research problem and shared goals.

J. Parapar
Centro de Investigación en Tecnoloxías da Información e as Comunicacións (CITIC), Universidade da Coruña, A Coruña, Spain
e-mail: javierparapar@udc.es

P. Martin-Rodilla
Centro de Investigación en Tecnoloxías da Información e as Comunicacións (CITIC), Universidade da Coruña, A Coruña, Spain
e-mail: patricia.martin.rodilla@udc.es

D. E. Losada (✉)
Centro Singular de Investigación en Tecnoloxías Intelixentes (CiTIUS), Universidade de Santiago de Compostela, Santiago de Compostela, Spain
e-mail: david.losada@usc.es

F. Crestani
Università della Svizzera italiana (USI), Lugano, Switzerland
e-mail: fabio.crestani@usi.ch

F. Crestani et al. (eds.), *Early Detection of Mental Health Disorders by Social Media Monitoring*, Studies in Computational Intelligence 1018,
https://doi.org/10.1007/978-3-031-04431-1_14

As organisers, these previous research efforts allowed us to provide this area with resources (collections, extraction and treatment strategies, evaluation methodologies, metrics, among others). On the other hand, participants have proposed diverse approaches to the challenges gradually improving the state-of-the-art.

In the immediate future, the eRisk 2021 edition intends to profound the tasks defined in the 2019 [33] and 2020 [34] editions to improve the results in the depression and self-harm challenges but also opening a new one: pathological gambling [39]. Specifically, we have released a new test collection for the early detection of signs of self-harm, making a total of three datasets (2019, 2020, and 2021). We have also provided the participants with new data for the depression level estimation task using standard questionnaires. An extra set of 80 individuals will booster the training and test capacity for the participants in the task looking to improve results from previous editions. Finally, the expansion of domains in eRisk (which will be systematically addressed later in this chapter) led us to propose in 2021 a new concerning early detection challenge: pathological gambling. Pathological gambling (ICD-10-CM code F63.0) [3] is also called ludomania and usually referred to as gambling addiction (it is an urge to gamble independently of its negative consequences). World Health Organization [6] reported in 2017 prevalence rates of gambling addiction in adults ranged from 10 to 60%. Following our usual methodology, the participant groups will interact with a dedicated server to obtain data sequentially and send their results.

This chapter looks beyond the 2021 edition and discusses the possible roadmaps for eRisk in the future as a multidisciplinary research space. Thus, all the work carried out should be analysed, and the lessons learned integrated for improvement, both in results (in detection and estimation) and in scope (addressing new challenges). This chapter summarises the plan for the future eRisk editions.

2 Future Outlines for Early Risk Prediction on the Internet

Over recent past years, eRisk has received a steady number of active participants, slowly placing the lab as a reference forum for early risk research. In eRisk past editions from 2017 [32], we have released many reference collections and proposed several early risk detection challenges using those datasets.

While analysing the lessons learned from previous editions, we missed a standardised approach to the eRisk problems. We have diversified eRisk in topics and challenges, while our primary focus is still the early risk problem. To promote a more comprehensive approach for eRisk, we designed an ambitious plan for future editions. This plan consists of three interrelated strategic lines.

First of all, it is necessary to re-define and broaden the concept of risk on the internet to address new risks emerging, which will arise in the future. For this reason, one of the strategic lines consists of the revision of the concept of risk on the internet, expanding the topic coverage and working on current and future internet risk domains and sub-domains we did not address so far. Closely linked with domain expansion is the need to explore early risk detection metrics that more realistically model the late warning penalty in detection. These metrics will allow us to get closer to detecting risk at an early stage. A fair assessment of the models' earliness is of particular interest in risks of mental disorders since diagnosis at initial stages is crucial in the disorder's evolution. Some studies even indicate that professionals' diagnosis may differ depending on the phase, complicating its detection and evolution [46].

Secondly, a systematic approach to risk detection on the internet involves studying the data and collections that eRisk released in successive editions in a diachronic and incremental way. This analysis will allow us to extract the added value of each edition results. To achieve that objective, we have defined a continuous improvement-based methodology for an eRisk trans-edition lab.

Finally, and in a complementary way to the efforts made in detection so far, eRisk will promote in the future more challenges related to the detection of risk levels through the automatic filling of standard questionnaires. This approach has been implemented in past editions in the specific context of depression, with tasks in 2019, 2020 and 2021 editions. In those editions, we used Beck's Depression Inventory (BDI) [8], a questionnaire which assess the presence of feelings like sadness, pessimism or loss of energy. The encouraging results achieved for this task on the specific risk of depression (despite the task's initial complexity) encourage us to broaden the range of standard questionnaires and risks to address in the future.

Next, we explain in detail each of these eRisk strategic lines.

2.1 Topic Coverage, Domain Expansion and New Metrics for Early Risk

The first strategic line of eRisk's plan focuses on expanding target domains for early risk detection on social networks. As we have previously said, the concept of risk on the internet has been expanding over time due to increased online human life activities where technology plays a central role. The recent changes towards a greater techno-mediation of our activities (i.e. remote working, e-health, a generalisation of virtual leisure activities, among others) allow us to anticipate a higher number of risks on the internet for the user. For example, due to the situations derived from the COVID-19 pandemic, patients and people in isolation use social networks as communication and support mechanisms. Among this greater amount of data, a more significant presence of mental disorders may be anticipated. Among these mental disorders, we may expect disorders derived from stressful situations [27] or related to the misuse of virtual leisure (gambling [21], compulsive behaviours in shopping [26], etc.). Besides, we can also foresee more activities that threaten users' security, privacy, reputation, or integrity.

In this context, eRisk uses all its resources and experience to expand its work scope with new internet risk challenges. Specifically, we believe it is necessary to work on some of these mental disorder challenges that may affect a large part of the population shortly, continuing with the challenge of pathological gambling initiated in 2021 [39] and treating anxiety disorders (whose diagnosis is increasing day by day) and, in the case of older people, the diagnoses of dementia.

These new challenges can be tackled from the two sub-approaches that coexist in eRisk: automatic detection and automatic estimation using standard questionnaires. About automatic detection, the shared task launched in 2021 on gambling will provide us with the initial resources to refine the automatic detection strategies for this pathology. Anxiety [1] (ICD-10-CM code F41.9) is defined as a mental disorder characterised by feelings of fear about current events and worry about future ones. The National Institute of Mental Health estimates a prevalence of 20% on the American Population [28]. Dementia matches several different ICD codes occur being the most prominent one dementia in Alzheimer's disease [2] (ICD-10-CM code F00). Recent studies in Spain estimate that dementia prevalence may scale from 5% on 75-year older adults to more than 20% when over 90 years [40]. The tackling of risk such as the development of dementia will impose new challenges given the lower use of social networks by older people, e.g. only between a 1% and 3% of Reddit user are estimated over 65 years [16]. In the case of anxiety and dementia disorders, it is necessary to make an initial effort to construct data collections from social networks to address the problem. Following the same methodology used in previous tasks, it is possible to identify from Reddit, for example, sources of information that allow building the necessary collections [4, 5]. We describe plans for automatic estimation of these new eRisk challenges in Sect. 2.3.

However, we do not want to forget about the initial broad understanding of risk that we considered when planning the first eRisk edition. Many other worrying non-pathological risks abound on the internet, and they are prone to be early alerted. Arguably, this joint effort's origin is on our work on sexual-predator detection at CLEF [24, 38]. Sexual predation on the internet [36] is a clear road were early alert models make the most sense. Similarly cyberbullying [43], the act of bullying over social media, is an increasingly worrying issue. Recent studies on Korean adolescents [29] reflect than more than 30% of individuals were involved in cyberbullying activities as victims, bullies or both. Such risks are also present in our planning for the near future.

Furthermore, it is important to note that the expansion of domains in eRisk will allow individual treatment of each disorder and allow us to make comparisons between traits and detection strategies in the future. This future possibility is especially relevant given that the biggest problem we face is the growth in the number of individuals who develop multiple pathologies. We did not address mental disorders co-existence detection in eRisk, due to its complexity, in-depth knowledge of the various cases can trace differentiating factors. For example, the presence of anxiety and depression disorders jointly [25], or situations in which anxiety lead to eating disorders or addictions in advanced stages [15] are increasingly common. In these cases, in-depth knowledge of these risks and their different detection characteristics can help us approach a multi-disorder detection model in the future.

Evaluation Metrics

The difficulty in finding and adjusting metrics for innovative tasks and new challenges has also motivated us to develop and incorporate new metrics for eRisk. Following the same approach, we plan to incorporate new metrics for automatic risk estimation tasks, specifically:

- MAE (Mean Absolute Error): MAE measures the average magnitude of the errors (expressed as a error vector y) in a set of predictions (starting in $j = 1$ to n predictions), without considering their direction. It is the average over the test sample of the absolute differences between prediction and actual observation where all individual differences have equal weight.

$$MAE = \frac{1}{n}\sum_{j=1}^{n} |(y_j - y'_j)| \tag{1}$$

- RMSE (Root Mean Square Error): is a quadratic scoring rule that also measures the average magnitude of the error. It is the square root of the average of squared differences between prediction and actual observation.

$$RMSE = \sqrt{\frac{1}{n}\sum_{j=1}^{n}(y_j - y'_j)^2} \tag{2}$$

MAE and RMSE are two of the most common metrics to measure accuracy for continuous variables [13, 14]. For example, they are widely used in rating prediction in recommendation systems and measuring accuracy in predictive forecasting systems, predicting natural disasters [14, 49].

Some attempts have been made to use those error metrics to measure mental disorders, especially depression, although in different research contexts than eRisk. For example, we can find MAE and RMSE metrics to measure depression prediction from modal multimedia information (audios, facial expression in videos, etc.) [31, 45, 48]. There are also some attempts to use them in detection from texts, especially using Topic Modeling [20], although the input texts used are not provided from social network sources.

In the future, we plan to introduce those and other new metrics both in the early risk prediction and level estimation tasks. On the one hand, MAE and RMSE are metrics widely used in prediction, which will help us evaluate with well-studied and standard measurements the prediction models developed in eRisk. On the other hand, as previously indicated, we must also explore metrics that realistically model the late warning penalty for the early alerts since adequately coping with the disorders' phases entails huge applications in diagnosis [46].

2.2 A Continuous Improvement of the eRisk Cycle

As a second strategic line, we have defined a continuous improvement-based methodology for an eRisk trans-edition lab. A Continuous Improvement process or methodology (hereafter abbreviated as CI) [10], is a meta-process model for describing the methodologies in business and project management that includes ongoing efforts for an incremental and sustained over time improvement of their services or products. It has been successfully and widely applied in project and business management, having its versions and applications in different sectors, such as in software development methodologies [37], education [7, 23], e-health and mental health systems management [11] or production chains.

We have applied this idea about always keeping in the main focus of any work the continuous improvement of the process carried out to define a work cycle for future eRisk. The ultimate goal is adopting a comprehensive approach that allows organisers and participants, as a research community, to maintain common goals in time, taking advantage of the results of the previous editions and performing diachronic and incremental research on each risk addressed.

Thus, it was necessary to design a balanced cycle in duration: a long cycle that allows us to receive some feedback from previous editions, but not too long to lose the participants' interest and researchers working on a specific challenge. Therefore, we decided to implement a 3-year cycle per task. Figure 1 shows the 3-year cycle defined for eRisk in BMNP notation [47]. Each year in the cycle present a particular goal: Risk Exploration, Learning Strategies and Results Improvement.

- First Year: Risk Exploration. We will not release training data in the first year (as it happened in the first edition of 2021's self-harm task). The objective is to foster research on methods that do not solely depend on the existence of training.
- Second Year: Learning Strategies. In the second year, we will see how participants may improve the systems' performance using training data, both in detection and estimation tasks.
- Third Year: Results Improvement In the third year, the main goal is improving the results achieved in previous editions, seeing how participants manage to improve and reuse their models after two years of experience.

It is essential to highlight that the design of the continuous improvement eRisk cycle is wholly or partially replicable. Our initial plan is to run each task for three years, but it is also possible to lengthen the improvement phases depending on the results obtained or the margin for improvement detected after the initial 3-year cycle.

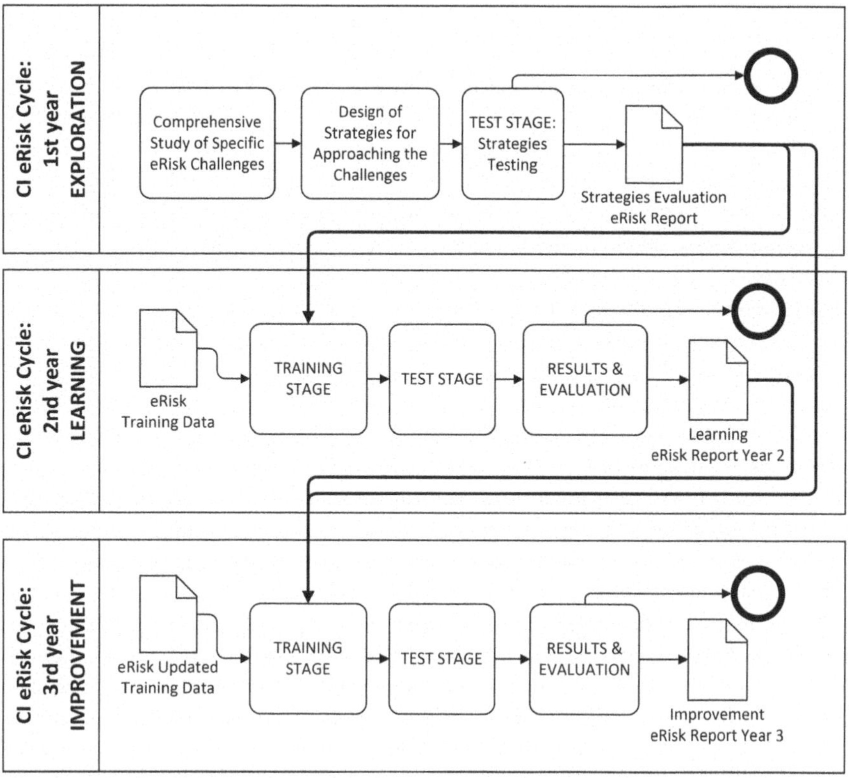

Fig. 1 3-year cycle based on continuous improvement methodologies designed for eRisk. Following BPMN notation [47], the diagram represents on each pool a year of the cycle with their tasks, sequence flow, inputs and outputs

2.3 New Challenges: Estimating Risk from Standard Questionnaires

The third strategic line continues the work started in the 2019 and 2020 editions of eRisk. Then we introduced a specific task to explore the viability and possible approaches for automatically estimating the occurrence and intensity of multiple well-known symptoms of depression. In this level estimation task, each participant group had to design an automatic method that processes each Redditor's writings' full history and fills a standard depression questionnaire based on the evidence found in the user's texts.

We chose a questionnaire derived from the Beck's Depression Inventory (BDI) [8], including 21 questions thematically related to some common depression signals with symptoms and their intensity (e.g., loss of appetite, sadness, and sleeping problems) according to four possible severity levels. In the 2019 and 2020 eRisk editions, a collection of questionnaires answers directly filled by social media users, together with their history of writings, constituted the ground truth. Due to the task's specific nature, it was necessary to introduce new metrics for evaluating the participants' estimations. We considered four metrics [33]: Average Closeness Rate (ACR), Average Hit Rate (AHR), Average DODL (ADODL) and Depression Category Hit Rate (DCHR). These metrics are clearly explained in previous chapters of this volume.

Following this approach that proved well received by participants, eRisk plans in the future to continue estimating risks on the internet using standard questionnaires. As we previously detailed, the standard way of measuring the degree of specific mental disorders by clinical professionals is commonly based on such validated psychometric tests, accepted by the practitioners' community. The medical community manages many such tests recognised for having satisfactory diagnostic results. Some examples are: the Beck Depression Inventory-II (BDI II) in the case of the depression [8]; the Self-Harm Inventory in the case of self-inflicted harm [42]; the SCOFF (Sick, Control, One, Fat, Food) [22], and the Eating Disorder Examination (EDE) [9, 18] in the case of eating disorders. It is also possible to find complementary information for developing new questionnaires in the Diagnostic and Statistical Manual of Mental Disorders-IV (DSM-IV) [17], which is not a questionnaire, but a manual which determines a common vocabulary and standard criteria to group and characterise the different mental disorders.

There are also other more recent questionnaires for pathological gambling (the South Oaks Gambling Screen, SOGS) [30] or anxiety (the Anxiety Screening Questionnaire, ASQ-15 and the Generalised Anxiety Disorder Questionnaire, GAD-7) [44, 50]. These questionnaires consist of the same diagnosis methodology and organisation: they ask different questions where the main symptoms of the disorder are analysed, both at cognitive (e.g., hopelessness, fears, worrying) and at physical levels (e.g., lack of appetite, loss of energy). Due to their satisfactory results in the diagnosis of these mental disorders, their systematic exploration in the form of new tasks in future editions of eRisk will allow: (1) contrasting the results obtained with BDI [8], (2) reevaluating the possibilities of estimation and automatic filling of this type of questionnaires, (3) measuring the level of dependency of the task of each specific questionnaire and the difficulty for each specific risk estimation and (4) evaluating the degree of generalisation achieved for estimation tasks.

These estimation tasks in eRisk establish a need to construct and validate ground truth collections for each specific risk. For example, in Fig. 2 we can see the GAD-7 questions and answers with the corresponding scores. Pfizer created the GAD-7 questionnaire which is free to use, and is indeed widely used for assessing the general population [35]. The *Likert* scale of GAD-7 goes from 0 points (*"Not at all"*) to 3 points (*"Nearly every day"*). We can observe how this particular questionnaire shares most of the BDI questionnaires' characteristics, but it also shows some differences that would promote new approaches for solving the level estimation problem. For instance, the different answers correspond to a total number of days when the question's circumstances are present; other questionnaires force a yes/no answer pattern.

In 2022 we will introduce a severity estimation task on eating disorders. Eating disorders (ICD-10-CM code F50) affect up to 5% of the population, most often

	Not at all	Several days	More than half of the days	Nearly every day
1. Feeling nervous, anxious or on edge	0	1	2	3
2. Not being able to stop or control worrying	0	1	2	3
3. Worrying too much about different things	0	1	2	3
4. Trouble relaxing	0	1	2	3
5. Being so restless that it is hard to sit still	0	1	2	3
6. Becoming easily annoyed or irritable	0	1	2	3
7. Feeling afraid as if something awful might happen	0	1	2	3

Fig. 2 GAD-7 questionnaire for screening of anxiety

developing in adolescence and young adulthood. For that, we will use the EDE-Q questionnaire (v6.0) [9, 18]. EDE-Q assesses the range and severity of features associated with the diagnosis of eating disorders. It is a 28-item questionnaire with four sub-scales (restrain, eating, concern, shape concern, and weight concern). It is free to use for non-commercial research purposes only, and no authorisation is required. In Fig. 3 we can see the structure of the EDE-Q. As can be observed, the structure of this questionnaire represents new challenges to the participants. First, it exposes a heterogeneous set of questions with diverse response types. Second, for some of the questions, it introduces the need to use some traces of temporal evolution on the severity estimation task, e.g. questions 1–12 must be answered regarding the number of days among the last 28 days where the individual expressed the symptom. Finally, questions 22–28 express graded assessments by the patient.

It is also essential to highlight the significant challenge at research-level that constitutes the estimation of mental disorders by automatically filling standard questionnaires. Individuals themselves, their families or friends are already using many self-assessment instruments to detect mental disorders [19, 41]. The generalised use of this kind of medical questionnaires reveals certain limitations of the questionnaire-based approach. The final score can be manipulated (either minimised or scraped) easily by individuals. There are investigations where the lack of objectivity of these tools is analysed. Because the questionnaires have straightforward questions, the answers may depend significantly on changing factors, such as environmental conditions or the patient's mood. For example, Bowling found significant differences in the BDI questionnaire scores depending on whether it is performed in the presence of a doctor or if it takes place in a domestic environment (i.e. the patient is at home) [12]. However, and despite these limitations, the results obtained in the detection of depression using these questionnaires within the clinical practice are positive, and it has been proven that they can work in different phases of the disease [46].

The promotion within eRisk of specific tasks that systematically study in-depth the strategy of estimation of mental health risks from information found in social media through the automatic analysis of standard questionnaires will also allow us to evaluate the possibilities and the impact of these limitations on the approaches' automation.

	NO DAYS	1-5 DAYS	6-12 DAYS	13-15 DAYS	16-22 DAYS	23-27 DAYS	EVERY DAY
1. Have you been deliberately trying to limit the amount of food you eat to influence your shape or weight (whether or not you have succeeded)?	0	1	2	3	4	5	6
2. Have you gone for long periods of time (8 waking hours or more) without eating anything at all in order to influence your shape or weight?	0	1	2	3	4	5	6
3. Have you tried to exclude from your diet any foods that you like in order to influence your shape or weight (whether or not you have succeeded)?	0	1	2	3	4	5	6
	. . .						

	TIMES
13. Over the past 28 days, how many times have you eaten what other people would regards as an unusually large amount of food (given the circumstances)?	
14. .. On how many of these times did you have a sense of having lost control over your eating (at the time you were eating)?	
. . .	

	NO OF THE TIMES	A FEW OF THE TIMES	LESS THAN HALF	HALF OF THE TIMES	MORE THAN HALF	MOST OF THE TIME	EVERY TIME
20. On what proportion of the times that you have eaten have you felt guilty (felt that you've done wrong) because of its effect on your shape or weight? ... Do not count episodes of binge eating	0	1	2	3	4	5	6
	. . .						

	NO AT ALL	SLIGHTLY		MODERATELY		MARKEDLY	
22. Has your weight influenced how you think about (judge) yourself as a person?	0	1	2	3	4	5	6
23. Has your shape influenced how you think about (judge) yourself as a person?	0	1	2	3	4	5	6

Fig. 3 Extracts from the EDE-Q questionnaire for screening of eating disorders

3 Conclusions

The results achieved so far motivate us to continue with the lab in the following years. We want to encourage the research teams working on the early risk tasks to continue improving their models and developing new ones for future challenges. Even when developing new resources is heavy lifting, we firmly believe that societal returns make it worthy.

We have planed our future work on three strategic lines around new early risk domains, new estimation level resources and a standardised three-year improvement cycle per task. However, the future is open; each year discussion session on the closing of eRisk serves us for getting feedback and ideas from the participants. We are thankful to them for their participation and for their help in shaping the future of this initiative. Their input is the real drive of the future of eRisk.

Acknowledgements This work was supported by projects RTI2018-093336-B-C21, RTI2018-093336-B-C22 (Ministerio de Ciencia e Innovación, Agencia Estatal de Investigación & ERDF) and PLEC2021-007662 (MCIN/AEI/10.13039/501100011033, Ministerio de Ciencia e Innovación, Agencia Estatal de Investigación, Plan de Recuperación, Transformación y Resiliencia, Unión Europea-Next GenerationEU).

The first and second authors thank the financial support supplied by the Consellería de Educación, Universidade e Formación Profesional (accreditation 2019–2022 ED431G/01, ED431B 2019/03) and the European Regional Development Fund, which acknowledges the CITIC Research Center in ICT of the University of A Coruña as a Research Center of the Galician University System.

The third author thanks the financial support supplied by the Consellería de Educación, Universidade e Formación Profesional (accreditation 2019–2022 ED431G-2019/04, ED431C 2018/29) and the European Regional Development Fund, which acknowledges the CiTIUS-Research Center in Intelligent Technologies of the University of Santiago de Compostela as a Research Center of the Galician University System.

The fourth and last author acknowledges the support of the Swiss National Science Foundation (SNSF) through the project "Early risk prediction on the Internet: an evaluation corpus" (IZK0Z2_160614), which in 2015 kick-started the whole idea of this long term initiative,

References

1. Anxiety disorder - ICD 10. Retrieved February 05, 2021.
2. Dementia in alzheimer disease - ICD 10. Retrieved February 05, 2021.
3. Pathological gambling - ICD 10. Retrieved February 05, 2021.
4. Subreddit on dementia. Retrieved February 05, 2021.
5. Subreddit on health anxiety. Retrieved February 05, 2021.
6. Abbott, M. (2017). The epidemiology and impact of gambling disorder and other gambling-related harm. In *Discussion Paper for the 2017 WHO Forum on Alcohol, Drugs and Addictive Behaviours* (pp. 26–28). WHO Headquarters Geneva.
7. Anderson, S., & Kumari, R. (2009). Continuous improvement in schools: Understanding the practice. *International Journal of Educational Development, 29*(3), 281–292.
8. Beck, A. T., Ward, C. H., Mendelson, M., Mock, J., & Erbaugh, J. (1961). An inventory for measuring depression. *Archives of General Psychiatry, 4*(6), 561–571.
9. Berg, K. C., Peterson, C. B., Frazier, P., & Crow, S. J. (2012). Psychometric evaluation of the eating disorder examination and eating disorder examination-questionnaire: A systematic review of the literature. *International Journal of Eating Disorders, 45*(3), 428–438.
10. Bhuiyan, N., & Baghel, A. (2005). An overview of continuous improvement: From the past to the present. Management Decision.
11. Birleson, P. (1998). Learning organisations: A suitable model for improving mental health services? *Australian and New Zealand Journal of Psychiatry, 32*(2), 214–222.
12. Bowling, A. (2005). Mode of questionnaire administration can have serious effects on data quality. *Journal of Public Health, 27*(3), 281–291.
13. Brassington, G. (2017). Mean absolute error and root mean square error: Which is the better metric for assessing model performance? In *EGU General Assembly Conference Abstracts* (p. 3574). EGU General Assembly Conference Abstracts.
14. Chai, T., & Draxler, R. R. (2014). Root mean square error (RMSE) or mean absolute error (MAE)?-arguments against avoiding rmse in the literature. *Geoscientific Model Development, 7*(3), 1247–1250.
15. Dokras, A., Stener-Victorin, E., Yildiz, B. O., Li, R., Ottey, S., Shah, D., Epperson, N., & Teede, H. (2018). Androgen excess-polycystic ovary syndrome society: Position statement on depression, anxiety, quality of life, and eating disorders in polycystic ovary syndrome. *Fertility and Sterility, 109*(5), 888–899.

16. Duggan, M., & Smith, A. (2013). 6% of online adults are reddit users. *Pew Internet & American Life Project, 3*, 1–10.
17. Edition, F., et al. (2013). Diagnostic and statistical manual of mental disorders. *American Psychiatric Association, 21*.
18. Fairburn, C. G., Cooper, Z., & O'Connor, M. (1993). The eating disorder examination. *International Journal of Eating Disorders, 6*, 1–8.
19. Giles, D. C., & Newbold, J. (2011). Self-and other-diagnosis in user-led mental health online communities. *Qualitative Health Research, 21*(3), 419–428.
20. Gong, Y., & Poellabauer, C. (2017). Topic modeling based multi-modal depression detection. In *Proceedings of the 7th Annual Workshop on Audio/Visual Emotion Challenge* (pp. 69–76).
21. Håkansson, A. (2020). Impact of covid-19 on online gambling-a general population survey during the pandemic. *Frontiers in Psychology, 11*, 2588.
22. Hill, L. S., Reid, F., Morgan, J. F., & Lacey, J. H. (2010). Scoff, the development of an eating disorder screening questionnaire. *International Journal of Eating Disorders, 43*(4), 344–351.
23. Hilliger, I., Aguirre, C., Miranda, C., Celis, S., & Pérez-Sanagustín, M. (2020). Design of a curriculum analytics tool to support continuous improvement processes in higher education. In *Proceedings of the Tenth International Conference on Learning Analytics & Knowledge* (pp. 181–186).
24. Inches, G., & Crestani, F. (2012). Overview of the international sexual predator identification competition at pan-2012. In *CLEF (Online Working Notes/labs/workshop)* (Vol. 30).
25. Jacobson, N. C., & Newman, M. G. (2017). Anxiety and depression as bidirectional risk factors for one another: A meta-analysis of longitudinal studies. *Psychological Bulletin, 143*(11), 1155.
26. Jaspal, R., Lopes, B., & Lopes, P. (2020). Predicting social distancing and compulsive buying behaviours in response to covid-19 in a united kingdom sample. *Cogent Psychology, 7*(1), 1800924.
27. Kar, N., Kar, B., & Kar, S. (2021). Stress and coping during covid-19 pandemic: Result of an online survey. *Psychiatry Research, 295*, 113598.
28. Kessler, R. C., Chiu, W. T., Demler, O., & Walters, E. E. (2005). Prevalence, severity, and comorbidity of 12-month dsm-iv disorders in the national comorbidity survey replication. *Archives of General Psychiatry, 62*(6), 617–627.
29. Lee, C., & Shin, N. (2017). Prevalence of cyberbullying and predictors of cyberbullying perpetration among korean adolescents. *Computers in Human Behavior, 68*, 352–358.
30. Lesieur, H. R., & Blume, S. B. (1987). The south oaks gambling screen (sogs): A new instrument for the identification of pathological gamblers. *American Journal of Psychiatry, 144*, 9.
31. Lopez Otero, P., et al. (2015). *Improved strategies for speaker segmentation and emotional state detection*. Ph.D. Thesis, Teoría do sinal e comunicacións.
32. Losada, D. E., Crestani, F., & Parapar, J. (2017). erisk 2017: Clef lab on early risk prediction on the internet: Experimental foundations. In Jones, G. J., Lawless, S., Gonzalo, J., Kelly, L., Goeuriot, L., Mandl, T., Cappellato, L., & Ferro, N. (Eds.) *Experimental IR meets multilinguality, multimodality, and interaction* (pp. 346–360). Cham: Springer International Publishing.
33. Losada, D. E., Crestani, F., & Parapar, J. (2019). Overview of erisk 2019 early risk prediction on the internet. In Crestani, F., Braschler, M., Savoy, J., Rauber, A., Müller, H., Losada, D. E., Heinatz Bürki, G., Cappellato, L., & Ferro, N. (Eds.) *Experimental IR Meets Multilinguality, Multimodality, and Interaction* (pp. 340–357). Cham: Springer International Publishing.
34. Losada, D. E., Crestani, F., & Parapar, J. (2020). Overview of erisk 2020: Early risk prediction on the internet. In Arampatzis, A., Kanoulas, E., Tsikrika, T., Vrochidis, S., Joho, H., Lioma, C., Eickhoff, C., Névéol, A., Cappellato, L., & Ferro, N. (Eds.) *Experimental IR meets multilinguality, multimodality, and interaction* (pp. 272–287). Cham: Springer International Publishing.
35. Löwe, B., Decker, O., Müller, S., Brähler, E., Schellberg, D., Herzog, W., & Herzberg, P. Y. (2008). Validation and standardization of the generalized anxiety disorder screener (gad-7) in the general population. *Medical Care*, 266–274.
36. Marcum, C. D. (2007). Interpreting the intentions of internet predators: An examination of online predatory behavior. *Journal of Child Sexual Abuse, 16*(4), 99–114.

37. Orłowski, C., Cygert, D., & Nowak, P. (2020). Continuous improvement process model for supporting the construction of internet of things system design environments. In Sitek, P., Pietranik, M., Krótkiewicz, M., & Srinilta, C. (Eds.) *Intelligent information and database systems* (pp. 424–435). Singapore: Springer.
38. Parapar, J., Losada, D. E., & Barreiro, A. (2012). A learning-based approach for the identification of sexual predators in chat logs. In *CLEF (Online Working Notes/Labs/Workshop)* (Vol. 1178).
39. Parapar, J., Martin-Rodilla, P., Losada, D. E., & Crestani, F. (2021). erisk 2021: Pathological gambling, self-harm and depression challenges.
40. Ponjoan, A., Garre-Olmo, J., Blanch, J., Fages, E., Alves-Cabratosa, L., Martí-Lluch, R., Comas-Cufí, M., Parramon, D., Garcia-Gil, M., & Ramos, R. (2019). Epidemiology of dementia: Prevalence and incidence estimates using validated electronic health records from primary care. *Clinical Epidemiology, 11*, 217.
41. Sanchez-Villegas, A., Schlatter, J., Ortuno, F., Lahortiga, F., Pla-Vidal, J., Benito, S., & Martínez-González, M. (2008). Validity of a self-reported diagnosis of depression among participants in a cohort study using the structured clinical interview for dsm-iv (scid-i). *BMC Psychiatry, 8*, 43.
42. Sansone, R. A., Wiederman, M. W., & Sansone, L. A. (1998). The self-harm inventory (shi): Development of a scale for identifying self-destructive behaviors and borderline personality disorder. *Journal of Clinical Psychology, 54*(7), 973–983.
43. Slonje, R., Smith, P. K., & Frisén, A. (2013). The nature of cyberbullying, and strategies for prevention. *Computers in Human Behavior, 29*(1), 26–32. Including Special Section Youth, Internet, and Wellbeing.
44. Spitzer, R. L., Kroenke, K., Williams, J. B., & Löwe, B. (2006). A brief measure for assessing generalized anxiety disorder: The gad-7. *Archives of Internal Medicine, 166*(10), 1092–1097.
45. Stepanov, E. A., Lathuiliere, S., Chowdhury, S. A., Ghosh, A., Vieriu, R.-L., Sebe, N., & Riccardi, G. (2018). Depression severity estimation from multiple modalities. In *2018 IEEE 20th International Conference on e-Health Networking, Applications and Services (Healthcom)* (pp. 1–6). IEEE.
46. Viinamäki, H., Tanskanen, A., Honkalampi, K., Koivumaa-Honkanen, H., Haatainen, K., Kaustio, O., & Hintikka, J. (2004). Is the beck depression inventory suitable for screening major depression in different phases of the disease? *Nordic Journal of Psychiatry, 58*(1), 49–53.
47. von Rosing, M., White, S., Cummins, F., & de Man, H. (2015). Business process model and notation-bpmn.
48. Williamson, J. R., Godoy, E., Cha, M., Schwarzentruber, A., Khorrami, P., Gwon, Y., Kung, H.-T., Dagli, C., & Quatieri, T. F. (2016). Detecting depression using vocal, facial and semantic communication cues. AVEC '16, Association for Computing Machinery.
49. Willmott, C. J., & Matsuura, K. (2005). Advantages of the mean absolute error (mae) over the root mean square error (rmse) in assessing average model performance.
50. Wittchen, H.-U., & Boyer, P. (1998). Screening for anxiety disorders. *The British Journal of Psychiatry, 173*(S34), 10–17.

The manufacturer's authorised representative in the EU is Springer Nature Customer Service Centre GmbH, Europaplatz 3, 69115 Heidelberg, Germany. If you have any concerns regarding our products, please contact ProductSafety@springernature.com

Printed and bound by CPI Group (UK) Ltd, Croydon, CR0 4YY
30/09/2026
02225493-0011